Dr. Runels

"Botulinum Blastoff" Course

Using Neuromodulators

(Xeomin®, Dysport®, Jeuveau®, or Botox®)

to

Change Lives

&

Increase Profit

by

Charles Runels, MD

ACKNOWLEDGMENTS

Cellular Medicine Association Members

Thank you for your bravery and for what you have taught me.

Dr. Mark Bailey

Thank you very much, Dr. Bailey.

The days I spent with you in Toronto learning your BoNT & filler techniques and (more importantly) how to think about cosmetic medicine in relation to medicine were life changing.

Drs. Jean & Alastair Carruthers

Thank you very much, Drs. Carruthers, for starting it all.

Dr. Stephen R. Marquardt

Thank you very much, Dr. Marquardt.

Your research and the resultant face maps you freely share (BeautyAnalysis.com) improved my patient outcomes tremendously by doing the impossible—quantifying beauty.

My Patients

Thank you very much if you are one of the thousands of people who have trusted me over the past two decades with those *most sacred of parts of your body*, the parts with which you interact with the ones you love—your face (giving me the info for this book and for my Vampire Facelift® procedure) and your genitals (helping me design the O-Shot® and P-Shot® procedures).

LEGAL DISCLAIMER

MODULES

Module I.
BoNT Parties & Other Events
A Sure Way to Boost Your Reputation & Double Your Practice Income

Module II.
Mixing and Injecting
Techniques to Avoid Hurting or Bruising Your Patients

Module III.
Twelve Injection Points to Create Gorgeous Results
These 12 Are All You Need to Know

Module IV.
How to Use BoNT to Help with Four Difficult-to-Treat Medical Problems
Depression, Migraines, Bruxism, & Erectile Dysfunction

ABBREVIATIONS

BoNT: botulinum neurotoxin; *for this course, a generic name for the brands Xeomin®, Dysport®, Jeuveau®, and Botox®*

CMA: Cellular Medicine Association

E2: estradiol

ED: erectile dysfunction

HIF: hypoxia-inducible factor

ICI: intracavernosal injection

IU: intraurethral

LiSWT: low-intensity shock wave therapy

PDE5i: phosphodiesterase type 5 inhibitor

PRP: platelet-rich plasma

PW-CBQ: people who cannot be quiet

SCT: stem cell therapy

VED: vacuum erection device

VEG: vascular endothelial growth factor

CONTENTS

ACKNOWLEDGMENTS 3

    CELLULAR MEDICINE ASSOCIATION MEMBERS 3

    DR. MARK BAILEY 3

    DRS. JEAN & ALASTAIR CARRUTHERS 3

    DR. STEPHEN R. MARQUARDT 3

    MY PATIENTS 3

LEGAL DISCLAIMER 4

MODULES 6

ABBREVIATIONS 7

CONTENTS 8

INTRODUCTION: WHAT'S IN THIS COURSE, HOW TO USE IT, & WHY I WROTE IT 19

    WHAT YOU WILL FIND IN THIS COURSE 20

    "SHOULD I USE BOTOX®, XEOMIN®, DYSPORT®, OR JEUVEAU®?" 22

    HOW TO GET YOUR MONEY'S WORTH FROM THIS COURSE 23

    A FEW WORDS ABOUT WHO I AM AND MY ROLE IN YOUR LIFE ... 24

    YOUR INVITATION 26

    FINAL WORDS 27

    REFERENCES REGARDING THE SAFETY OF BONT 28

1. WHY BONT PARTIES (& OTHER EVENTS) GROW YOUR PRACTICE FASTER THAN ALMOST ANYTHING 31

    THE PARTY PROFIT MODEL: WHERE DOES THE MONEY HAPPEN? 31

    MORE ABOUT CONNECTORS & HOW TO FIND THEM IN THE WILD 34

    CONNECTORS, BONT PARTIES, & OTHER EVENTS—HOW THEY WORK TOGETHER FOR EXPLOSIVE GROWTH OF YOUR PRACTICE 35

    THE MONEY-MAKING, RELATIONSHIP-BUILDING HEART OF A PARTY ... 37

    THE MONTHLY PRACTICE THAT BRINGS YOU GOLD 38

    REFERENCES 39

2. HOW TO DO A BONT PARTY (OR ANY OTHER EVENT) & BE SEEN AS THE MISSIONARY & HEALER THAT YOU ARE 40

    IMPORTANT LIFE QUESTION: WOULD YOU PREFER THE COMPANY OF THE PRIG OR THE PROSTITUTE? 40

    THE PERSON WHOM YOU NEED THAT YOU WILL *NEVER* SEE (EXCEPT AT A PARTY) 42

THE 2% SHOCK.. 43

ELON MUSK TEACHES YOU ABOUT BUBBLES 43

THE KEY MENTAL SWITCH THAT CHANGES YOU FROM A STARVING SALESMAN TO AN
ALTRUISTIC MISSIONARY AT ANY EVENT 44

HOW DARLENE HELPED ME HELP THOUSANDS 46

THE MAIN PRINCIPLE 49

ASSIGNMENT.. 49

WHAT REALLY HAPPENED AT CHURCH................................. 50

FROM "SWEET HOME ALABAMA" TO "HOTEL CALIFORNIA" 50

YOUR NEXT STEP TO PROFITABLE & FUN BONT PARTIES 51

3. THE ETHICS OF BONT PARTIES & WHY DOING THEM IS GOOD FOR YOUR
PATIENTS 52

THE ORIGIN OF BONT PARTIES 52

IS IT ETHICAL TO KEEP YOUR CURE A SECRET?..................... 53

WHAT UBER CAN TEACH YOU ABOUT MARKETING YOUR PRACTICE............................. 54

USING BAIT SO YOU CAN HELP 55

WHO IS RESPONSIBLE?.. 57

4. SAVING TIME AT YOUR PARTY & YOUR OFFICE...................... 58

START WITH THIS CHECKLIST... 58

FIRST, YOU NEED BONT (BUT YOU DO NOT BRING MOST OF IT IN THE BOTTLE) 60

5. BRING THESE TO THE PARTY: ATTITUDE, RULES, & TWO BAGS 61

THE BONT PARTY "TOOL BAG" 61

THE PRIZE BAG 64

ATTIRE AND ATTITUDE TIPS 65

PARTY RULES ABOUT ALCOHOL, FOOTPRINTS, & MUSIC.......... 66

PARTY RULES THAT GROW YOUR PRACTICE 69

CONCLUSION 70

6. SPECIAL TOOLS FOR YOUR BONT PARTY BAG & YOUR OFFICE 71

THE AMOUNT OF PREFILLED BONT SYRINGES 71

THE BONT BOARD 72

BOTTLE OPENER... 72

ICE PACKS 73

ICE CUBES 73

7. ORGANIZATION OF THE BONT BOARD FOR SPEED, PROFIT, & ACCURACY 75

8. SIMPLE DOCUMENTATION AT PARTY & OFFICE 76

WHERE DOES THE TIME GO? 76

THE MAP THAT I DRAW & THE FLOW 77

MORE ABOUT THE ORDER OF INJECTION 80

HOW THE PREFILLED SYRINGES SAVE TIME 80

REVIEW OF THE MAIN TIME TIP 81

SAVE EVEN MORE TIME, SEE BETTER RESULTS, & KEEP YOUR MEDICAL LICENSE 82

NOTE ABOUT HOW TO LOSE YOUR LICENSE TO PRACTICE MEDICINE 83

9. CHARGING PEOPLE AT THE PARTY—HOW MUCH & HOW TO COLLECT 84

WHAT I LEARNED FROM A MAN WHO MADE A FORTUNE COOKING FISH 84

THE CASHIER AT THE PARTY (THE REST OF THE STORY) 85

THE PATIENT FLOW 86

MOVING MONEY FROM THEIR BANK TO YOURS...................................... 86

AFTER THE PARTY 87

10. STARTING BONT PARTIES & CONSENTING (PART 1 OF 2) 89

INTRODUCTORY SPEECH 89

CONSENTING SPEECH 91

11. CONSENTING & EXPLAINING BONT (PART 2 OF 2)................................ 94

PASS OUT THE CONSENT FORMS... 94

CONTINUING THE CONSENT SPEECH 94

STARTING THE TREATMENT 97

THE ONLY TWO WAYS TO FIND THE BONT VIRGINS 97

WHY YOU NEED BONT VIRGINS TO GROW YOUR COSMETIC PRACTICE 98

PRIZES 98

TWO AT A TIME 99

REFRESHMENTS (THE HOSTESS' COST) & FREE BONT (MY COST)................ 99

HOW MANY AT THE PARTY? 100

12. START YOUR OWN BONT CLUB TO KEEP YOUR PATIENTS LOYAL & INCREASE INCOME 101

WHY CLUBS MAKE MONEY 101

FURTHER EXPLANATION OF HOW TO SET UP YOUR CLUB, INCLUDING EMAILS YOU CAN SEND.. 102

WHERE TO SEE A VIDEO DEMONSTRATION 104

THE DETAILS OF THE SHOPPING CART, WEB PAGE, & OTHER ASPECTS OF A CLUB 104

TRANSCRIPT.. 105

STANDARDIZATION OF PROCEDURES-ACCOMPLISHED BY THE CMA 106

A WHOLE NEW CLASS OF OPTIONS FOR HEALING 108

PROFIT: THE DOCTOR'S FOUR-LETTER WORD & "CRABS IN A BUCKET"...................... 110

CHARLES DICKENS & DOCTORS 114

HOW TO CREATE YOUR OWN CLUB 115

A STEP-BY-STEP PROCESS TO MAKE YOUR CLUB 117

SOCIAL MEDIA MAKES ME NEED A BATH 126

EMAIL 126

OTHER "CLUSTER CLUB" IDEAS 127

EXAMPLES OF PRODUCTS I SELL INDIVIDUALLY AND AS A CLUB.......... 128

13. HOW TO TURN THE INFO YOU LEARN AT A PARTY INTO A GROWING LIST OF FANS WHO WANT EVERYTHING YOU OFFER....................... 129

WHAT A BONT PARTY REALLY IS... 129

WHAT YOU "TAKE HOME" AFTER THE PARTY AND WHY................ 129

WHAT TO DO THE NEXT DAY AFTER THE PARTY 131

THE DOLLAR VALUE OF A NAME 131

NOW THAT YOU HAVE A GROWING LIST OF PEOPLE, WHAT DO YOU DO WITH IT? 132

THE TWO MAIN SUBJECTS OF EMAIL, & "VALIDATE THE VOYEUR" 133

YOU DO NOT HAVE TO DANCE FOR YOUR MONEY................... 134

WHERE TO FIND TODAY'S TRUTH 135

EDUCATIONAL & MOTIVATIONAL FORMAT (NOT PRETTY)........... 135

RINSE AND REPEAT 136

THE MAIN POINT 136

14. WHY YOU LOSE IF YOU ONLY DO WHAT YOU PROMISED, & HOW TO GROW YOUR PRACTICE LIKE AMWAY.. 137

KNOW YOUR PATIENT BETTER EVERY TIME THEY GET BONT.................. 137

YOU BECOME PART OF THE MOST IMPORTANT EVENTS IN ANOTHER PERSON'S LIFE 138

DO MORE THAN WHAT THEY PAID YOU TO DO 139

TURN YOUR OFFICE INTO MLM.. 141

START YOUR OWN CLUBS 142

15. OFFICE ENVIRONMENT AS A WAY TO LESS PAIN & MORE HEALING...... 144

A CELLPHONE ON THE TABLE POISONS DINNER—SO, NO SIGN 144

DEEPER INSIDE THE OFFICE... 147

BE AT LEAST AS CAREFUL AS STARBUCKS IS ABOUT THIS............ 148

WHY YOUR MASSAGE THERAPIST MAKES MORE DOLLARS PER HOUR THAN YOU......... 149

MY STRICT OFFICE RULES THAT HELP MY PATIENTS FIND PEACE AND PERCEIVE VALUE . 151

PW-CBQS WASTE YOUR TIME (TWO WAYS) AND KILL THE PEACE........... 153

THROW AWAY THE MAGAZINES & DISPLAY THIS INSTEAD 154

JUNK COMES IN THE FRONT DOOR AND GOES OUT THE BACK DOOR 155

IF YOU TURN RED, YOU CANNOT WORK WHERE WE TALK SEX................... 156

IMPORT THE ORIENT (THEY THOUGHT ABOUT THIS FOR 4,000 YEARS)................... 156

How to Measure You (Because You are Also Part of Your Office Environment) 158

Music Magic: Never Underestimate It nor Neglect It 158

Extra Tips for Healing: The Sheets, the Clock, the Thermostat 160

The Walls...161

Synergy of Environmental Ingredients 162

Easy Assignment 162

16. INTRODUCTION TO MIXING BONT 163

Diluent Matters...163

Rifle vs. Shotgun 163

How to Mix BoNT 164

17. MIXING BONT FOR MORE ACCURACY & LESS PAIN 165

The Math of Dilution—Use a Small Volume 165

Summary...165

The Needle Touches Nothing Until It Touches the Patient.............................166

Use the Needle No More than Three or Four Times 167

Summary...168

18. EXTRACTING THE LAST DROP WITHOUT DULLING THE NEEDLE 169

19. THE "ONE THING" YOU MAY BE DOING THAT *DOUBLES* THE PAIN 171

When You Hold the Syringe, Think Smoking 171

20. A MARKETING METHOD WITH SOUL 174

Same-Day Appointments or Lose the Patient 174

Snacks Get You Out of Jail 175

A Question That Gauges Patient Treatment..175

A BoNT Patient Who Died...176

Summary of a Marketing Method with Soul..178

21. NEEDLE SECRETS TO AVOID PAIN & BRUISING 179

More about How to Extract BoNT from the Vial 179

Bubbles Make You Inaccurate..179

A Tiny Injection Demands a Small Syringe & No Bubble 181

Lighthouse 182

22. THE "HOLDING BOARD" FOR SAVING TIME & AVOIDING PAIN 184

Making & Loading the "Holding Board" 184

23. FOUR GUIDING PRINCIPLES OF PROVIDING GREAT BONT 188

Guiding Principle #1: Follow a Consistent Sequence 188

Guiding Principle #2: Facial Muscles Attach Skin to Bone 189

Guiding Principle #3: Muscles are Belts that Make Pleats 189

Guiding Principle #4: Before Injecting, Watch the Face Move........................ 190

A Common Mistake that Can Cause Either a Lack of Effect or a "Crazy" Effect from BoNT 191

Example of Using the Principles.. 192

Lighthouse... 193

24. FACE CONSULT: CLEAR THINKING & ACCURATE PROMISES.................. 194

How to Swap Brains (and Why You Must).. 194

Your Patients Are Not Looking for Compliments 198

Why You Should Study Faces in Movies 200

What Every Patient Wants 200

My Favorite Aesthetic-Consult Question 201

If You Are Trying to See Better, Use Less Light.. 204

25. "LITTLE SPEECHES" THAT HELP YOU IMPROVE YOUR TECHNIQUE & MAKE MORE MONEY 206

The "It Didn't Work" Speech 206

My Little "Go-Home" Speech that Can Help You Become a Better Injector and Keep You from Losing Patients 207

How to Become Excellent at Anything 208

Becoming the Expert for Each Patient 209

The "Free Offer" Speech I Make after Every BoNT Treatment........................ 210

Nobody Dies... 210

The "If-You-Can-Do-This" Speech to Help You Improve 211

The "Reassurance" Speech 212

The Forever Challenge 213

26. BEFORE & AFTERS, AN OVERVIEW, & A FRONTALIS WARNING 214

A Prize for the Patient 214

A Frontalis Pearl that Saves Two Units of BoNT... 215

Short-Hand Notation for BoNT 216

A "Disclaimer Speech" that Brings Them Back.. 217

What Makes BoNT Valuable? 219

Time to Inject 219

27. INJECTION POINT #1: FROWN LINES, THE DASH & THE NUMBER 11'S .. 220

First, a Word About Gloves.. 220

Skip Betadine & Alcohol... 221

Go Into Your Peaceful Space 221
Glabella = (Procerus + Corrugators) 222
1a. Injecting the Procerus (Erasing the Dash) 223
To Avoid Bruises, Follow the "Full-Minute" Rule..................225
A Note on Music 226
1b. Injecting Left & Right Corrugators (Erasing the 11) 227
Gentle Massage After Injection in Two Places 230
A Fast & Accurate Record 231

28. INJECTION POINT #2: BROW LIFT 232

The Muscles & Vectors that Control the Brow 232
How to "Tailor-Make" Brows 233
Where to Inject to Lift the Brow 235
Can't Touch This 237
Documentation of the Brow Lift 238

29. INJECTION POINT #3: SOFTENING CROW'S FEET 239

Smile Lines vs. Eye Lines...239
Where to Put the Needle 240
More About the Amount 242
Avoid the "Crow's Feet Catch" 243
"Don't Touch This" 243

30. INJECTION POINT #4: THE FOREHEAD SMOOTHER 244

Where to Inject Frontalis...244
Three Frontalis Treatment Traps & How to Avoid Them 248
A Tip About Those Who Have Had a Surgical Facelift...........252

31. INJECTION POINT #5: EYE OPENER 253

Why Open the Eye? 253
Give This to Make Your Patients Happy and Your Profits Grow......................254
Ectropion & A Warning About Treating Eyes.........................255
Exactly Where to Put the Needle 257
Important: to Keep from Injecting Too Much 258

32. INJECTION POINT #6: BUNNY LINES ERASER 260

Facial Muscles Allow You to Read Minds 260
Finding the Nasalis Injection Point 260

33. INJECTION POINT #7: GUMMY SMILE ERASER...................... 263

What is a Gummy Smile?...263

EXAMPLE OF GUMMY SMILE YOU SHOULD NOT TREAT..............................263
THE QUESTION TO ASK TO DISCOVER IF YOU SHOULD TREAT A GUMMY SMILE............264
WHERE TO PUT THE NEEDLE & HOW TO INJECT 265
WARNING (TO AVOID MAKING YOUR PATIENT LOOK AS IF SHE HAD A STROKE) 266
HOW VALUABLE IS THIS SIMPLE LITTLE TRICK?.....................................266

34. INJECTION POINT #8: FROWN ERASER 268

SCULPTURE OR ENGINEERING?...268
THE TRIANGULARIS CONNECTIONS..268
WHO WANTS THEIR FROWN FIXED?..269
WHERE TO PUT THE NEEDLE...270
WHAT TO SAY & DO TO KEEP YOUR PATIENTS FROM LEAVING AFTER A TRIANGULARIS
TREATMENT 272

35. INJECTION POINT #9: ORANGE PEEL CHIN................................... 275

"CRINKLE, PLEASE"..275
WHOM SHOULD YOU TREAT? 275
WHERE TO PUT THE NEEDLE..276
A TIP FOR INJECTING MENTALIS 277
WHY DO YOU NEED A MENTALIS MUSCLE ANYWAY?! 278
MENTALIS WARNING 278

36. INJECTION POINT #10: WEBBED NECK 279

PLATYSMA BANDS 279
WHAT ARE PLATYSMA BANDS? 279
THE TREATMENT OF PLATYSMA BANDS: TWO METHODS 280
WHERE TO PUT THE NEEDLE: "SAVE STRATEGY" 280
DILUTION CHANGE FOR THREE PLACES 280
WHERE TO PUT THE NEEDLE: "SURE STRATEGY" 281
DOCUMENTATION: WHY I PREFER PAPER & PEN (NOT IPAD) 283
A MOTHER IS GLAD TO SEE ME WRITE ON PAPER 284
YOUR SECOND HUSBAND & YOUR COMPUTER..285
MUCH GRATITUDE TO THE AUTHORS 287

37. INJECTION POINT #11: NECKLACE LINES.................................... 288

NECKLACE LINES..288
WHERE TO PUT THE NEEDLE...288
COMBINE THESE WITH BONT FOR AN AMAZING RESULT..............................289

**38. INJECTION POINT #12: LIP GLAMORIZER ("LIP FLIP") & SMOKER'S LINES
ERASER 291**

The Orbicularis Oris & the Definition of a Kiss 291

Lip Strategies: Understanding the Why of the Where 292

Reconstitution Variation 294

Deciding If to Inject for Shape 295

My Mouth Goes from Caucasian to African (& My First Experience of Medicine's Malice) 295

The Moral of the Story 299

Teaching the Woman (or Man) About Her Face 301

Where to Put the Needle 302

Pain Control 304

The Homunculus Predicts Your Bedroom Behavior 304

Where to Put the Needle to Inject the Lower Lip 305

A Beauty Clue 306

What if you Miss 306

Where to Put the Needle for a More Aggressive Smoker's Lines Treatment 307

Another Peek at the BoNT Board 307

References 308

39. TREATING MEDICAL PROBLEMS WITH BONT 311

She Did not Cry Because of Pain 311

The Insurance-Tail Wagging the Doctor-Dog 311

Can You Do a Double-Blind, Placebo-Controlled Study of Parachutes, Birth Control Pills, or BoNT? 312

What to Do for a BoNT Treatment Covered by Insurance if You Do Not Accept Insurance 313

Never Keep the Money If the Patient Does Not Love the Result 313

40. TREATING DEPRESSION WITH BONT 315

Holy Serotonin—And the Hindrance to a Better Way....................................315

Not a "Magic Bullet" 316

Darwin & Depression...316

Cold Emotions & Warm Emotions 317

"Selective Blocking" ...A Hypothesis for Why SSRIs Increase Suicide & BoNT Does Not 319

The Warming of an Emotion & the "Facial Feedback Hypothesis" 319

BoNT Blocks the Facial Feedback Loop 320

Facial Feedback Can Cause a Death Spiral...321

Summary of How BoNT Helps the Depressed 321

BoNT, Depression, & the CNS..322

Should Insurance Define Standard of Care? 324

Profit Governs Altruism 324

WHERE TO PUT THE NEEDLE 325

A REQUEST & AN OFFER FOR YOU 326

REFERENCES 327

41. TREATING MIGRAINES WITH BONT **331**

THE THEORY OF MIGRAINES 331

HOW DOES BONT HELP MIGRAINES? 331

A WONDERFUL SIDE EFFECT OF TREATING MIGRAINES WITH BONT 332

A SIMPLE SECRET ABOUT TREATING MIGRAINES WITH BONT 332

SETTING EXPECTATIONS 333

MIXING BONT TO TREAT MIGRAINES 334

HOW TO INJECT SEVEN MUSCLE GROUPS TO TREAT CHRONIC MIGRAINES 335

1. INJECTING PROCERUS 337

2. INJECTING THE CORRUGATORS 337

3. INJECTING FRONTALIS 339

4. INJECTING OCCIPITOFRONTALIS (OCCIPITALIS, FRONTALIS, FRONTO OCCIPITALIS) 340

WHERE TO PUT THE NEEDLE 342

5. INJECTING TEMPORALIS 343

6. INJECTING TRAPEZIUS 344

7. INJECTING SPLENIUS CAP 345

THAT WAS THE LAST OF THE SEVEN 347

AN EXTRA INJECTION TO KEEP IT PRETTY 347

ANOTHER WORD ABOUT CASH VS. INSURANCE AS IT SPECIFICALLY APPLIES TO MIGRAINE
TREATMENT 349

FURTHER HELP TO MAKE IT EVEN EASIER THAN EASY 349

REFERENCES 350

42. TREATING BRUXISM (& ASSOCIATED HEADACHES) WITH BONT **352**

A QUICK & EASY MIRACLE 352

HOW TO SPOT THE PERSON WHO NEEDS YOU 353

WHERE TO PUT THE NEEDLE 355

HOLLYWOOD TIP 356

FURTHER HELP 357

REFERENCES 357

43. TREATING ERECTILE DYSFUNCTION WITH BONT **358**

BONT FOR ED—WHY & WHY NOT? 358

A SUGGESTED ALGORITHM FOR COMBINED THERAPIES (HOW BONT FITS IN THE
TREATMENT PLAN) 365

THREE WAYS BONT IMPROVES ERECTION (MECHANISM OF ACTION) 366

Two Questions You Answer Every Time You Treat Erectile Dysfunction (Even if You Do Not Know the Questions) 371

How to Prepare for the Treatment of ED with BoNT 371

How to Inject BoNT into the Penis for ED 373

Frequently Asked Questions 378

Further Help with Both *Injection Technique* and *Marketing* BoNT for ED 381

References Regarding BoNT for ED 382

Research Regarding the Regenerative Effects of BoNT 384

References Regarding BoNT for Fibrosis and Scaring 385

Representative References Regarding the P-Shot® Procedure 386

References Regarding PRP for Peyronie's Disease 389

References Regarding PRP for Neovascularization....................................... 389

References Regarding PRP for Neurogenesis 390

References Regarding the Use of PRP for Muscle Repair 391

TABLE OF FIGURES 393

INDEX 408

ABOUT THE AUTHOR 413

FURTHER HELP 414

Introduction: What's in this Course, How to Use It, & Why I Wrote It

I wrote this course with one purpose in mind: to help you use botulinum neurotoxin (BoNT) to safely improve the lives of your patients while dramatically increasing your practice profits.

This is not an idle promise.

For two decades, I have proven this promise in my own practice of medicine.

Also, I have proven this promise for twelve years by teaching physicians how to increase their profits and help their patients using BoNT; I have trained over five thousand physicians in over fifty countries. In my

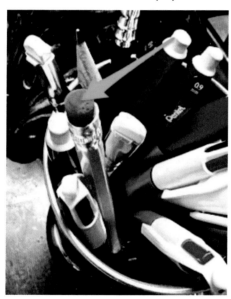

Figure 1. If you can stick a needle into an eraser, you can become a BoNT injector.

online courses and hands-on workshops, I have helped family practitioners, internists, gynecologists, urologists, and their nurses learn to use BoNT to provide excellent patient results.

Too often, physicians will attend hands-on workshops and read multiple textbooks and still feel confused and afraid to offer cosmetic injections to their patients. This should not be the case. Even if they have previously attended multiple classes before mine and still struggle to get started, doctors confidently inject their patients to achieve beautiful results after attending my classes.

Unless you suffer a tremor that makes it difficult for you to accurately stick a needle into a spot the size of a pencil eraser, you can learn to provide excellent BoNT. I have proven over and over in my classes, at least once a month, every month (but for three) for the past 12 years, that one can easily and quickly learn how to do cosmetic BoNT injections.

You can also use BoNT to help your patients with some difficult-to-treat medical problems—all with minimal risk.

You never lose sleep because you treated someone with BoNT.

What You Will Find in This Course

This book is divided into forty-two chapters that are grouped into four modules. But don't worry; you do not need to read every chapter before offering your patients excellent BoNT.

Let me explain what's in each module, and you will know how to get started quickly.

Module 1
The first module tells you how to easily find all the new patients you could ever want by becoming the star of events hosted by others. And, importantly, how to be the featured guest at an event in a way that improves your reputation. You never look like a desperate salesperson.

Most people who already receive BoNT are not looking for another provider; they already have their provider and are no more likely to change their BoNT provider than to swap their gynecologist. But many people (around 98% of adults) do not yet have a BoNT provider, and that is a huge opportunity for you (if you know how to find and communicate with that person about what you can do for them). You will find that person at events.

Also, suppose you are a primary care physician and already have an office full of charts. In that case, there is a way to introduce your new BoNT capabilities to your current patients in a way that encourages them to see you and enhances your reputation.

So, whether you have been in practice and have many charts or are just getting started, if you want a steady stream of new patients who will love you (and what you do) and want to pay you, then Module 1 will show you how.

This module is dear to me because I lived it. As an internist in a small town, Fairhope, Alabama, I used cosmetic injections and events (using exactly the methods I teach in Module 1) to create an income stream that both improved my lifestyle and gave me time to spend with my very sick patients—without worrying that insurance would not pay me enough to cover my overhead.

Module 2

One of the best ways to always have patients is to be very good at what you do; if you are so good that people cannot help but talk about what you do for them, you will always have people calling for appointments.

An essential part of being excellent at cosmetic BoNT is knowing how to inject faces without hurting or bruising. Even if you know the anatomy and know the science and know exactly where to put the needle, if you cause bruises and pain, your cosmetic practice will die.

The techniques I show you in Module 2 will keep you from bruising and hurting your patients—helping to distinguish you as an expert.

Nothing is difficult in this section (or anywhere in this course), but do not let the simplicity cause you to underestimate the effectiveness and power of the techniques.

Follow my simple instructions, and no one will hurt or bruise their patients less than you.

Module 3

Anyone can complicate; my goal (and the goal of any good teacher) is to take what looks complicated and simplify it.

In Module 3, I simplify whole textbooks about BoNT injections down to just twelve injection points. Then I tell you how to use variations of those twelve to create excellent results for your patients.

For each of the 12 injection points, I show you the anatomy and the reasoning, exactly where to put the needle, and how much to inject.

Use this section as a reference whenever you need it. If you already inject BoNT, use this section to fine-tune your current techniques, and you will confidently and safely create gorgeous results for your patients.

Module 4

In Module 4, I show you how to use BoNT to help your patients with four medical problems: (1) depression, (2) bruxism, (3) migraines, and (4) erectile dysfunction. People will gladly pay you (and you deserve to be paid) to help them with these common problems using your BoNT injections. And you can do so without losing sleep—worrying that you hurt someone.

Nothing works for everyone. But these treatments have a very high success rate. And *I even tell you how to make more money by giving people their money back (all of it) when they are not helped.* So, do not worry; you are not going to be keeping money unless people feel like you profoundly changed their life for the better.

Some of your most grateful patients will be the ones who come to you for BoNT. Module 4 shows you ways to make that happen.

"Should I Use Botox®, Xeomin®, Dysport®, or Jeuveau®?"

Regarding neuromodulators, use any one of them.

I have used them all. They all work.

Botox

Botox was first to market and has been the gold standard. You should familiarize yourself with it. And if you live in the US, you should buy it only from Allergan in the US (do not look for discount suppliers that ship from other countries unless you are interested in losing your license to practice medicine).

Xeomin

I also like Xeomin because it (in theory) is less immunogenic. You mix and inject it with the same dilution and injection technique as with Botox®. So *everywhere in this book where you see the word "BoNT," you could* substitute the word *"Xeomin,"* and all would be the same and beautiful and safe.

Important: Xeomin has the advantage of not needing to be refrigerated before you use it.

Jeuveau

Jeuveau® has also been a wonderful product for some of my students. I have less experience with it. The company offers a handy app that makes ordering easy. Again, mix it and use it like you would Botox® and Xeomin®.

Dysport

Dysport also has a solid history. To use Dysport, mix it and use it as you would the other three. The only difference is that *when you record what you did, multiply the number of units on your syringe by 3.*

For example, when you inject two units (as measured on the syringe), you really injected 2 x 3 = 6 units.

Summary of How to Choose

Try them all and make up your own mind. When the products are similar, then much depends upon the attention and courtesy of your local sales representative and on the price. The main point is to understand your product, whichever neuromodulator you choose. Know it as well as anyone knows it; do not settle for less. Become an expert at everything you do in medicine, or if not, decide not to do it.

The great news is that you can very quickly become an expert at injecting neuromodulators.

In short, *be an expert with your chosen product and be sure to keep the final dilution volumes the same as what I teach, or else you risk inadvertently affecting muscles you did not intend to treat.*

How to Get Your Money's Worth from This Course

This book will do little for you if you scan through it, put it on your shelf, and forget it.

Instead, *if you want to fill your practice with people who love you (and what you do) and who want to pay you, people who are grateful for the ways you have dramatically changed their life for the better, then keep this book on your desk, in a place where you see it every day, and follow this plan...*

Every day,
read one chapter from this course,
And implement at least one tip
From what you read.
Go through the book in this way two times,
and it will change your practice (and maybe your life)
for the better
in dramatic ways.

Some chapters may be a review for you. In that case, you will be reminded and encouraged to continue your current best practice.

But most chapters will offer at least one new idea that warrants action. If the recommended action involves the internet or computer work that you do not want to do, then at least you know what needs to be done— *hire someone to do it for you* (I'll tell you where to find them).

If you follow this plan and go through the book in this way, your life will become dramatically better, as will the lives of thousands of people who come to see you.

A Few Words About Who I Am and My Role in Your Life

At heart, I am an internist and a chemist.

Before medical school, I worked for three years as a physical chemist at Southern Research Institute (Birmingham, Alabama), which gave me a way of thinking mathematically; if you watch carefully, you will see the math appear throughout this course. The math helps with the injections, and it helps with the marketing (the money).

Marketing could be defined as psychology combined with math. And the best marketing educates and persuades people to do what is best for them. So, I love marketing, and I love the math in marketing, and I love to see physicians change their lives (and those of their patients) for the better after learning marketing from me.

Why an Internist Needed to Learn Cosmetic Medicine

Twenty years ago, as a busy internist, I noticed that my patients often did not want to lose weight because it made their faces look older (which it does). So, I grew interested in cosmetic medicine, and after I learned how to use BoNT and fillers, I encouraged my patients to lose weight for their health and then to reward themselves for the weight loss with BoNT and fillers. And that strategy worked! People lost weight (for a younger and healthier body), and I helped them keep a younger face.

After I immersed my brain in cosmetic medicine as a way to encourage weight loss, the discipline expanded my thoughts and my medical practice in ways I had never imagined. *My cosmetic work has been as rewarding as anything I have done in medicine and has led to helpful ideas outside of aesthetics.*

Using ideas that I learned in cosmetic medicine, I developed all the following cosmetic procedures: the Vampire Facelift®, Vampire Breast Lift®, Vampire Facial®, and the Vampire Wing Lift® as well as techniques with hair growth.

But, surprisingly, some of *my best ideas in the arena of disease also came from what I learned in cosmetic medicine; I developed all the following by combining what I know from internal medicine with what I learned in cosmetic medicine:*

- I was the first to inject platelet-rich plasma (PRP) into the anterior vaginal wall and into the clitoris, inventing the O-Shot® procedure, which has been shown to help with dyspareunia, stress urinary incontinence, lichen sclerosus, and interstitial cystitis (see OShot.com).

- I was also the first to inject PRP into the penis, inventing the Priapus Shot® (P-Shot®) procedure, which has been shown to help with erectile dysfunction, Peyronie's disease, and penile rehabilitation post prostate surgery.
- Bocox® to help with erectile dysfunction also evolved out of my work in both cosmetic and internal medicine.
- The Cellular Medicine Association and the Institute for Lichen Sclerosus and Vulvar Health both evolved out of working in the combined cosmetic and internal medicine spaces. By becoming a facilitator and organizer of the many brilliant physicians and their extenders who make up these groups, I have become blessed to see much accomplished that I could have never done alone.

Your Invitation

At sixty-three years old, I have spent over thirty years thinking about medicine and about the subject matter of this book. My strong desire is that your life and that of your patients will be dramatically improved by this course and by the ongoing research and teachings of our organizations.

For that reason, I invite you to contact me and let me know how this book helps you and the people who trust you with their health.

Please go to Runels.com and CellularMedicineAssociation.org and subscribe (for free) to my email updates. If you would like further training, you will find options there.

Also, write to me (DrRunels@Runels.com) or call me (1-251-648-7704) and let me know your questions. If I am writing or seeing patients when you call, you may reach my staff; but if I miss you, I will be eager to return your call and help where I can.

If the answers to your questions are in one of my online courses, I may refer you there; if not, I will help you personally. Fair enough?

Final Words

After you have studied this course and implemented what you have learned, after you have seen a huge boost in your income, and after your patients have cried in your office out of gratitude for what you have done for them (using what you learned in this course), I hope that you will write to me and let me know.

I have seen the tears in my own patient's eyes when someone has felt a new level of wellness and a new depth to their love relations because of my BoNT practice. It will thrill me to hear that you have seen the same.

Medicine can be difficult, and it can be lonely. But it can also be glorious!

Reach out.

I will be honored to congratulate you for the work you will do and for the positive change in lives that you will cause, especially if that change is partly because of this course.

Sincerely,

Charles

Charles Runels, MD
Fairhope, Alabama
June 2023

P.S. You can learn all you need to know to become excellent at neuromodulators from this course alone. But the videos at BoNTClass.com can clarify and greatly accelerate your learning process.

P.P.S. This course offers an occasional rhyme. Like a corny dad joke, they may not touch your soul, but if cringe helps cement an important point in your brain, that's a good thing. I have no illusion that these rhymes belong in a book of poetry along with Walt Whitman and Emily Dickenson. But I am glad to sacrifice my dignity to make important ideas less forgettable.

References Regarding the Safety of BoNT

1. BOTOX 100 Units - Summary of Product Characteristics (SmPC) - (emc). Accessed September 1, 2022. https://www.medicines.org.uk/emc/product/859/smpc#gref

2. Nigam PK, Nigam A. BOTULINUM TOXIN. *Indian J Dermatol.* 2010;55(1):8-14. doi:10.4103/0019-5154.60343

3. Arnon SS, Schechter R, Inglesby TV, et al. Botulinum Toxin as a Biological WeaponMedical and Public Health Management. *JAMA.* 2001;285(8):1059-1070. doi:10.1001/jama.285.8.1059

4. Omprakash HM, Rajendran SC. Botulinum Toxin Deaths: What is the Fact? *J Cutan Aesthet Surg.* 2008;1(2):95-97. doi:10.4103/0974-2077.44169

5. Dhaked RK, Singh MK, Singh P, Gupta P. Botulinum toxin: Bioweapon & magic drug. *Indian J Med Res.* 2010;132(5):489-503. Accessed September 1, 2022. https://www.ncbi.nlm.nih.gov/pmc/articles/PMC3028942/

6. Frevert J. Content of Botulinum Neurotoxin in Botox®/Vistabel®, Dysport®/Azzalure®, and Xeomin®/Bocouture®. *Drugs R D.* 2010;10(2):67-73. doi:10.2165/11584780-000000000-00000

7. Bhatia KP, Munchau A, Thompson PD, et al. Generalized muscular weakness after botulinum toxin injections for dystonia: a report of three cases. *Journal of Neurology, Neurosurgery & Psychiatry.* 1999;67(1):90-93. doi:10.1136/jnnp.67.1.90

8. Stephens ML, Balls M. LD50 Testing of Botulinum Toxin for Use as a Cosmetic. 2005;(2):5.

9. Naumann M, Jankovic J. Safety of botulinum toxin type A: a systematic review and meta-analysis. *Current Medical Research and Opinion*. 2004;20(7):981-990. doi:10.1185/030079904125003962

10. Hefter H, Samadzadeh S. The Necessity of a Locally Active Antidote in the Clinical Practice of Botulinum Neurotoxin Therapy: Short Communication. *Medicina*. 2022;58(7):935. doi:10.3390/medicina58070935

Module I.

BoNT Parties
A Sure Way to Boost Your Reputation & Double
Your Practice Income

1. Why BoNT Parties (& Other Events) Grow Your Practice Faster Than Almost Anything

When I was a teenager, I would watch my mom come home from a Tupperware® party. Her car, a station wagon that she had won selling Tupperware, would be full of Tupperware bowls.

Our garage was full of Tupperware. And the phone constantly rang because her customers and the 35 women in her downline (it's a multi-level marketing business) would call.

All of it was about Tupperware.

The main promise was that Tupperware bowls were guaranteed for life. And after dinner, you can put your leftover food in those bowls, and your food will be fresh the next day. And they also sold planters with plant food, orange peelers, toys, and all sorts of things (other than bowls), all made of plastic.

People made fortunes selling plastic bowls in the USA in the 1960s and 1970s.

They still do!

But, in the USA, you can now buy your Tupperware in Target® stores (which helped kill the Tupperware parties here); but in Asia and Latin America, the Tupperware party still thrives and makes loads of money.

So, what does a Tupperware party teach you about how to grow your BoNT practice?

The Party Profit Model: Where Does the Money Happen?

There is a secret business idea embedded into the Tupperware party that can blast off your whole medical practice more powerfully than can a huge marketing budget. As you read the next section, see how long it takes for you to see it.

When I was sixteen years old, I asked my mother to recruit me as a "Tupperware Lady" so that I could understand her business. I did not sell much (I had other jobs and school and mostly wanted to understand the business more than to understand bowls), but I got to see how the Tupperware business works.

Tupperware parties in the USA are less popular now, but perhaps you have been to a clothing party (where someone brings a trunk of clothes to sell at someone's house) or to a sex toy party; they all work the way the Tupperware party worked back in the 1970s when my mother was a "Tupperware lady."

The hostess of the Tupperware party would invite her friends to a party, and my mom would show up on the appointed night. Then my mother would demonstrate bowls, and the hostess' friends would buy them.

The hostess would get free Tupperware bowls because she connected everyone (my mother with the hostess' friends).

But so what?

Here's my question to you, "How and why does a party make money?"

When I ask that question, most people answer, "Because you get many people there at the same time to buy stuff. That's how it makes money."

Yes, that is true, but that is not the critical part of the answer. If "lots of people in the room" is the heart of the party model, you could save gas money and just ask a bunch of your own patients to come to your office next week for a party. But then, after one party, whom do you ask to come to your party next week, the week after, and every week for the next five years? You exhausted your friend list with the first party.

The answer is more subtle: *the way the Tupperware party makes money is through the "connector."*

Connectors Are the Key

Imagine that my mother had a party for her friends (the same as if a doctor had an event in his own office). Her friends will not want to hear about bowls the very next week.

So, now imagine that my mother spends $25,000 to run a television ad that says, "Come to my house next Wednesday night, where I can sell you plastic bowls."

No one would show up, and if they did, *the cost of the ad would be more than could be made selling the plastic bowls.*

But Mary can ask her friends to a party at *her* house. And my mom can show up on the same night, at the same time.

And Mary can say, "Hey, you should buy these bowls."

And her friends do. My mom makes money selling bowls; Mary gets free bowls. Then, one of Mary's friends, Jane, can then host another party next week—because Jane has friends that Mary does not have.

That is the concept of party profit.

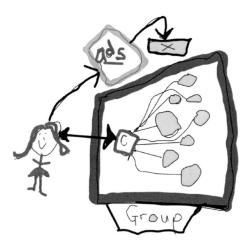

Figure 1. The (1) connector invites (2) you and the (3) members of her group to a party. You come to the party (enter their group) and meet people you could have never reached with paid advertising. The people receive your services. The connector receives a higher standing with her group.

And *the reason it makes a profit is that the person showing up with the goods to sell is leveraging the relationships of the hostess*, who is the connector to all her friends, some of whom are also connectors. That is a perpetual motion marketing machine.

The best explanation of "connectors" is in *The Tipping Point.* (Gladwell, 2000) Read it to really understand party profit. I read that book at least four times, trying to understand how connectors work and how things go viral before I came up with the Vampire Facelift® procedure (which I invented and named, and it went viral).

More About Connectors & How to Find Them in the Wild

If someone talks continuously, but no one cares what they say, that is a "bore," not a "connector."

The opposite, if someone is insightful, and people want to hear their ideas, but the person never talks, that is a "guru" in a cave of solitude, not a connector.

To be a connector, a person must have both qualities: (1) they like to talk, and (2) people want to hear what they say.

Connectors make things go viral, and they grow your business.

So, my mom used a connector (the hostess) to put her in the hostess's living room with *people with whom my mom had no previous relationship.* Then, the connector tells her friends how great my mother is and to buy plastic bowls from her, so they do.

NOTE: Where does the profit happen?
With a party, the marketing cost to make hundreds of dollars selling plastic bowls while drinking Kool-aide® for an hour in someone's living room is near zero—the marketing cost is only a few plastic bowls given to the hostess, traded for the hostess's introduction to her group. That is where the profit happens—the *almost free connection.*

But that is not the whole story.

The hostess gets something else more valuable than the free plastic bowls. Because she brings something to her group who makes their life better (a fun party and a deal on some bowls), she increases her standing with her group.

So, to make that happen for the hostess when my mother showed up, she had to bring value to the hostess's group and make the hostess proud that she introduced my mom. Mom had to make the life of the hostess's group better, and not on a future date; she had to make their life better the night of the party with a fun event, even for those who did not buy bowls.

Connectors, BoNT Parties, & Other Events—How They Work Together for Explosive Growth of Your Practice

When you are the speaker at an event, your service to the group must make the connector glad she invited you; so she invites you back. And others in her group will want to invite you to their group! This nonlinear expansion becomes multilevel marketing on steroids: not one gets two, and those two get four; instead, one gets ten, two of those ten get twenty, and four of those twenty get eighty!

With the BoNT party, your best connector is the person who owns a hair salon or the person who lives in a house that gives them pride; and they like to host social gatherings. That person will ask their friends over to their salon or to their house and host an event for you. That event could be a BoNT party (or something else, as you will see).

The hostess gets free BoNT, but those in her group who show up get a free consult from you (even if they do not want BoNT), and they get a fun social outing. You give away door prizes, she puts fun people in the same room at the same time, and (only those who want it) get BoNT at $1 less per unit than what you charge in your office.

So, the hostess, in addition to the free BoNT, also gets increased standing in her group for bringing something of value to her group—you and your party.

A Surgical Version of the "BoNT Party"

I know a prominent surgeon who sells liposuction by the party model in cities and states other than where he does surgery. A woman will invite her friends to her home. He will show up and give a free consult for her friends.

Then if the attendees want to book liposuction surgery with him, they can do it at the party for a slight discount; then, they will fly to see him (in the state where he is licensed) on a future date that is booked at the party. The hostess gets free or greatly discounted surgery, and her friends have fun at the party and get a free consult even if they do not schedule surgery. He sells surgeries in the same way my mother sold Tupperware and in the same way you can sell BoNT.

Other Party Examples

Places I have used the party profit concept includes the following (and more):

Seventh-day Adventist Church

At the invitation of the minister's wife, I lectured at a Seventh-day Adventist Church because she knew that I was living a vegetarian lifestyle. I spoke to her church congregation about how vegetarian food can help control blood pressure (which it does). And some of those people followed me back to my office, so I became their internist.

The Palms Hotel, Las Vegas

A husband and wife who had received a P-Shot® and an O-Shot® (from a physician whom I trained) invited me to a convention of swingers that they hosted at The Palms in Las Vegas. The couple owned the email list that generated the event.

I lectured to their group about the O-Shot® and the P-Shot®. Larry Flint also lectured there, giving the most motivational talk I have ever heard about freedom of speech. Hundreds of people attended the event, and in the evening, after lectures, there was a huge orgy.

When the attendees went home, they knew about the O-Shot® and P-Shot® procedures, and many of them sought treatment from one of our licensed providers (which they could find on the directories at OShot.com and PriapusShot.com).

Hotel California

When I started teaching other physicians the procedures that I had invented and wanted to meet physicians in California, a prominent plastic surgeon there invited thirty-four of his friends to a hotel in Los Angeles, and we demonstrated the Vampire Facelift® procedure. His friends got to learn the Vampire Facelift®. And afterward, he and I talked in private about intellectual properties (trademarks and patents) in relation to some of his inventions—that was his "free bowls" reward for hosting the party.

He wanted to learn how I was developing and protecting intellectual properties; he knew his group would be interested in the Vampire Facelift® procedure; and I wanted to meet people he knew in Los Angeles. So, it worked for all of us.

That's the idea of a "Tupperware party."

The Best Part is After the Party

In this course, we will talk more about BoNT parties and you are going to make money at your parties. But, *most of the money happens when the people at the party follow you back to your office and get other procedures and products from you—all of them.*

Everything.

Just remember, as we continue to talk about BoNT parties, *the concept applies if you travel to any group to bring them something of value for the opportunity to meet the people there*; parties are definitely not just about BoNT.

The Money-Making, Relationship-Building Heart of a Party

To review (because this idea is so valuable if you implement it), the more important concept about party profit that allows you to make money and to help people in profound ways other than providing BoNT is that you go to a group, and you are introduced to the group by a connector. You were invited because you bring to the group information or services *while you are there*; it could be consultations, it could be only information, or it could be services—for example, BoNT injections.

You go to the event. You are introduced to the group by the connector. You bring something to them, and *what you want is the names and emails of the people at the event and for them to know who you are.*

That is it.

Nothing more and nothing less.

Never show up if you are not bringing something of value to the group that they receive *immediately (while you are there), even if they choose never to contact you after you leave.*

Never show up if you are not allowed to collect names and email addresses *while you are there.*

I spoke in India and Serbia and Greece and Spain, New Zealand, Great Britain, and other countries and traveled throughout the U.S.; I was introduced to groups by device manufacturers and by other physicians, but I never took money for speaking, never, not for the plane or for the hotel—not even for a meal, because I feel like that makes me biased.

I won't take it.

What I want (that is more valuable than a plane ticket) is for the connector to introduce me to people I do not know. If I can go home with the names of people who now know me and something about my expertise, that is worth getting on an airplane. It is even worth me buying the ticket and taking time away from my practice.

That is a Tupperware party.

For example, if someone who sells a centrifuge (needed to do the Vampire Facelift®, O-Shot®, and P-Shot® procedures) wants to put me on stage in Las Vegas to talk about PRP (and they do), I buy the ticket. I buy a hotel room. I go on stage. I talk about PRP—all at my expense.

All I want is the names and contact info of the people in the room.

The Monthly Practice that Brings You Gold

The main suggestion of this chapter is this (whether you want to do BoNT parties or not): *Once a month, leave your office and bring something of value to a connector's group for the chance to meet people who may need you and to collect their names and email addresses.*

That is enough about the concept of parties. Next, we will consider the mechanics of how to have a profitable party.

And what about this idea of leaving your office? Does that make you less respectable? Does that make you look like a desperate salesperson? We will answer that in the next chapter.

References

Gladwell M. *The Tipping Point: How Little Things Can Make a Big Difference*. 1st ed. Little, Brown; 2000.

2. HOW TO DO A BONT PARTY (OR ANY OTHER EVENT) & BE SEEN AS THE MISSIONARY & HEALER THAT YOU ARE

Maybe you have seen the movie, *The Boy in the Plastic Bubble*, with John Travolta, about a teenager who lived in a bubble because he could not risk exposure to bacteria, or he would get sick and die. His immune system was inadequate, so he lived in a plastic bubble. Unfortunately, many physicians do the same thing. Their office is their bubble, and they believe that if they take off their white jacket and leave their office bubble and walk into someone's home or hair salon, then they may catch "cooties of disrespect" because they left their "sterile ivory tower bubble" and entered the domain of the "unclean."

Important Life Question: Would You Prefer the Company of the Prig or the Prostitute?

Whatever you think about what happened 2000 years ago, even history says that people criticized the Christ healer for hanging out with tax collectors and thieves, and murderers instead of hanging out in the marble temple with priests and "holy people."

In *Mere Christianity*, C.S. Lewis notes that Christ would think the prostitute on the back row of the church better than the prig on the front row.

What do you think?

Maybe not a great metaphor for physicians, but would you prefer to sit on the front row with the prig or the back row with the prostitute? Would you prefer to be in the doctor's lounge at the hospital or in a living room filled with people who are curious about what you could do for them if you were their doctor?

Do you fear you will be thought unclean if you leave your office and enter someone else's home or office?

I met some of my wealthiest, most private, most elitist patients, and my most kind and gracious patients at events; because at an event, I went into their bubble (which overlaps with that of their connector) instead of requiring them to enter the sterile temple of my office.

For example, there is a smart, wealthy lady in a city near mine who worked as an anchor on one of the news shows. Recently she quit doing that full-time (but still enjoys those connections) and does TV as a part-time gig. Now, she works full-time on two radio stations.

She is a celebrity in her city. If she goes to the store, people recognize her. When I first met her, she didn't walk into my office because she knew that if she walked into anyone's office, she was going to be seen and recognized (and maybe hassled—maybe even have her visit tweeted for the world to see by one of her fans).

She is not going to want to hang out in someone's waiting room, but she came to one of my parties where she knew the hostess and knew that her privacy would be respected within her friend's bubble.

The party she attended was at a hair salon, which sounds not so private; but it was a private after-hours event at a hair salon with only a handful of people who responded to a private invitation—her bubble, not mine.

She came to that private event and met me.

Now, she has been coming to my office for almost a decade after that party. She knows that when she comes to my office, she will not sit in a room with 50 other people, nor will she need to write her name on a sign-in sheet for others to read for the rest of the day. She learned about my office at a party (within her bubble, not mine); now she visits my bubble.

She can slip in, get her BoNT, and leave without being seen by anyone other than my nurse and me.

Every time she shows up, she tells me, "Anytime you want to be on the radio or TV, just let me know."

She smiles in the comfort and privacy of my office, and we talk about our families and medicine and the politics of our city while I do her cosmetic treatments, then she goes.

I would have never pulled her into my office with a newspaper. Even a word-of-mouth recommendation would probably not have worked because she needed to meet me (which could only happen in her friend's bubble) before she would feel safe coming to see me.

The Person Whom You Need that You Will *Never* See (Except at a Party)

This next tip is HUGE; please do not skip over this: *there is a person who will likely never see you unless you do parties—that person is the one who has never had BoNT.*

She is the one who will say, "Well, it's got poison in the name, right? 'Bo-*tox-in* [botulinum toxin]'".

She will NEVER go to your office.

Even if you show her a $100,000 TV ad, she will not go to your office. But she will go to *her* hair salon where *her stylist* (connector) does *her hair*, and she will hang out with *her friends* if she's coming for a free consult with no obligation to buy or do anything. She is only there in her friend's hair salon to get a free consult from you and drink some Kool-Aid and eat a carrot stick and *support her friend's party. She would like the party better if you were not even at the party. But she will tolerate you for the benefit of her friend.*

She will show up at the party, but she will never come to your office, and *when she comes to the party, she has already decided that she is not going to get BoNT.*

But, while she's at the party, she has the chance to be introduced to BoNT and see that it doesn't hurt and to hear your explanation in person—to hear you explain why BoNT is safe and fun.

In summary, with an ad on TV, you have an almost zero chance of meeting the woman who has never had BoNT; but if she comes to her friend's party, and you explain BoNT the way I will teach you, she has an almost one-hundred percent chance of getting a BoNT treatment from you. And, after meeting you at a party (where you are paid money rather than spending money to find her), she will likely spend thousands of dollars with you for the rest of her life.

The 2% Shock

Here is something that may shock you: *only 2% of the population (who might get BoNT) gets BoNT*; 98% of BoNT-eligible people have never had BoNT—*98%!*

Moreover, of the 2% of the eligible who are already happily receiving BoNT, the appreciative ones (not the constant bargain shoppers) are very attached to their BoNT doctor. That person is not likely to ever swap providers and come to see you even if you are a better injector.

So, *to grow your practice, you are much more likely to find a new and loyal patient if you engage with one of the 98% who has never had BoNT instead of trying to seduce someone (who is already getting BoNT) to leave their current provider and come to see you.*

And, *the best way, once again, to find this BoNT-Virgin, who has never had BoNT, who is the key to growing your practice, is at a party. He will not go to your office; at least not yet.*

Elon Musk Teaches You About Bubbles

I recently read that someone showed up, just someone off the street showed up and managed to say "Hello" to Elon Musk as he was walking into one of his offices. This was not someone whom most would consider wealthy enough or important enough to warrant spending hours hanging out with a busy billionaire, but he managed to just say "Hello" to Elon Musk.

But, this "unknown" person was interested in electronics, so Elon Musk spent half a day with him, talking with him about batteries and electric cars—not to do market research or to sell anything to him or to make a YouTube video, just to hang out with him because they shared interests.

Mr. Musk is not trapped in his geographical bubble or in his known engineer's and billionaire's bubbles by the fear of looking common.

Are you?

You may say, "My ivory temple office [your bubble] is where I best heal, and when people come to my office, I can do things for them I cannot do on the street or in someone's hair salon."

No doubt, you will be most effective at most treatments when you work at your office. For this reason, you always do difficult and time-consuming procedures (like surgery or even hyaluronic acid fillers) at your office. But being willing to leave your bubble to introduce yourself will bring people back to your office for the more difficult procedures—people whom you would have never met for the first time at your office.

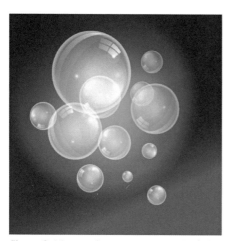

Figure 2. Most patients want to stay in their friend-bubble and most physicians want to stay in their office bubble. The smart doctor finds ways to enter the patient's bubble and does not spend a fortune trying to "get" people to leave theirs to enter hers.

The Key Mental Switch That Changes You from a Starving Salesman to an Altruistic Missionary at Any Event

I am not suggesting that you take an attitude of overt familiarity. It is very true that "familiarity breeds contempt."

If you leave your bubble with the attitude, "I'm a starving doctor, and I'm looking for patients because I do not have enough people coming to see me at my office," that obviously will not help your reputation; that should not be your mentality.

Your mentality when you leave your office to do an event must be that it is not even about BoNT (or whatever service or product you discuss at the event). *Yes, people benefit from what you provide at the event, but that is not the reason you go.*

When I went to speak with a Seventh-day Adventist Church congregation about using vegetarian cuisine as medicine to control blood pressure, it was not even about blood pressure, and it sure was not about selling groceries even though the topic was food.

When I went to Vegas and spoke about the P-Shot® for erectile dysfunction to a room full of hundreds of swingers, it was not even about the P-Shot® procedure, at least not about me providing them with a P-Shot® procedure.

What it is about is this: if you are a healer and you are in your office, you have spent years reading and years hanging out in the hospital with people bleeding and dying and vomiting on your shoe; and you stayed up all night, many nights learning how to take care of people; you have been to classes, and you are studying this class now; you know how to do many wonderful things for people, but *your own patients do not even know all that you can do.* People who have never met you certainly do not know what you can do. All they know is what they read in Cosmo or saw on the news.

They do not know what you know or what you can do until you teach them!

Think about it again, *if you know how to help people (and you do), it is not your patient's responsibility to know what you are able to do for them. It is your responsibility as a physician, healer, and teacher to teach them what you can do.*

So, *to teach them your capabilities and to motivate them to seek your help, if they will not come into your bubble so that they may learn, then you must go into theirs.*

When you show up at an event, you are not a starving doctor begging people to come to see you; you are a missionary teaching people about how you can help them.

How Darlene Helped Me Help Thousands

As an example of elevating a BoNT party (or any event) into a missionary trip to teach people what you can do, the following was my usual way of doing a BoNT party when my main practice focus was 40-year-old women who struggled with the effects of carrying 40 pounds of extra weight—diabetes, hypertension, fatigue, increase risk of breast cancer and stroke, and shortened life expectancy.

My practice focus is no longer weight loss as I have become more involved in researching sexual medicine. Still, you can use the following way that I elevated BoNT parties as a model for how you can elevate any of your events:

I would always bring with me to the BoNT party, Darlene. I'll explain why I brought her.

In the beginning, as an internist, I ran a weight loss program as a big part of my practice. Of course, the weight loss was not just about buying a smaller dress. Weight loss is also about becoming healthier.

Darlene, one of my patients, was an amazing woman who lost 100 pounds with me—100 pounds exactly.

When she got exactly to the 100-pound mark, she told me, "I'm going to work for you for free until you hire me."

So, she would work the night shift in labor & delivery at a hospital in Mobile, Alabama (her usual job). Then, she would come to my office straight from work, and she would bring with her the picture she took when she started my program, her "before picture." She didn't need an after picture because she would be standing there, in the flesh, in the "after" when she worked in my office.

She would show that before-picture to people who came through my office for a sore throat or whatever. When they would see her "before" and then look at her "in the flesh after," they would sign up for my weight loss program.

So, I hired her, and she was a blessing to me and motivated many people to become healthier.

Back to the BoNT party.

I would take Darlene with me to the party, and when I got there, I would say the following (I recommend you craft a similar opening statement for your events):

"Thank you very much for having me here tonight. I love doing BoNT parties. We're going to have fun. My mom was a Tupperware® lady, so I think I have a gene for enjoying parties. But the real reason I'm here is that almost half of you are struggling with your weight and the side effects of that—fatigue and low sex drive, and maybe hypertension and diabetes. I'm going to trick you into coming back to my office, and I'm going to change your life. That is really why I'm here; but if you want to know more about that, talk with Darlene on the way out. For now, let's have a party."

And that's it.

That's all I would say about my weight loss program.

Later in this course, we will discuss how to do the BoNT injections at the party and how to consent the patients, and how to explain BoNT; but first, I'll fast forward to what happens after each patient receives her BoNT, as they leave the party.

An Inspiring Cashier

After I've done each person's BoNT, as she's paying, Darlene (as she's taking their money) would have (in front of her on a table) her "before" picture.

Remember, she's standing there, in the flesh, looking happy and healthy, usually in a beautiful red dress; the "after" is visible without a photo.

They look at the before picture, then look at Darlene and say, "Wow, how'd you do that?!"

She wouldn't explain it—never!

In answer to their question, she would hand to them an audio CD on which I explained how I think about obesity, how to be done with it forever, and live a life of energy and clarity. The CD had my photo, website, phone number, and email address on it.

On the CD, it took me 82 minutes to explain how I thought about weight loss and hormone replacement and how they worked together with exercise and diet. The explanation was long. This was before Suzanne Summers wrote her first books on hormone replacement, so the hormone part of it was new to almost everyone.

The whole explanation was much too long to tell right there at a party, so Darlene would hand the CD to the BoNT party attendee and say, "Listen to this; if you are still interested, then go to the website; and if you're still interested, call us."

She would never offer any more explanation. If someone is not motivated enough to listen to an 82-minute CD, what are the chances they will be motivated enough to stick with a weight loss program for weeks? The CD was both educational and a test of whether this person would be accepted as a patient in my practice.

We knew that for every 50 of those CDs that we handed out, either in that way or to current patients as a way refer others or to people who came to see me for other things who also suffered from obesity, we would get one new patient.

It cost me $2 a piece to make the CDs, so it cost me $100 in CDs (and none of my time) to find one new patient who would come to me for life-changing treatments for which they would pay thousands of dollars.

That's how you do it; that is how you elevate an event.

You may want to carefully reread this section and think about what and whom you would substitute for the elements in the story because this is the best way I know for you to elevate an event from looking like you are begging for patients to becoming a true missionary for health—going out into the community to help spread the word about how you can help people change their lives for the better. Your event is simply the ticket that puts you in front of the people who need your highest-value product or service.

The Main Principle

In other words, when you go to an event, you are going out there to bring to the group something that may be helpful to them that day, but while you are there, you are letting them know your highest value so that if they (or someone they love) needs your best, they know where to find it. If you are a surgeon, it's the surgery you do that makes lives change for the better in the most dramatic, most soul-satisfying way. It is also usually the procedure or service that helps your bank account grow the most.

That is how you avoid looking like what you are not, which is someone out begging for patients, and how you legitimately become something more: you are educating people, outside your office, about what you are able to do for them when you are doing your best work.

That's how you elevate it.

Assignment

Now do the following:

Go back and reread that little speech I gave at the beginning of the BoNT party (or watch me say it on my online version of this course, BoNTClass.com). Then you decide what procedure or service you want to offer the person if they follow you back to your office (usually your highest-level use of your time); then bring with you to your next party someone who has received and enjoyed the benefits of that intended offer. Now, that person will collect the money, checks, and credit cards at the party.

Notice, I never explained the details of the weight loss program at the BoNT party—never. I only let people know that I did it. I had someone with me who had it done, who then handed out something that explained it.

Of course, I also collected emails from everybody at the BoNT party and sent them an email immediately after the party that also took them to something that told them about other things that I do—including the top offer that was the feature of the party.

The most important nugget of an event of any kind is that you are bringing to the group something of value to the people at the party in return for them learning (by your teaching them) about your highest value.

What Really Happened at Church

With the purpose of an event in mind, let's review my visit to the Seventh-day Adventist church (see previous chapter in this course):

Living as a vegetarian is something I knew because I was practicing it, but what I was doing at their church was introducing myself to that group and letting them know that I could take care of their medical concerns. If they had hypertension and would come to my office, I could help them with their hypertension and know how to integrate diet and lifestyle changes into that treatment. They still may need medication, but I would not limit my abilities to throwing pills at them without thinking about their whole organism and strategies that might integrate pharmaceuticals with lifestyle practices.

From "Sweet Home Alabama" to "Hotel California"

To revisit another example from the previous chapter, when I left my office in Alabama to speak to a group of physicians at the introduction of a plastic surgeon from Los Angeles, I went there to speak to his friends about PRP and the Vampire Facelift® procedure.

They found it helpful and left knowing something new to offer their patients; but what was my higher value there, and what did the host receive?

I introduced the attendees to our group, the Cellular Medicine Association (https://CellularMedicineAssociation.org), and how we sponsor research, host a weekly journal club, and how we support the group with continuing education, legal support, and group buying power for their practice, and with educational programs to improve their outcomes. By bringing instructions regarding the Vampire Facelift® procedure (the immediate delivery), through the introduction of the plastic surgeon who lived there (the host/connector)—I gained the chance to educate them about the Cellular Medicine Association and offer them membership.

Your Next Step to Profitable & Fun BoNT Parties

In the next lessons, we're going to explain the mechanics of a BoNT party (and, by extension, any other event that follows this model).

We will cover the details of how to consent the attendees of the party and how to set up for the party—exactly how to get ready.

Thank you for following along with me this far. I hope this will prove helpful to you and your patients.

In the next chapter, we will discuss the ethics of parties.

3. THE ETHICS OF BONT PARTIES & WHY DOING THEM IS GOOD FOR YOUR PATIENTS

Someone may ask you the following question: "Is it really okay to go to someone's house and do BoNT?"

When someone asked me that question (which hardly ever happens now, but a decade ago, it happened occasionally), I would look at them with a facial expression that said, "Did you really just ask me that?"

And then I would look away and then look back at them and laugh and say, "Hmm. So, it's okay to do home dialysis, and it's okay to do home chemotherapy, but you're wondering if it's okay to do cosmetic BoNT?"

And then I would laugh and walk away.

You do not have to answer the question that way, but it can be a fun way to answer not-so-smart questions.

If your medical license covers you to go to someone's home and do a house call and function as their physician and change a foley catheter or administer IV antibiotics or IV chemotherapy or dialysis (all of which are riskier than a BoNT treatment) and if your license covers you to do BoNT in the office, then it should be okay for you to do BoNT in someone's home.

The Origin of BoNT Parties

The original purpose of BoNT parties was that in the package insert that comes with the Botox, it says that once you mix it, you should use it that day. BoNT is good for at least a few weeks (if keep it in the refrigerator). But if you had that erroneous idea that once you mix it, you must use it that day, and if you do not need a whole bottle of it for one person, then you might gather two or three people so that when you do open a bottle, you can use it all without having to discard remnants.

So that was one of the reasons people started doing parties when cosmetic Botox was first brought to market. Now we know that you can store BoNT in the refrigerator for weeks after you mix it. So, there is no reason to use the whole bottle every time you mix a new bottle; which means if we have a party, we do so for other reasons.

Is it ethical to keep your cure a secret?

The other ethical part about BoNT parties involves the simple idea that if you have something valuable to offer the world, then it is ethical for you to do what you can to let people know. The corollary would be that if you have this highest value (your surgery or our consultation that changes people's lives in the most dramatic way) that you offer the world, then is it ethical for you to keep that skill or knowledge a secret?

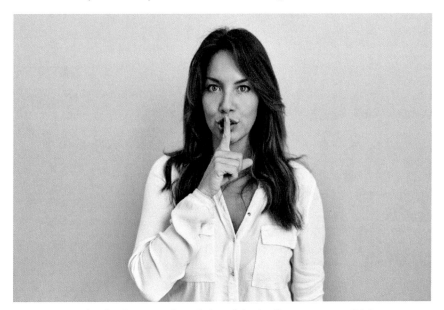

*Figure 3. Is it ethical to keep your knowledge of the healing arts a secret? Is it your **patient's** responsibility to know what you are able to do? Or is **it your** responsibility to teach people what you can do for them?*

To understand a question, I like to think about the extreme, so to help with understanding, pretend that you have the cure for anyone with breast cancer—you can snap your fingers, and you have magic fingers, and you can make breast cancer go away. Yet you don't tell anybody about it, and you just stay in your office and hope they will figure it out and make an appointment. Of course, the extreme is the extreme, but I think the extreme helps the understanding of the actual. And the actual is that *you know what you are able to do, and what you can do is valuable; but people do not know what you can do unless you tell them.*

People who live within 200 miles of your office live in your "neighborhood." If they can get there within a three-hour drive, that's your neighborhood. If those people don't know what you're able to do, it is your responsibility to let them know. And as we talked about in a previous lesson, having an event allows you the most excellent chance of doing that.

What Uber Can Teach You About Marketing Your Practice

Next time you are in a room with many people, ask them, "Who in this room has used Uber?"

Most of the hands will go up. I have done this experiment repeatedly, and it always ends the same way.

Then ask them, "How many of you first learned about Uber online?"

Almost no hands will go up. I have only seen one person's hand go up after asking those two questions of hundreds of people (at my workshops).

The point is that, even in these days of a mature internet, there is still such a thing as "word of mouth," as in someone tells by their tongue wagging in the same room that you're in, and then vocal cords create sound that travels to your ear (not by Tweeting you). That is word of *mouth* before the internet, and it still works.

And *even with internet-based businesses (like Uber), the best advertising is often still word of mouth.*

So if you know something you are able to do, and it is of help to people, then hopefully you are finding connector people (which we talked about in the previous lesson) who will put you in a room full of other people so that you can move your tongue and make sounds come out of your throat (word of mouth), and let people know what you can do.

And if you don't do that, to me, that is an ethical dilemma; not actually going out into the community and delivering your message of hope means that people you could help may not receive help. Moreover, there is nothing wrong with using bait to bring someone to what may benefit them.

So, if I must use BoNT as bait to get someone in the room to teach them how I can make their life better, I will do it.

Using Bait so You Can Help

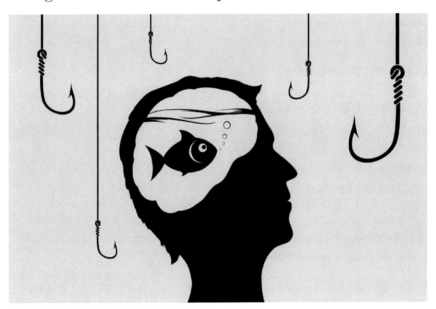

Figure 4. Is it ethical to use bait to lure people to something of great benefit?

At the beginning of this course, you heard me say that I used BoNT as bait to introduce people to a nurse who lost 100 pounds with my weight-loss plan and to what we were able to do for them. After I came up with the O-Shot® procedure (research is growing about how it helps dyspareunia, urinary incontinence, lichen sclerosus, and sexual function), I would go to BoNT parties and bring with me a nurse who had had the O-Shot®; she eventually wound up having 14 O-Shot®'s while she worked for me because they made her sex so fun; now she's moved on to another job, but it changed her life.

So, I would bring her with me and start the party with a statement something like this:

"Thank you for having me at your party. We're going to have fun; I love doing BoNT (here, say the name of what you are injecting, Xeomin, Botox, etc.); but the real reason I'm here is that somewhere around 40% of you (if the stats are the same in this room, as they are to in the rest of the planet) are psychologically distressed because of your sexual dysfunction. And it's more prevalent in younger women. And I'm going to trick you into coming back to my office, and I'm going to change your life, even change your relationships, with my understanding of how to treat sexual dysfunction. But if you want to know more about that, talk with my nurse on the way out; let's have a BoNT party."

When I first started doing the O-Shot® procedure, I thought, "I have this way of helping incontinence for women who don't want surgery yet, but Kegel's didn't work, and they don't want to be constipated and stupid on anticholinergics drugs that are prescribed for urinary incontinence—then, is it ethical for me to stay home and hope that someone knocks on my office door or is it more ethical for me to use BoNT as bait to go out into the community and teach people what I can possibly do for them?"

The side effect of teaching people in this way, using a BoNT party as a way of spreading the word about your highest value, is that you make money while you spread the word.

So should I use parties as advertising (which I hate to use that word, "advertising," because really it's education) and get paid, or should I just stay in my office and hope people see my website, or somehow just hear about what I can do? Or, should I spend trainloads of money on ads that do not work?

I decided that it is better for me to get paid to go out and educate people about what I can do to make their life better.

Who is Responsible?

That is the reason why it is ethical to have a party and the reason why it is unethical to stay in your office all the time and hope people find you and figure out what you are able to do for them.

Find the suffering and teach them what you can do;
It is not their responsibility to find you
and figure it out.

Next, let's examine a checklist that will help you do the party in an efficient and easy way.

4. SAVING TIME
AT YOUR PARTY & YOUR OFFICE

One of the main ways to save time at a BoNT party is by the way you prepare.

Start with This Checklist

I will give you the "BoNT-Party Checklist" that has worked for me for almost two decades.

You can download a printable, pdf version of the list as part of the online (with videos) version of this book found at BoNTClass.com. But, without going to that website, you can still see the complete checklist here:

Bag #1: The *Tool Bag* (a soft, insulated picnic cooler) :

❏BoNT Cosmetic (100-unit bottles) - order BoNT according to guest count

❏Bottle opener

❏Large ice packs - 3

❏Large ice cubes in a zip-lock bag- 10

❏Large gloves - 1 box

❏Hand towels - 4

❏Gauze Sponges Medi-Pak™ (4" x 4", 12 ply) - 1 pack of 200

❏Alcohol Prep Pads (1.25" x 2.5", single-use) - 1 box of 200

❏BD Insulin Syringes (3/10 ml, 8mm, 31G) - 2 boxes of 10 packs

❏1ml Syringes BD Luer Lock Tip - 10

❏18G x 1 ½ BD PrecisionGlide™ Needles - 10

❏ Bacteriostatic 0.9% Sodium Chloride (20ml) - 2 bottles

❏Hand mirror

❏Headbands - 3

❏BoNT board

❏Facial muscle chart

❏Individual plastic cups marked for syringes of 5, 6, 7, & 8 units

Bag #2: The *Prize Bag* (a soft shoulder-carrier bag):

❏O-Shot® books - 10 (or the book about whatever highest-value product or service you intend to promote)

❏O-Shot® t-shirts - 10 (or other free marketing materials about your highest-value product or service)

❏Altar® cream - 5 bottles (or 5 bottles of your favorite cream you like your cosmetic patients to use)

❏BoNT consent forms

❏Business cards

❏Notecards (more about what to do with these when we talk about how to document your treatments)

❏Pens

❏Cash to make change - $100 divided into $5s, $10s, & $20s

❏Square to take credit card payments

❏Sharps container (1.4 qt or 6.9 qt). In a pinch, you can use an empty water bottle after you chug one at the party. The insulin syringes will fit through the top of the bottle.

First, You Need BoNT (But You Do Not Bring Most of It in the Bottle)

In the previous checklist, here's how you calculate how much BoNT you need: Let's say someone tells you they will have three people at their party. For most parties, you'll have some people who don't get that much BoNT and some who want everything injected. Usually, *I need at least one BoNT bottle of one hundred units per three people who will attend the party.*

So, if you are going to BoNT six people at the party, then you should bring two bottles of BoNT. But *if all you do is show up with bottles of BoNT, and you haven't drawn it up already into syringes, you are going to go very slowly.*

So, if you just show up with the BoNT still in the bottles, unless it is a small party, people will become restless and leave the party before you have the chance to treat them.

In the next lesson, we will discuss more about preparation for the party. The main idea here is to *not spend time at the party drawing up the BoNT into the syringes—prefill syringes before the party. This is the main time-saving tip.*

Later, we will discuss exactly how to fill the syringes.

5. BRING THESE TO THE PARTY: ATTITUDE, RULES, & TWO BAGS

Preparing for the party Involves all the following:

- The Tool Bag
- The Prize Bag
- Attire & Attitude
- Other Rules that Grow Your Practice

The BoNT Party "Tool Bag"

Bring an insulated picnic bag with one box of large gloves.

Bring hand towels.

If you want to be fancy, you can bring blue surgical towels. But I prefer white towels that I Clorox like crazy between uses. I spread them out to create a surface on which to work at the party where nothing on the actual table contaminates my syringes or other supplies, and I leave nothing behind from having been there when I gather my towels at the end of the party.

I just lay the towels out and make a space on the counter next to wherever I am.

If I am in someone's home, the towels might go on the kitchen counter. The patient sits on a bar stool pushed up against something sturdy, say a refrigerator, with a bright light overhead. The guests are in the living room, while I'm doing the treatments in the kitchen.

If I'm in a hair salon for the BoNT party, then the towels go on their version of a Mayo stand—the rolling stand where they put their brushes. Then my BoNT board and other tools go on top of the towels. This feels cleaner to me than putting my supplies directly on the kitchen counter or the hairbrush stand.

I bring gauze/sponges. Some people like 2 x 2 sponges. I prefer a stack of 4 inches x 4 inches. The larger sponge feels more luxurious. When I'm doing BoNT, I use the sponge to hold pressure. I prefer a gauze over an alcohol wipe to hold pressure.

I use alcohol wipes to clean any dots of blood left on the face after I finish; I do not want to send anyone home with dots of blood on their face. So, I bring a stack of around twenty alcohol prep pads.

I bring insulin syringes. And the only brand that I recommend you use is BD-brand, insulin syringes, 30 units, 31 gauge, with five sixteenth (8mm needles). Even a 30-gauge needle hurts noticeably more than a 31-gauge needle.

These insulin syringes are sold at my local pharmacy, and they're also sold on Amazon. Even right after COVID, when everyone was running out of everything from baby formula to toothpaste, I could still get these syringes on Amazon.

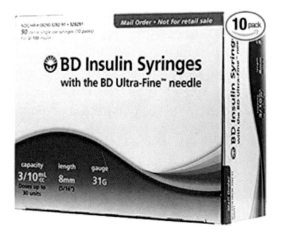

Figure 5. My favorite syringe to use with BoNT treatments: 31-gauge, 30-unit, 8mm, BD-brand, insulin syringe.

I also bring a one-milliliter syringe with a luer lock, and I use those with an 18-gauge needle to mix the BoNT by adding the bacteriostatic saline.

I bring cough drops because sometimes, when I talk a lot at a party, I will start coughing; cough drops keep my throat moist to avoid coughing when talking.

I bring 18-gauge needles (to attach to the one cc syringes) to mix the BoNT with the bacteriostatic saline. So, I have some 18-gauge needles, and I'm not going to mix that many bottles of BoNT (because I will prefill syringes before I go). But I have some extras in there in case extra guests show up and to fill syringes with odd amounts in them (amounts not usually part of my pre-mix routine).

I fill up plastic cups with syringes prefilled with the amount of BoNT that I think I will need (more about that elsewhere in this course), but I also always bring two or three extra bottles of BoNT. And I'll go ahead and add the saline to them. I put all the BoNT into the insulated picnic bag so they're ready. And then if I need to draw up some other amount, not a seven or a six or an eight or a five, for example, if I need to draw up a ten unit or a twelve, I'll have it with me.

I don't normally actually need this, but sometimes if I'm in a hurry, I'll just throw some unmixed bottles in there. And if I have the unmixed bottles plus an 18 gauge and one cc syringe, I can mix new BoNT because you're going to see when I mix it, I just put one cc of bacteriostatic saline in there. It's not a bad idea to always bring two or three extra bottles because extra people show up sometimes. If you don't have a busy practice, maybe you are not using this frequently, and maybe you don't want to mix it until you need it. But if you do, you will have what you needed. A one cc syringe, 18-gauge needle, and a bottle cap opener to take the cap off.

Then you have bacteriostatic sodium chloride, which is what you need to mix it.

I also bring a hand mirror. The reason I have a hand mirror is that you need the person to be able to directly point to their face and show you what they would like to "make better." And they can't do that accurately without a mirror. So, it gives you a way to talk about their face.

And I bring headbands so that I can push their hair away from their face while working and for the before photos. I usually either let them keep them or throw them away just for sanitary reasons. I don't guess many people are going to come get BoNT with lice, but it just feels better to me. After I use it, I throw it away, or I let them take it home, like a prize.

I also bring the facial muscle chart. I know where the muscles are, but I bring the chart because I talk about the muscles when I'm consenting everyone and explaining what I do; I use the chart as teaching tool. Every time I see a person in consult about their face, as I'm explaining what I'm doing and why, it helps to have this chart to use as a teaching tool. You will find yourself pointing to it frequently if you have it with you.

I also bring the cups in which I put the prefilled BoNT syringes, as we talked about, marked for five-unit prefilled syringes, sixes, sevens, and eights.

The Prize Bag

Now the second bag that you bring is the "Prize Bag." Your bag may differ from mine, but mine will give you ideas. The tool bag contains what I will use at the party. The Prize bag contains what my staff will need to help me. We bring books about what I am going to talk about that's my higher value (my reason for being at the party). These days, that's the O-Shot® procedure book.

Whoever is taking your money at the party needs to have experienced the life-changing procedure that you plan to offer to those in attendance to the BoNT party—the procedure, as we talked about previously, that you want to do to change lives (other than your BoNT). It's basically your up-sell, but it's also your soul up-sell.

So that's what you need, and you need to have that with you for them to hand out. We also bring t-shirts to give away.

We bring five bottles of our Altar® cream because that's a very good product. If you're doing the Vampire Facial® procedure and don't have that, you should get it. We have a good markup on it, and people love it. So, we bring that, and we give them away as door prizes.

We have consent forms, my business cards, and the note cards (later in this course, you will see how I use the note cards to make notes both on paper and electronically, using only index cards and my iPhone).

I bring pens to write with and cash to make change: one hundred dollars: 4 five-dollar bills, 4 tens, and 2 twenties.

You are also going to process credit cards. We use a little square thing. PayPal makes its own device, which I use often in the office. But when we do the BoNT parties, we use Authorize.Net, and they have a scanner too. So, it doesn't matter which device you use, but you need something that connects to the phone that belongs to your person taking the money and that puts the money into the business bank account.

I bring sharps container, but a water bottle can double for that.

And that's it.

Attire and Attitude Tips

I always dress nicely for the parties. If you are the main attraction at any event, you should be a little overdressed (compared with the attendees) out of respect for the people who invited you.

Mark Twain was known more as a speaker than an author during his day; he was like our modern version of a standup comedian and storyteller. He would travel and speak. Some wrote that if you walked into the room where he was speaking, you knew who was the guy who was going to be talking just by looking at him; he had enough presence, and his attire also distinguished him.

So, I recommend that you dress (and behave) such that if a stranger walked into the room, they could look around the room without you speaking and know that you are the person who is there to do the speaking or to do the service.

And your staff, you should demand the same thing from them. They should be dressed a little bit more formally (or sexy) than how your guests would be dressed.

I don't mind sexy.

When you are selling BoNT, you are selling sex. Not sex in a pornographic way; sex sells relationships—Emerson said, "Beauty is the scaffolding of

Love." I make no apologies about my staff being somewhat sexual in their dress. They do not come in there in G-strings, but I have no problem with them looking *attrac*tive and desirable because desirable and sexual are what we are selling.

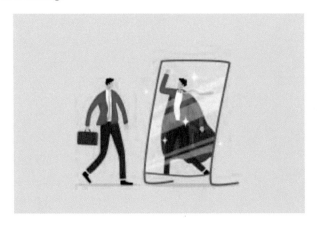

Figure 6. A stranger should be able to walk into the room and know by your attire and demeanor that you are the speaker. It is a show of respect to be dressed up (slightly more formal than your attendees) for the occasion.

I know most people like to get to an event a little early, but I think being early for a BoNT party can be awkward. I like to be ready early, but I like to arrive right on time and maybe even five minutes late, never more than five or ten minutes early.

Get there early and wait down the road or in the parking lot until it's time to walk into the party.

Party Rules About Alcohol, Footprints, & Music

Alcohol

If there's alcohol, I don't drink it. I don't drink alcohol anyway, even at home (I never understood a reason for drinking something that makes me less smart, sleepy, and wanting sex all at the same time); but if I did drink alcohol, I still would not drink it at a BoNT party, even on the way out.

If I partake of the refreshments, it's a cracker or two as I'm leaving (to be social), but I leave very soon after the party's over, after the hostess has been treated since she went last; *I'm gone within 5 minutes* after that.

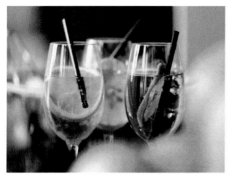

Figure 7. It is not my job to become the sobriety police.

If other people drink alcohol, it is their business, not mine. When someone signs a consent form for BoNT in my office, for all I know, they had two beers and LSD on the way to my office. I do not do a drug screen and a sobriety test before getting a consent form signed. So, if the hostess serves alcohol at the party, it is her business and that of her guests; I am not going to worry about mental status due to alcohol before I get a consent form signed at a party any more than I would at my office.

Trail of Zero

I don't leave anything behind, not even a scrap of paper. I bring my own garbage bag. And I bring a red bag for gauze with blood, I bring my needle disposal; and when I leave, everything at the party site is back such that you cannot tell I was there. I do not put anything in their garbage cans.

Nothing.

I leave no footprint. If the FBI came in afterward, since I'm wearing at least one glove, they would find it difficult to show I was there unless it would be from DNA from the non-gloved hand. That is how careful I am not to contaminate or even leave the impression of contamination of the space where the party occurred.

Music

I might use my phone for music (if they don't have music). I like to play George Winston—his *December* album—the most relaxing and inspiring album ever recorded. I just play it through the speaker on my iPhone. If the hostess plays music, then I let her pick what she wants.

Short Goodbyes

In the end, I always express my most sincere and deepest gratitude to the hostess. Remember, she trusted me to take care of some of the people she loves most—that deserves gratitude.

She gets her BoNT, the very last thing. Remember, the host/hostess gets all the BoNT she wants if she gets three people to pay me for BoNT. If she does not get three people to pay me (very rare), then she just pays me $7.50 a unit for at least trying.

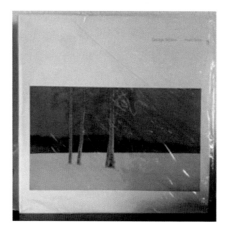

Figure 8. George Winston's December Album is full of magic that will calm your patients.

By the time everyone has been treated, including the hostess, the guests will have mostly left. There might be a few lingering socialites, but for the most part, everyone will have left. And it gives us (the hostess and I) a chance to do our niceties and plan the next party. So, I often help her pick a date and time for the next party before I leave, but sometimes that appointment is made with a phone call a week or so later.

I never let the goodbye take longer than five minutes—literally. I abhor long goodbyes unless it is with a family member going away for a long time. It was just a BoNT party.

Grab your stuff, eat a cracker, say, "Thank you," and go.

Party Rules that Grow Your Practice

When I'm at a party, it is not a secret that the hostess receives her BoNT for free. Everyone knows it.

Pretty commonly, probably at one out of three or four parties, someone there will want to do their own party. So, you will have a party that springs off a couple of other parties. And those parties spring off parties, and you can even suggest and encourage such offspring.

For example, you may see a cosmetologist or hairstylist, or personal trainer (those are great connectors) show up at someone else's party.

When they do, there is nothing wrong with saying, "Hey, you should host your own party."

And your hostess will be okay with that. She understands how you make your living. She does not care that one of her guests found a way to get their BoNT free too. If she gets eight people at this party and six at the next, she still gets free BoNT at both parties, even if one of her attendees decides to have their own party. So, I have no problem with saying to someone at a party that they could do their own party and get their BoNT for free too.

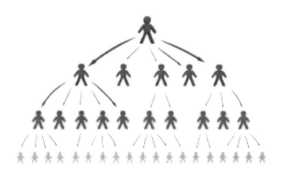

Figure 9. Parties grow your practice like multi-level marketing on steroids.

Important: Never succumb to the temptation to do fillers or any procedures other than BoNT at your BoNT party. One of the main reasons for doing the party is to persuade people to come to your office for other products and services. To learn where your office is, to meet your staff, to have time alone with you—to develop a deeper relationship. So, do not create the opportunity for a visit to your office and then squander it by doing anything other than BoNT at a BoNT party.

The honest reason I give (from a physician's view) about why I do not do fillers at the party is that my light and my environment at the office are necessary for the best outcomes when injecting fillers. If you use time as the reason for not doing fillers at the party (even though time is part of the reason, since fillers take longer than BoNT), it implies that you are busier than your patients—not good.

Conclusion

You just read, in this chapter, the mechanics of packing for the party and running the party.

The how and why of parties (events) are some of the most valuable pearls that I am bringing to you in this course.

Of course, it is also valuable to know an elegant and simple method of injecting BoNT, a method that is effective but simple and easy. But the value of BoNT only manifests *when you have a bus full of people showing up at your office every day to get the BoNT, people who then discover YOU and want everything you know how to do.*

In the next lesson, we will talk more about exactly what goes in the bag that you bring with you to the party.

Videos of all these lessons can be viewed at BoNTClass.com

6. SPECIAL TOOLS FOR YOUR BONT PARTY BAG & YOUR OFFICE

To help you move faster and easier, it will help to examine more closely a few special items on the checklist of what you bring to a BoNT party.

The Amount of Prefilled BoNT Syringes

For BoNT parties, I fill syringes using the following formula:

Assuming the number of people expected at the party is 6, then I bring the following.

6 x 1 = 6 syringes with 5 units (for the procerus of 6 people)

6 x 2 = 12 syringes with 7 units (for each of the two corrugators of 6 people)

6 x 3 = 18 syringes with 6 units (for brow lift and crow's feet)

6 x 1 = 6 syringes with 8 units (for some frontalis and for some with a stronger corrugator)

For whatever number of people you plan to have at the party, substitute that number for the number 6 in the above example. So, if you expected 10 people at the party, then you would bring the following:

10 x 1 = 10 syringes with 5 units (for procerus).

10 x 2 = 20 syringes with 7 units (for each of 2 corrugators in each attendee).

10 x 3 = 30 syringes with 6 units

10 x 1 = 10 syringes with 8 units

Don't worry; the number of syringes with each of the aliquots of BoNT will make more sense after we discuss each injection point.

The BoNT Board

In your tool bag, you also bring your BoNT board—see the following screen shot from the video version of this course (BoNTClass.com).

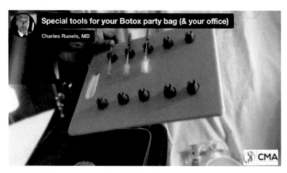

Figure 10. The BoNT-Board

The grey syringe holders are the rubber stoppers of BoNT bottles; the stoppers have been inverted and glued with "Gorilla Glue" to a cutting board like you would use in your kitchen for slicing cheese. The board allows you to organize the syringes and to keep them organized when you carry them around (without them falling onto the floor).

You can also see (at the bottom of the photo) the red, insulated picnic bag in which I carry all the tools I need for the party (including the board).

Bottle Opener

Keep a bottle opener on your key chain so that you never lose it or waste time looking for it in your bag.

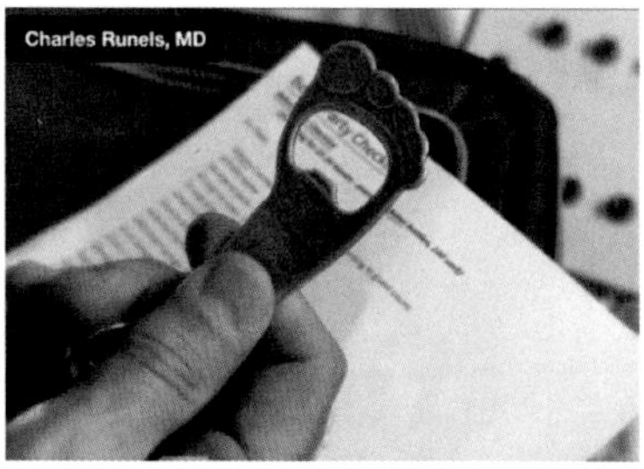

Of course, when you live near the beach, you always have a barefoot bottle opener.

This works perfectly to open the caps of the BoNT bottles, to remove the rubber stoppers, so that you do not dull the needles before putting them into the face of your patient.

Figure 11. Bottle opener to remove the caps from BoNT vials.

72

You don't need a fancy $100 tool to take the stoppers off (they do make one) that gets misplaced and takes up room in your bag. The BoNT top comes off easily (once you get the knack for it) with a beer bottle opener.

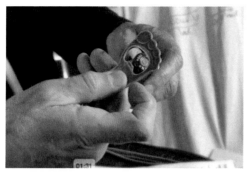

Figure 12. Removing the cap from the BoNT vial.

If you do lots of BoNT, you will learn that it saves loads of time to never be without your beer-bottle opener in your pocket.

Ice Packs

Plastic ice packs go into the top of the cooler to keep your BoNT cool.

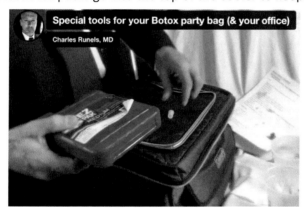

Figure 13. Insulated picnic bag is the BoNT toolbox. Frozen blocks go into the bag.

I bought my insulated picnic bag at Walmart.

Ice Cubes

I bring large ice cubes which I make with an old-fashioned ice cube tray that goes in the freezer.

I bought the ice tray on Amazon.

When you see how I do BoNT in the mouth, you'll know why I bring ice.

You put the ice cubes in a Ziploc bag, and that bag goes into your toolbox.

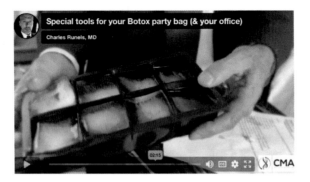

Figure 14. Large-cube, ice cube tray.

When numbing the mouth, some like to apply small, reusable, plastic, freezable blocks that have ice in them. I like regular ice cubes (even though they drip) because you can throw them away when you are done (more sanitary), and I think bare ice gets the mouth colder than the plastic blocks—you get better anesthesia when you use bare ice directly against the skin.

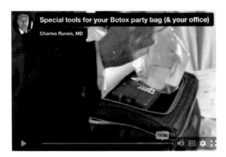

Figure 15. Plastic bag with ice cubes goes into the tool bag.

To keep the dripping from dampening the clothing of the patient, I bring small terrycloth towels (these also go in the bag).

When I use ice, I drape the towels like a baby's bib across the lower neck and upper chest of the patient before I do their treatment.

7. ORGANIZATION
OF THE BONT BOARD
FOR SPEED, PROFIT, & ACCURACY

Take a closer look at how my BoNT board works because it will save you time (money).

I learned about this board over a decade ago from Dr. Mark Bailey and his nurses in Toronto, Canada. It saves me loads of time, so I use it both when I do BoNT parties and when I do BoNT in the office.

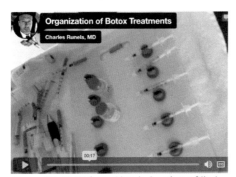

Figure 16. BoNT board loaded with prefilled syringes.

In the following photo, you can see that I've drawn up BoNT into several syringes. After I draw up a syringe of BoNT, I put it onto my board in the same place every time. Procerus, left corrugator, right corrugator, and so on, always in the same order.

Some syringes will be held in place by the rubber stoppers.

Sometimes, I put the syringe directly flat on the board, but the needle stays clean because the barrel of the syringe elevates the needle, so it does not touch the board.

After I use a needle/syringe, it goes immediately into the needle disposal and never back onto the board.

You will understand more about how the board works when we talk about the individual injection points on the face. Once you form the habit of using the board, you will never want to do BoNT without it.

8. SIMPLE DOCUMENTATION AT PARTY & OFFICE

Now that you have seen the tools, let's talk more about how to prepare for a BoNT party and how to document your treatments.

Where Does the Time Go?

Most of the time spent doing a BoNT treatment is time spent drawing up the BoNT into the syringes.

Let's say you're going to do four different injections. How long does it take to touch the skin and push a plunger? Almost none!

Imagine touching your face four times: count 1, 2, 3, 4.

That's how long it would take you to do a BoNT treatment with four injection points, about four seconds—if it only involved doing the injections, because the actual injection involves simply touching the face with a needle followed by pushing the plunger.

So, most of the time involved in doing a BoNT treatment is not in doing the actual injections; most of the time involves (1) speaking with the person and deciding what you're going to do, (2) taking the before pictures, (3) getting the consent form signed, and (4) drawing up the BoNT into the syringes.

Of these four tasks, other than the actual injections, drawing up the BoNT into the syringes takes the most time.

Also, to decrease pain, I always draw up a separate syringe for each muscle group (so no needle is used more than three or four times). For example, one syringe for the procerus, another for the left corrugator, another for the right corrugator. And I draw up the BoNT so that the needle does not touch anything, not even the side of the bottle, so the needle stays sharp and hurts less. All of this takes extra time but is worth it because it leads to more precision and less pain.

So, the best way to keep the party moving is to fill most of the syringes you will use at the party before you go to the party.

The Map that I Draw & the Flow

Note: *Come back to this chapter after you study the individual injection points later in the course, and it will make more sense to you.*

You will easily learn, later in this course, exactly how to do each injection point; what I'm showing you now is my shorthand notation for recording exactly what I do when I treat someone with BoNT. The photos are screen shots from the video version of this course—found at BoNTClass.com

The following are the 12 principal injection points sketched the way I quickly document them at a party or on a paper chart. When I am at a party or even in my office, I find that paper is quicker than any software. So, I make sketches like the one you see here to document the treatment.

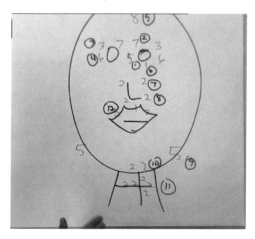

Figure 17. A simple drawing to document injections.

After I take a photo of the patient's face and discuss what can be done (with her looking in a mirror), then I sketch on an index card a plan that looks like the above photo.

I draw an oval for the head and a column for the neck. Then, I add a circle for each eye, then the nose (a capital "L"), and the mouth.

On the sketch above, I numbered the injection points consecutively with black numbers in the order in which I would normally treat a patient. The red numbers represent the amount of BoNT, in units, that I would normally use on a repeat BoNT treatment of most women.

When I do my sketch, I only write the red numbers. The black numbers are there to show you a possible order of treatment.

You should also *establish an order in which you always do your BoNT so that you don't forget a spot and so your procedures flow automatically,* freeing up your mind to think about where you are going to put the needle and about your conversation with the patient.

To document my injection plan, I simply write the number of units that I intend to inject onto the diagram on the place where I plan to do the injection. So, in the following sketch, only the red numbers would be written on my patient chart.

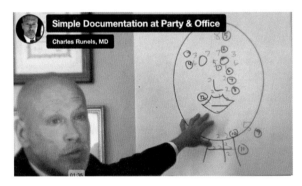

Figure 18. The red numbers indicate the number of units usually given for repeat visit for a female. Black numbers show order of injection.

Remember, at a party, the "chart" is an index card on which I draw the diagram and the photos that I take of her face and of the consent form.

Then I show the patient the card and the plan, I talk about what I have planned, and I have the price for the BoNT written on the card as well.

So, I ask her, "Does that look OK?" while pointing at the price on the card.

If she says that it's too much money, then I leave off one of the muscle groups and offer her a new price. Never do I treat a muscle group with less than what it would take for a good relaxation of the muscle.

If we don't reach a price that agrees with her, it's OK. Maybe she needed a Vampire Facelift® or a facial peel or surgery or no treatment at all. She's still glad for the free consult, and I'm still glad to have met her. I get her name and email on the card so I can "send her more information," and we say goodbye.

Then the hostess brings to me the next patient.

But usually, we reach an agreement on the price and the plan (it is BoNT, not open-heart surgery). After we agree, I then hand the card to the patient and ask her to write her name, email address and birthday on the card at the top, above my sketch.

While she is writing her info on the card, I pull the BoNT needles out of the cups; I have a cup for syringes prefilled with 5 units, one for 6's, one for 8's, and one for 10 units). I place the needles/syringes on the board in the proper order.

I take photos of the index card (which now has my plan and her contact info) and of her consent form.

Then I do the injections.

After the injections, we say goodbye, I send her to see my cashier (who will sell her my higher-level services), and the hostess brings to me the next patient.

After the party, all the photos are stored in the business version of Dropbox (which is HIPPA compliant). I make a separate folder in Dropbox for each patient.

The folder in Dropbox is done when I get home. At the party, I just draw the sketch, and snap photos of the sketch (after she's added her name, birthday, and email), of her face, and of the consent form.

More About the Order of Injection

I usually do the glabella first (number "1" on the map) because I treat it in everyone, and it seems to hurt the least for most people.

Next, I inject both corrugators (number 2), which hurts more but still not much if you follow my methods and do the brow lift (number 3 on the map).

The brow lift would be the third thing that I do; the "crow's feet" is the fourth.

The fifth injection area is the frontalis.

The sixth injection area (if done) is to help open the eye (only if they need it).

The seventh injection point is for the bunny lines.

The eighth (only if needed) is for a gummy smile.

The ninth is for the frown to lift the corners of the mouth.

The tenth area is for an orange peel chin.

The eleventh is for the necklace lines or a webbed neck.

The twelfth is for a glamorous mouth or to even out an asymmetric mouth.

So those are the 12 injection points.

Most of the variation in the numbers of units is when treating the corrugators and procerus (the glabella, which forms the frown lines). There will be some variation in the other injection points, but 80 to 90% of the time, the other injection points will involve the numbers of units shown in the diagram.

How the Prefilled Syringes Save Time

When at a party, if you had ten syringes already drawn up with five units in each of them (collected in a plastic cup labeled with the number

5). Then when you get to the party, for the procerus you only have to pull one of those out for a five, add it to your board, and you are ready to treat the procerus.

And, if you're going to have ten people, you might have 20 sevens' already drawn up (one for each of two corrugators x 10 people). So, before you even go to the party, you sit there and draw twenty syringes with seven units, or your helper draws up twenty of these syringes with seven units in each.

Maybe someone needs more than this, and you don't use as many sevens. That's fine. You just bring the cups of unused prefilled syringes back with you after the party, and store them in your refrigerator to use in your office the next day when you see patients.

Review of the Main Time Tip

You could use this same system every day in your office (not just for parties) and have cups with prefilled syringes sitting in the refrigerator.

Always load the syringe for each muscle group in the same place on the board.

I always load my board with each syringe filled with the amount I want to inject on the designated holder on the board in the following order: glabella, left corrugator, right corrugator, brow lift (usually one syringe with six units, and I inject 3 units on each side). Then, two more syringes, one for each side, to treat crow's feet, then whatever else I do.

If you are at a very busy party, you can draw a sketch of what you plan to do, then you can have a helper look at the sketch and load your board for you using the prefilled syringes you brought—always loaded in the same order.

To save time in the office, I draw the sketch and then simply walk to the fridge and pull out prefilled syringes and load my board (instead of drawing up BoNT at the bedside).

Always, nothing dirty or used goes onto your board.

Of course, you will have people that need something different than what you may bring in your prefilled syringes. That's OK. You simply draw up what you need at the bedside when this happens. But, you still save loads of time by having most of the syringes prefilled.

Save Even More Time, See Better Results, & Keep Your Medical License

To save more time at the party, and to avoid making people feel like I am trying to collect their last dime, if I see someone at a party and they have never before had BoNT, then I tell them (as part of their free consult) everything I think would make their face look younger including Vampire Facelifts®, creams, and maybe even surgeries or light therapies. You should know about all the most used therapies for decreasing the age of the face, even the ones you do not do—not just where to put BoNT. Give them a true consult, telling them everything you think may help them look younger.

But no matter what I think may help, for someone who is getting BoNT for the first time, I only treat the glabella (corrugators and procerus), do a brow lift (you will see how in a later chapter), and maybe treat their crow's feet. Nothing else for a first-time BoNT treatment.

I never treat the forehead on the first visit.

I will not treat bunny lines on the first visit either. I might treat a gummy smile because that's such a big crowd pleaser, but I don't treat bruxism on the first visit. I don't treat orange peel chin. I don't treat the neck. I only treat the frown, brow lift, and crow's feet on the first trip, never frontalis on the first trip.

Do Not Try to Take Every Dime You Can Take
Limiting what you treat on the first visit helps you go faster (at the party), and it reassures the patient that you are not trying to take all their money since you choose to not do everything you know how to do.

If You Droop Them, You Lose Them
The other reason that you do not treat the frontalis on the first visit is that you may droop them. Remember, *the frontalis is the only muscle that*

lifts the brow. So, if they have very strong corrugators and you weaken the frontalis but do not weaken the corrugators enough, then their brows fall, they look droopy, and they will never come to see you again—you lose them forever.

So, you only treat the pull-down muscles (frontalis, procerus, and orbicularis oculi), which creates a lifting of the brow (because you weakened the vectors opposing the lifting effect of the frontalis); and then see them in follow up in two to four weeks in your office and treat the frontalis (aggressively, lightly, or not at all) based on where the brow rests after full effect of treating all the pull-down muscles.

All this will make more sense after you learn each injection point. The main idea now is that you never treat the frontalis on the first visit, and your party goes faster, you do not risk dropping them. You see a better result because you tailor-make their frontalis treatment on the second visit, and you have a reason to bring them to your office.

After the first visit, and *after you see them in follow up between two and four weeks and tailor make how much you put into their frontalis, from then on, you do the frontalis and all the rest in one trip.*

If you feel like you must treat the frontalis on the first visit, then limit it to eight units; that lower dose will decrease your chances of drooping their brow.

Note about How to Lose Your License to Practice Medicine

WARNING: If you live in the United States, always buy your Botox, Xeomin, Jeuveau, and Dysport from your sales rep in the United States. They charge you more in the US than you would pay in Canada and other places, but it costs them more to do business here (your politicians at work).

Here's the trap to avoid—you will receive emails where online companies tempt you to buy your BoNT from outside the country. Don't, or you could lose your license; unless something changes, *it is illegal to buy BoNT from outside the US if you practice medicine in the US.*

9. CHARGING PEOPLE AT THE PARTY—HOW MUCH & HOW TO COLLECT

When I finish a BoNT treatment at the party, I have an index card that has the person's name, their birthday, and their email address (which they wrote on the card while I pulled BoNT syringes from the cups) with a sketch of what I just did to their face. *I also have the price of the treatment written on the index card.*

When I finish the treatment, I say, "Thank you very much," and I give the person their card.

The patient then takes that card to my checkout person, which in some places, may be in the same room. I may be in the same room doing the next BoNT treatment. For example, if I'm in a hair salon, the checkout person could be in the same area where I'm treating them, or that person could back in the lobby.

My person does need to be by the door.

What I Learned from a Man Who Made a Fortune Cooking Fish

There was an amazing Greek restaurant (Niki's in Birmingham, Alabama) that I used to go to with my dad when I was a child.

My dad always said, "If you want to find good food and you're in a town where you don't know anybody, find a Greek restaurant and order fish because they've been cooking that stuff for several thousand years, and they got the recipe down."

So, he would take me to this Greek restaurant when I was a kid, and the man who owned the restaurant would usually be at the door by the cash register.

And I remember my dad asking him once how he had built his successful business, and the man told him, "If you own a restaurant, you should have one cash register by the door, and you should stand by it."

You want your person collecting the money at your BoNT party to be by the door.

Not that people are going to *try* to sneak out on you, but they do *forget* to pay sometimes. So, your cashier needs to be stationed between you and the door.

The Cashier at the Party (the Rest of the Story)

Let's pick up where your patient, whom you just BoNT'd, is leaving.

Your cashier, remember, is the person who had the thing done that is your highest value; this person collects the card (with the treatment documentation and the price) as the patient walks toward the door.

When I first started doing BoNT, my cashier was my nurse, who had lost 100 pounds on my weight loss plan. Later, it became a nurse who enjoyed the results of several O-Shots given to her by me; her orgasms were galactic.

The cashier should have on a table (as they collect the card and then the money) something to hand the BoNT client that talks about the higher lever service. When it was Darlene, my nurse, who lost 100 pounds, she would have stacked (next to her on the table) CDs on which I explained how I help people lose weight. When it was my nurse who had an O-Shot® procedure, it was a stack of books about the O-Shot®.

So the person is leaving and paying—they pick up the thing on the table (our your cashier hands it to them) and talks with your person about the higher-value service--THIS IS WHERE THE MONEY HAPPENS (NOT THE MONEY FROM BONT, BUT THE REAL MONEY)--AND WHERE YOU FIND THE PERSON WHO NEEDS THE THING MOST VALUABLE TO YOUR SOUL AND TO THEIR LIFE--IT'S WHERE THEY LEARN ABOUT IT.

Warning: *Do not do BoNT parties if you do not want more patients because you will get them.*

The Patient Flow

To review the flow; they come to the party; they hear the consenting speech (discussed in the next chapter); they get the consult including "before" photos; you make the card with the sketch of what you plan to do; they fill in their contact info; they get the treatment; they take the card to the cashier.

The flow works best if the cashier is in as private a place as possible, at least not in earshot of the other conversations. Then the person is more likely to say, "Yeah, what about this O-Shot thing?" or, "What about the surgery she does?" or, "What about [whatever the higher level service you are upselling]?"

Then they take the book, or they take the CD (or whatever you are giving that talks about the higher-level service), and they pay for the BoNT.

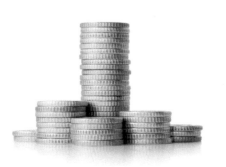

The price of BoNT should be $1 less per unit than what you charge in your office. So, if you live in a city where you're charging $15 a unit, it should be $14 at the party. In

Figure 19. BoNT parties bring you new patients who give you stacks of money.

Alabama, where it's $10 a unit, I charge $9 at a party. I think the most in our group is New Zealand, where it's around $24 a unit.

So, it depends on where you live but charge a dollar less per unit at the party.

Moving Money from Their Bank to Yours

A decade ago, we just took checks and cash, and if they wanted to pay with a credit card, my helper would write down the credit card number and charge their card when we got back to the office. I have only had one check bounce for BoNT in over a decade. For some reason, people always make sure their check is good when they pay for BoNT.

Now, my nurse brings her iPhone, and I have her plugged into my account (to collect but not to withdraw money) so she is able to slide a credit card and charge it at the party, and it goes into our account.

Then when I leave, the cards (with the sketches and charges) associated with each treatment are numbered. So, for example, if I had ten patients, the cards are numbered as I do them, one through 10; and when I leave, I will have ten cards, each with a sketch of what I did, the contact info, and how much was charged.

The cashier stacks them numerically, with a check or the cash collected on top of each card, or she will note "credit card" for the cards where they paid with their credit card.

When I get back to my office, I have the person's contact information and a sketch of their face. But the card is also in my pictures since I took a photo of the card before I did the treatment. So, the photo of the card (with the contact info) is in my phone next to a photo of the person's face.

I also have a picture of their consent form in the camera, all together with the photo of the person's face.

After the Party

When I get back to the office. I put their name, their email, and their birthday into my computer.

Now they're going to start getting my emails.

They will receive an email the week before their birthday, telling them to come to see me to get $100 off (any time from a week before to a week after their birthday). This email is sent automatically.

And they're going to get every email (about aesthetic medicine) that I send until I die, or they unsubscribe.

You could also send them an email the next time you do a party at the location where they saw you. You could create a list of just the people at

Mary Jo's hair salon. And then, two weeks before your next party at Mary Jo's hair salon, you could send them all an email and say, "Hey, I'm going to be at Mary Jo's; come see us," at whatever time the party is.

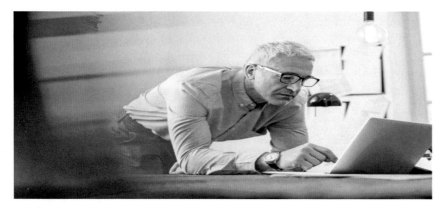

Figure 20. After the party, go home and put each name, birthday, and email into your computer. Their face photos go into a file with the photos of (1) the consent form and (2) the diagram of their treatment plan.

That is how you collect the money; it's how you keep track of the money; and it's what you do with their information.

Now, let's talk more about how you consent everyone at the party.

10. STARTING BONT PARTIES & CONSENTING (PART 1 OF 2)

I'm going to walk you through the beginning of a BoNT party, up until the consenting for the BoNT. We will do a group consent.

Introductory Speech

I come to the party with my entourage. If it is a smaller party (10 people or less), I might only bring one other person. I prefer (when there is over 10 people in attendance) to bring two people to help me; I routinely do parties for 20 or 25 people and have done parties for 35 or 40 people. But, in the beginning, keep your numbers between 8 to 12 people at the party so that you can move quickly without rushing and finish your party at a reasonable time.

I try to follow what John Wooden used to tell his basketball players. "Move fast, but don't hurry."

You come to the party, and let's say the party starts at 5:00. I prefer around 5:00. That way, the people who get off early or work at night or work from home can come earlier. And those that are getting off work at 5:00 can show up at 6:00, and it can be sort of a walkthrough thing, but 5:00 or 6:00 is a good time. Depending on the event, it might be a daytime party depending on the crowd.

You do want to start the party when most everyone can be there from the start so you can do a group consent.

So you come at the start of the party, let's say it's 5:00. You show up on time. And there are some people there, probably just about everybody that will show up. You may have to consent individually some people that show up late. But most everyone is there when you arrive, and you bring your entourage.

Now, you say the following [comments in brackets give you reasons and thoughts behind what is being said]:

"Thank you for having me here tonight. I love doing parties."

[Remember my little talk because you must elevate it immediately if you want to love it. And you will not do parties or much of anything at work for long if you do not love doing it.]

"I love doing parties, but the real reason I'm here is that..."

[We'll use the O-Shot® as an example.]

"The real reason I'm here is that 40% of you are suffering with your sexuality. To be counted as suffering from sexual dysfunction, as a woman, you must have psychological distress from it. And the latest numbers show that around 4 out of 10 women suffer from sexual dysfunction, and sexual problems are worse and more common in younger women. So, that's my real reason for being here is that 4 out of 10 of you are having that problem, and I'm going to trick you into coming back to my office, and I'm going to change your life. But if you want to know more about that, talk with Mary Jo [my cashier] on the way out. For now, let's have a party."

That's my introduction. Notice that it is about something other than BoNT.

Now *I have gone from being a doctor who's out begging for patients to someone who is sincerely looking for people whom I can help.*

And remember that person that you just introduced (that will be taking the money) must have had, personally have had that thing that you really want to do—that thing that is your highest, best use of your time, the thing that gives you the most soul satisfaction and maybe the most coins in your bank.

If your cashier has not experienced the higher value service, her effectiveness will be near zero because she will be using a script instead of giving her personal story when she explains your higher value service.

Consenting Speech

After the first part of your introductory speech, where you elevate your purpose for being there, then you go into the consenting process. So I'm back on stage now, and here is what I say:

"So, if you want to know more about that [your higher value service], talk with Mary Jo on the way out. Let's have a party."

"Now...[pause for transition and suspense, then you go into the actual explanation of BoNT]... *BoNT was discovered when some people died*."

[I like to start off with this bold proclamation because a lot of the people that have never had BoNT[1] have not had it because they think it is poison. And so, I just go ahead and bring it right out into the light of the hair salon. By talking about the scariest worst part first, you earn their trust.

If you want to read more about why to talk about the worst part first, read the book, *Influence* by Cialdini; he will explain it better than I can. Read the entire book if you want to understand the best ideas ever written about sales and marketing.

[I will continue with my consenting speech...]

"BoNT was discovered when some people died from food poisoning. And the way botulism works, which is what killed them, is the bacteria creates a toxin that blocks acetylcholine. That's a chemical that allows your nerve to tell your muscles to contract. And when botulism blocks that acetylcholine, now the nerve cannot tell the muscle to contract. So, you can't breathe. You fall over, and you die. That is botulism."

[Now, at this point, the people who've never had it before are saying, "Yep, that's right. BoNT is poison. That's why I'm not going to get it."]

---

[1] During your speech, you can use the name of your product in place of the word "BoNT."

[But they're also thinking, "Well, this guy will not try to lie. He's obviously being openly honest with me."

So, now, they will be more likely to believe the next thing you say.]

"But the toxic dose of BoNT, the LD 50, or the toxic dose that would kill 50% of people is literally close to $100,000 worth. For a 100-pound woman, it is around 100 full bottles of BoNT injected iv; that would be 100 pounds x 100 units per bottle, or 10,000 units. At $10 a unit, that would be $100,000 worth. And doses 10 to 100 times more than what we would use on the face are used to relax the muscles of children with cerebral palsy or relax the muscles of adults with back pain."

"The muscles in the face are so tiny. Think about the size of a facial muscle. It's this long in your forehead [pointing to my forehead]; compared with the thigh muscle of even a small child [pointing to my thigh], this [pointing at my forehead] is minuscule. So the amount of BoNT needed to relax facial muscles is so tiny that no one dies from cosmetic BoNT. They just don't.

"But you shouldn't have it if you're pregnant because we don't want to have to worry about babies. We don't know of any ill effects that have happened to children or in utero from BoNT, but we don't want to be doing that experiment on you. So if you're pregnant, or think you could be, then don't get BoNT."

"You should not get it if you have myasthenia gravis. If you don't know what myasthenia gravis is, you don't have it. So, you shouldn't have it if you have those two things."

"You could get a bruise. You could get a droopy eyelid. If that happens, you get Visine with the red letters. That's the kind that has a little epinephrine-like stuff in it, and it'll open your eye. There are fancier things to take, but that works well. Use it every two or three hours when you're awake and out in public, and your eyelid should not be as droopy until the BoNT wears off. I've only had three of those events, by the way, in the past, over a decade. So it doesn't happen often, but it could happen. If it does, it wears off in two or three months. Use the Visine until it does."

"With most people who get droopiness, however, it's not from their eyelids. It's because someone over-treated their forehead, and it droops their entire brow (not the eyelids). So, in the beginning, or if you've never had BoNT before, I prefer not to treat your brow at all. Because that's the only muscle, your forehead muscle, or your frontalis, that's the only muscle holding your brow up. So, if I relax it too much, your brow falls."

"If you have never had BoNT before today, if you're a BoNT virgin, just treat your frown (the number 11's). Nobody likes a frown. It's been shown to help depression if you treat that. Maybe get a brow lift, crow's feet, nothing else today."

"I don't do fillers ever at the BoNT parties. It takes too long, but we can talk about it. I'll do a free consult for you. You don't even have to get BoNT. I'll do a free consult. Look at your face; tell you what might help you most to look younger. Maybe you need surgery. Maybe you just need a bodyguard. I don't know what you need, but I'll look at your face and tell you what I think in my honest opinion about what might help you most. It may not be anything I know how to do, but I'll tell you about it. And if you want BoNT, that's good too."

"BoNT starts to work in a couple of days. The full effect is two weeks. Wears off in two months. But if you get it repeatedly, if you get it about every three months for a year, it starts to last longer. So, it will last the full three months, or it'll start lasting four or five months, or you may be able to go down on the dose because you get out of the habit of using those muscles. So that's a good, easy practice to do (every three-month injections). And it saves you money in the long run. You just go every three months for a year and then stretch it out or go down on the dose."

11. CONSENTING & EXPLAINING BONT (PART 2 OF 2)

We're still doing the consent process. In the previous chapter, in the consenting process, I described what bad could happen, who should not have it, and what to do if you get a droopy eye. With most of the people that say they drooped, it wasn't their eyelid; they got their forehead over-treated.

Now I'm back on stage to finish the consenting process.

Pass Out the Consent Forms

At this point, I will ask the hostess to pass out the consent forms.

Now everyone has a consent form in their hand. I haven't asked them to sign it yet. They just have it in their hand.

Then I will go through very quickly the things I can do with BoNT, even the stuff I may not be planning on doing to the virgin BoNT people.

I bring with me a picture of the muscles, and I explain to them that wrinkles are like pleats on your belt.

Continuing the Consent Speech

[I'll take my belt, and I'll tighten the belt, and I'll say the following]:

"See, your belt goes this way, but the pleats go that way—perpendicular to your belt [pointing at my belt]. If you look at the muscles of the face, for the frown muscle, the muscle goes this way, and the wrinkle goes this way [pointing at the corrugators]. Or with the frontalis, the muscle goes this way, but the wrinkles go this way."

"All you can do with BoNT is you can relax these belts and, in the process, pull out the pleats. You can't tighten anything with BoNT."

[Though the skin does get tighter, you are actually loosening the belts-muscles.]

[Many people don't know the difference between BoNT and fillers, so the next part of your consent speech explains].

"Think about BoNT as something that pulls the wrinkles out of the sheet, and fillers and PRP fluffs up the mattress. And so does Retin-A; collagen-building creams can fluff the mattress. BoNT tightens the sheets."

"When you think about the appearance of something, you have only four traits: size, shape, color, and texture. And shape contributes a lot to the youthfulness of the face, and so does texture. I can change the shape with fillers and PRP, the Vampire Facelift® procedure. I can change the texture with BoNT and the Vampire Facial® procedure."

[If you do the Vampire Facelift® or Vampire Facial® procedures, bring brochures to give to people who ask questions; you do not have time to explain them at a party.]

"Let's just go through some of the things I can do with BoNT. I can take the frown lines out. I can soften the brow. But again, I don't want to do that for your first trip. We just do the frown today, and then come see me in the office just this one time between two and four weeks before it wears off and after it's full effect, so between two and four weeks, and I will tailor make the way I do your forehead based on where your brow is."

[If you treat the forehead on the first visit and you droop the brow, they're never coming back. But if they come in (on the second visit) and you droop them, they'll still come back; they'll just tell you not to BoNT their forehead next time. Many people have never seen how high you can lift the brow.]

[When you don't treat the forehead, and you just lift the brow with the other treatments, they're glad that you did it. Don't treat the forehead, even though oftentimes this is the main thing they want. If you just treat the forehead, so you relax the frontalis but you haven't relaxed all the pull-down muscles, the glabella, the corrugators, when you relax the frontalis, it's going to droop them.]

[You explain that to them using the diagram of the facial muscles as a teaching tool, and then you always treat the pull-down muscles first, bring them back two to four weeks later, treat the frontalis. Then after that, you can do it all in one trip.]

[But if they come in and their brows aren't up very high, maybe you don't treat the frontalis. You do it very lightly. If you come in and they're spiked out, you can go more heavily. Even in young people, I split it up.]

"Okay. Other things I can do."

"I can open one eye like my left eye is a little smaller than the other, so I could open it."

"If I have narrow eyes that I want to be more almond shape. Oftentimes either hereditary or often a Caucasian woman who just squints when she smiles, I can open the eye more so it's more open when she's smiling."

"I can treat bruxism."

"I can treat a gummy smile where the mouth goes up too high when someone smiles or high enough that they're self-conscious when they smile really big for the camera."

"I can treat bunny lines, which is where people scrunch up there. We'll talk about all this later."

"I can treat orange peel skin."

"I can help lift the corners of the mouth, and I can create a more glamorous shaped mouth by treating the edges of the mouth."

"I can treat the smoker's lines, too."

"Those are things you can do with BoNT. But again, if you've never had it before, let's just do the frown brow lift and some crow's feet."

[All right, so I think that covers everything about consenting the person. At this point, I would stop, and I would BoNT one person while everyone was watching. Preferably someone who's had it before, so they're not nervous about it, and everyone sees that they're not being hurt. If I were at a hair salon, I might do that in the lobby. If I'm at someone's home, I may do that in the living room.]

Starting the Treatment

Then in the hair salon, I move to the treatment or the stylist area, and I have one of those tables like the cosmetologist puts her brushes on, and pull that up next to the treatment chair, and use their brush stand like a Mayo stand.

The hostess brings her guests to me in the order she thinks they should be treated. She knows who's in a hurry and who wants to hang out all night.

So, she brings them to me in whatever order pleases her.

I snap a picture of their face. I snap a picture from front and each side, obliquely, and I snap a picture of their consent form.

But first, I do a consult.

Show them the mirror, and I say, "What would you want to make better?"

I look at their face while they look at their face in the mirror.

If the thing they want to make better is something to do with a collapsed shape, I tell them they need to come to the office where I can do fillers. But almost everybody at least wants their frown done, and the hostess is there cheering them on. They get caught up in the mentality of the party, and they've heard an explanation, and they see everyone else getting it.

So, they go for it.

The Only Two Ways to Find the BoNT Virgins

Of the people who have come to me who've never had BoNT before seeing me, probably 99% of the time, that's how I found them—at a party.

Occasionally, I will see someone in my office who has never had BoNT when someone who is my current patient brings a friend with them. But those are the only two ways I see most BoNT virgins: (1) brought by a friend to a party or (2) brought by a friend to my office.

I do not find new BoNT patients by advertising to people who've never had it. Never. I don't think I've ever had one of those people. It's always at a party, or their friend brought them to my office.

Why You Need BoNT Virgins to Grow Your Cosmetic Practice

The reason you NEED to create a system of finding people who have never had BoNT and persuading them to become your BoNT patient is that it is very difficult to take another person's BoNT patient unless you offer a lower price, which you do not want to do because you now have a "bargain" hunting patient instead of someone WANTING to pay top dollar for the BEST (which you will be if you follow my system).

Also, BoNT is one of the best ways to introduce people to other cosmetic and sexual medicine procedures. BoNT gets them in your door, then they trust you with the rest of your treatments if they can afford them.

So, the KEY to growing a cosmetic and sexual medicine practice is knowing how to attract people who have never had BoNT.

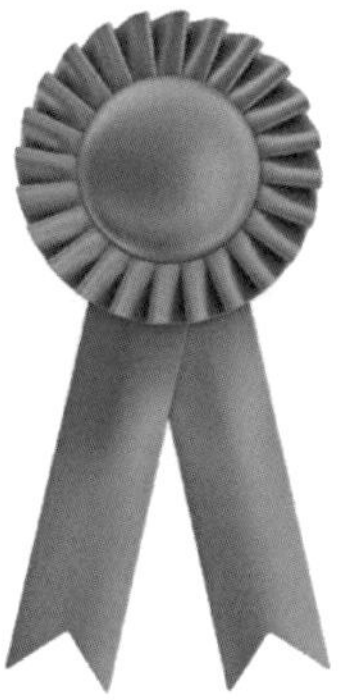

Figure 21. Give away door prizes at the party and bring extras to sell to those who do not win the prize.

Prizes

You will have more fun at the party if you bring some door prizes and you let the hostess give those away. Three prizes seem to work best. It is always fun to give things away.

The prizes should be a cream or something that people who get BoNT would want to buy from you anyway. Bring two or three more than you plan to give away because some people will want the prizes when they see others excited about winning them, so they will buy the prizes from you.

Two at a Time

The hostess may bring to me two or three people at a time. Sometimes girlfriends come together. That's okay. They'll come to cheer each other on. I especially like it when mothers and daughters come together; when they do, you are looking at a mother and daughter who are emotionally close and having fun, and they are making you a part of it—that's a great privilege for me to cherish.

Even though the hostess may bring people to me in pairs, I want to be out of earshot of all the others when I'm injecting (though people do not expect extreme privacy at a party, you can still achieve some intimacy).

At the salon where I currently do BoNT parties (it's the only one where I still do parties), it's a very small space; but they have a porch. So, most of the ladies and men wait outside on the porch, enjoying refreshments, while the person I'm treating is on the inside. But it may be two of them at a time in front of me when they are close friends or family.

Refreshments (The Hostess' Cost) & Free BoNT (My Cost)

I tell the hostess not to spend a lot on refreshments, or else she will fall in the trap of spending more money on refreshments than it would have cost her to buy her BoNT from me. Simple snacks, simple drinks work best.

The deal is the hostess(es) gets to receive from me all the BoNT she wants (or he wants) for free, but they go last. Not fillers, just the BoNT, and they get all they want for free.

Since there may be more than one chair at the salon, and so more than one person wanting free BoNT, they need to each persuade at least three people to pay me in order for each of them to receive the free BoNT.

For example, if a salon has two people working there who want free BoNT from me and Jane has six of her people pay me and her coworker, Mary, didn't bring anyone to me; then Jane gets free BoNT, but Mary does not. Jane needs to bring me three, and Mary needs to bring me three. And then they would both get all the BoNT they wanted for free.

Remember, you're not just making profit on the BoNT; you're going to make profit on all the people who follow you back to your office, but you should still make profit at the party, and that will happen if at least three people pay you for BoNT for every one hostess that you treat for free. If you want, and Mary brings 6 and Jane brings none, you may treat them both for free, but I encourage them both to bring 3, and it works better (when both are talking about you, the party will be overall more attended).

I think that covers all the rules of the party.

How Many at the Party?

Following my suggestions, you can easily treat 20 to 25 people in a couple of hours at a BoNT party. If you have 3 to 3.5

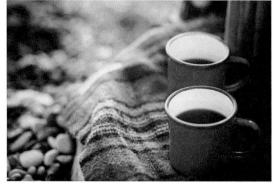

Figure 22. The hostess should have simple refreshments or else she will spend more on refreshments than her BoNT would have cost.

hours, you should be able to treat 40 people and keep good records of your money and of what you've done.

Until you do a few parties and practice the flow, I would tell the hostess to limit the number in attendance to around eight to ten.

Even though you will make money and have fun at the party, most of the money happens after the party. One of the ways you can increase the income from the party and better help your patients is by creating your own BoNT club. In the next chapter, I will show you how.

12. START YOUR OWN BONT CLUB TO KEEP YOUR PATIENTS LOYAL & INCREASE INCOME

Important: This chapter discusses some technical skills of building websites. You can learn to do these things yourself (it is much easier than what you learned in medicine). But, rather than becoming discouraged by the aggravation and time needed to implement the technology, you can simply go to UpWork.com and hire someone to do the work for you. Just show them this chapter so they know what it is that you want them to do.

This chapter includes a transcript of a video about clubs (with explanatory notes and links). You can watch the video and access the links at BoNTClass.com.

- Video Transcript
- Further Explanation of How to Set Up Your Club (including emails you can send)
- The shopping cart, web page, and other aspects of a club

Why Clubs Make Money

I run my BoNT club like a way to put BoNT on layaway, the way mothers did back in the nineteen-sixties when I was a kid. Your mother didn't have a credit card. So, if she couldn't pay for Santa Claus or somebody's birthday gift, she "put it on layaway."

She put a little money down, the store stored the item she wanted back in the closet somewhere, and then she paid a little on her item whenever she had some extra money, and after she paid it off, she got to take it home.

The way I do my BoNT club is similar. A person pays me $25 monthly; their credit card is billed automatically. After three months, they paid me $75, but they get $100 off their BoNT treatment. After four months, they paid me $100, and they get $135 off their BoNT treatment. It is a simple system that bills them every month for as long as they are in the club; and they can drop out anytime they wish.

They pay monthly and cash in whenever they get their BoNT. Some people paid me monthly for over a year, during the COVID pandemic, without receiving BoNT. Then they came in and cashed in with free BoNT until I had paid them back, plus an additional 20% or so of what they prepaid. It works out since you are paying them back in BoNT—the dollar you give them in BoNT costs you less than a dollar.

I have people who have been in my club for over a decade; it is beautiful. And they are not shopping on Groupon for BoNT because not only are they in my club but also, I have their recipe. I treat them special, genuinely.

You can see the page that advertises and enrolls people in my club here: http://www.runels.com/botoxclub.html

Feel free to model your club after mine.

Further Explanation of How to Set Up Your Club, Including Emails You Can Send

Ways "Your-Office" BoNT Club Helps You and Your Patient
Your BoNT club may offer more benefits than are first apparent. Here are a few of them:

- They have already paid part of the fee for the BoNT, so they are more likely to come to your office instead of shopping for a lower price (so they do not lose their investment and where you know their tailor-made BoNT recipe).
- Since they will pay less for the BoNT, they have more money to spend on something else when they come for the BoNT treatment but often need to add more money to the pot to purchase the extra product or service.
- Having your own club keeps them out of Allergan's club where they can cash in their points at another doctor's office.

- The club is automatically handled by your shopping cart, so there is money coming in for each member of your club—even in the months when the patient may not be coming to see you.

Here are more specifics about how it all fits together (emails, shopping cart, BoNT club, websites, & recipes)

1. A person gets BoNT for the first time from you—in your office or at a BoNT party.
2. You mention joining your club as a way to save money. Tell them, "You pay $25 a month; so, after 3 months, you've paid $75 but you get $100 off of your next BoNT[2] treatment. If you wait 4 months, you've put in $100, but you get $135 off your next BoNT treatment."
3. When you get back to the office (after a BoNT party), or after their first treatment at your office, you put them into your series of 3 emails that tell them about BoNT and about your BoNT club (more about these emails later).
4. Set up an autoresponder to send the following 3 emails (see #5). The autoresponder messages should deploy (without you having to do anything after putting the person's info into your computer) as follows: On the day of treatment; the next one at 2 weeks after their treatment; & the last one at 3 months after their treatment.

   Do not worry, your software can do all of this for you. You can see pick up a free book about email and selling online at: *CellularMedicineAssociation.org/email*

5. The three emails previously mentioned encourage your patient to keep getting BoNT, to join your club, and to bring a friend to see you. Write the emails, tailored to your practice, using the following checklist associated with the content of each email:
   a. The first email (that goes out the day of their treatment) tells them about the club and encourages them to tell

---

[2] Substitute the brand name of the BoNT you inject.

their friends about your BoNT offerings and your practice.

    b.   The second email (which goes out ten days after their treatment) reminds them to see you again in 2 weeks after the first treatment—so you can fine-tune their results and reminds them of your BoNT club.

    c.   The third email (which goes out three months after their treatment) reminds them to see you for another BoNT treatment in 3 months after the first treatment—and reminds them of the BoNT Club.

6.   The person gets the 3 emails and signs up for the club.

7.   Each of the 3 emails has a link to the web page where you talk about your BoNT Club.

Where to See a Video Demonstration

I demonstrate, on video, how to set up the club in 1ShoppingCart (including making a link for a web page or a button) at *BoNTClass.com*. I also give you the three emails to copy and paste into your software (just change the contact info from mine to yours).

If you are offering BoNT to your patients, you will also find one or more of the Vampire Procedures® will help your patients (and bring more profits to your business). Application for online and hands-on training for the Vampire Procedures® can be found here:

VampireFacelift.com/members/procedures

The Details of the Shopping Cart, Web Page, & Other Aspects of a Club

This chapter is a modified transcript of a video that shows how to set up a club. If you prefer to watch a video instead of or in addition to reading, you can find the video demonstration of exactly where to click on the software to set up your club at BoNTClass.com; but *you have all you need to know what to do right here in this book.*

Here's an outline of this transcript for one of our private meetings of the Cellular Medicine Association's *Journal Club with Pearls & Marketing*:

- Intro
- Standardization of Procedures—Accomplished by the CMA
- A Whole New Class of Options for Healing Disease
- Profit: The Doctor's Four-Letter Word & "Crabs in a Bucket"
- How to Create Your Own Club
- A look at my BoNT Club
- A step-by-step process to making your club
- Other "Cluster Club" Ideas
- References
- Relevant Links

Transcript

Welcome to The Journal Club tonight. Tonight's club meeting will be mostly focused on marketing, but I want to relate it to a review article that came out this past week, let me just show that to you, because it brings up a point that needs to be discussed more. And it's one of the biggest criticisms of anyone who's using platelet-rich plasma and many of the surgeries that are being done.

And remember a good critic or even a smart enemy is good because it makes you smarter. It makes you remember to think about things more deeply. And without people looking at us and criticizing us, we have less motivation to get better. And this is mostly a friendly article, but it brings up a common thread in those who would criticize us. And so I'll just go ahead and get to it.

By the way, this article is open source, so I have it where you can download it in the handout section if you click on that. And I have links to everything we're going to talk about. The marketing piece will be about how to set up your own club or your own click and subscribe the way Amazon does. And it's much easier than you might think. And even if you don't want to do this yourself, you will know what to request if you hire someone else.

Standardization of Procedures-Accomplished by the CMA

But first, look at this article in JAMA because here's the thing that I want to bring up. It talks about the need for standardization; that's what I'm getting at. If you read this whole introduction, our main criticism, for those of us who use platelet-rich plasma (PRP) as part of our practice of medicine, is always that there is no standard way of doing things, or standard definition of PRP.

Here is a quote from the article that delineates the main point of the article, "Despite the advancements made in this field [PRP treatments], it lacks regulatory guidelines and standardized procedures, which imposes one of the biggest challenges of the field."

This is the reason I started our group (the Cellular Medicine Association). And I should emphasize this more because I think we see it as a way to share ideas, and it serves that purpose. We pool our money and finance research; it serves that purpose. But when I first started doing this, what I had noticed as a cosmetic physician is that there was no regulation of cosmetic injections. And that seemed to be a problem. And as far as I know, to this day, no medical board exam regulates how cosmetic fillers are done or how cosmetic BoNT is done.

Think about that, what else in medicine even comes close to the equivalent frequency of use and yet is not standardized by any specialty board? Unless something has changed recently that I do not know about, cosmetic BoNT is not part of any regulatory standardization process (except for the few FDA, on-label indications that make up minority percentage of its use). Also, BoNT crosses all these different specialties: dentists, plastic surgeons, family practitioners, urologists, gynecologists. It seems everyone is doing BoNT and fillers. Some cater to more than one indication for BoNT than another, but it still crossing multiple specialties. And what is everybody's business, becomes nobody's business.

So, the way one person is doing Juvéderm, for example, in the same neighborhood as another person, their technique may vary widely. Twelve years ago (2010), seeing that inconsistency and starting to use

PRP for sexual treatment purposes, I thought, "There is a need for a way of standardizing how PRP is used."

Also, PRP is not a drug, so there are no FDA regulations of PRP use (only of the devices used to prepare PRP), and there is no board regulation. So, there should be some way to agree upon some standard procedures and formally define a group of doctors who agree to follow specific guidelines. Then that defined way of doing things becomes as respectable as the group becomes by the results achieved.

So, there is a standardization of PRP procedures within our group (the Cellular Medicine Association). There is no standardization (as of the time I am writing this) among and group of providers who are not part of our group; PRP methods are not being regulated by any board, just as no board regulates BoNT and filler use.

So, there is really nothing that keeps anybody from buying a centrifuge, some tubes, and saying they are doing a Vampire Facelift® or an O-Shot®, using either of those names, except for our group, we own the names and require training and an agreement to our protocols before advertising of the procedures. That allows us to regulate who uses our names to communicate with potential patients.

Note: in no way is the Cellular Medicine Association (CMA) a medical board. I realize medical boards are a different stratosphere of requirements and history, and the CMA is not a comparison, except in the idea that the CMA is a strong way of regulating how things are done if things are advertised with a particular name. And that is why I formed the group. And that is why I trademarked the procedures; with a trademark you, can enforce who can use and who cannot use a name for marketing purposes—which means you can regulate quality by regulating who can advertise to potential patients.

So, we are indeed doing the standardization of protocols that the paper under consideration suggests is needed. This is one of the main purposes of our group and we have done it well. And it has not been easy or cheap. You guys know that we have spent literally millions of dollars to enforce our quality standards. Our biggest budget item by far is not me or my staff or even our research. Our biggest budget item is legal expenses, just fighting back against the infringers who want to pretend like they're doing something when they don't even know who we are, much less how we have standardized our procedures, which are laid out in detail on our membership websites.

So, we (at the Cellular Medicine Association) do finance research, and we do things to help educate patients, but this criticism of our procedures (lack of standardization) IS being done and is being addressed daily at the costs of many thousands of dollars a month and multiple attorneys. A big part of what I do daily is deal with attorneys about how to keep it tight and keep people from using our names who do not know what we are doing (and, therefore, may be putting patients at risk).

A Whole New Class of Options for Healing

Part of the reason that there is less understanding about why PRP is not regulated—*PRP is part of a whole new class of therapies*. Previously, we had, for treating patients, only surgery, antibiotics, and vaccines. We also have autoimmune attenuators like prednisone, and we have mechanical ways of treating disease (stents, and the surgical removal of cancer for example). We also have nutritional and endocrinology strategies. But *the idea of injecting something or waving a wand that has energy (radio frequency or laser) to trigger tissue to become healthier, that is a more recent development in medicine.*

So, because the idea is new, the medical institutions are wrestling with how to regulate and standardize a whole new category of medicine-- making the body healthier by doing something to directly make the tissue healthier.

As an example of the fact that making tissue healthier as a way of healing disease is a new idea, consider the following: Until we started doing PRP in the penis, there was nothing that a person could buy and no procedure he could undergo that would actually make the penis tissue healthier. Viagra, penile implants, Trimix, vacuum devices that is what we had for erectile dysfunction. None of those therapies, not one of them, makes the tissue of the penis healthier. People were doing and are still doing, thankfully, research with stem cells, but that treatment is not available for practicing physicians in the US (for now), because the FDA has classified stem cells as a drug. Currently, physicians in the U.S. cannot use stem cells unless under the umbrella of an IRB study. I will not try to explain the political and scientific reasons for the rules of the land, but that is the rule.

So, what do we have available to make the tissue healthier, as far as something you can currently do in a medical office? You can go running and you can take vitamin E, and you can do things that make the whole body healthier and, secondarily, make the tissue of the penis healthier; but there is nothing in *Harrison's Textbook of Internal Medicine* that directly makes the tissue of the penis healthier.

It is not there.

So, along comes PRP. Well, that therapy offers a whole new class of *helping erectile dysfunction by improving tissue health*. And now we know BoNT, used in the penis, also actually helps the tissue of the penis become healthier, *Bocox™*. And there is going to be a combination of BoNT with PRP very soon that we're going to be doing (we are doing this now and call it the P-Shot 100™ because we use 100 units of BoNT). And then you'll have two ways that make the tissue healthier combined into one procedure that you can legally (within the guidelines of the FDA) do in your office.

We are living history, I think; we are living to watch a whole new branch of medicine developing—regeneration of healthier tissue as a way to heal disease—"regenerative medicine."

This new branch of medicine is in its infancy, and it is having growing pains. Of course, the dentists and orthopedic surgeons were a decade ahead of us on this; in regard to sexual medicine, are only a decade into regenerative sexual medicine, using tissue health enhancers like the P-Shot® and Bocox®.

Profit: The Doctor's Four-Letter Word & "Crabs in a Bucket"

I was brought up in a conservative Southern Baptist home, and as I grew up, my heroes were Moses and St. John out in the wilderness eating grasshoppers. In my teens, I slept for a year on the concrete basement floor of my parent's home (I allowed myself a sleeping bag) to experience a spartan way. In my twenties, I read about Gandhi, who died owning only a pair of spectacles and a loin cloth, yet was wealthy in other ways; and, I read Thoreau's *Walden*; I decided to live out of my car for a year to come close to owning nothing (I still needed the car to get to class and allowed a storage room for my books and a post office box for mail).

When I was a kid, my dad took me to see this little statue in Birmingham. It was some guy that help found the University of Alabama in Birmingham School of Medicine. And the inscription under the statue said (it's still there as far as I know) something to the effect, "He would've been known as a statesman and successful businessman (and two or three other things), but instead, he was known as a physician."

My dad showed me that, and I thought, "Okay, that makes sense. So, I'll go be a doctor."

But my dad warned me, even as a kid, he said, "People will always want their doctor to be poor and their lawyer to be rich. It's always been that way. It will always be that way."

So, I just decided, "Okay, I'm just going to be broke my whole life." I did not really strive for money; my heroes were about something else.

So, I said, "I'm just going to be like a St. John and eat grasshoppers and wear camel skins, and I will be financially poor, but I will be a good doctor, and the system will provide necessities for my family and me."

The system did not provide.

And when I quit the ER after 12 years and opened a private practice, I just went broke because I was doing so much for free (whether I wanted to or not), but I kept thinking that if I were a good doctor, insurance would take care of me. And you know about how far that lasts if you're doing primary care. You can't live on 140 bucks for a 90-minute, level-four visit (out of which you must give $14 to the insurance billing company, $70 to overhead, and 1/2 of the $36 that's left over to taxes—leaving you with $18 an hour on a good day—and that's for the visits for which insurance actually pays you (and you get the money 3 months after services rendered). So, you do tricks to survive (a procedure or a test) to bring in cash or extra insurance income. But, as far as diagnosing sick people and figuring out the best medicine or advice to help them get well or stay well, you cannot survive on it.

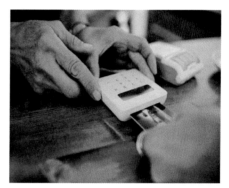

So, eventually, I had to learn a dirty word, "profit."

Enter the Dirty Word "Profit"

Most *doctors* cringe when you say the word "profit."

Figure 23. The part of medicine that makes doctors squirm with guilt.

I used to cringe; it was a dirty word.

"You should *not* try to make profit if you're a doctor," I thought.

Most of your patients do not want you to make a profit. They want you to live and be St. John and do it only because you want them to be well. They definitely do not want you to be rich, and that is okay; it is not their fault. It is just the way the world is. My Dad was right.

Surprisingly, most of your colleagues do not want you to make profit either. They will allow you some profit, but if you make too much profit, they will despise you for it, and will think you unethical both in business and in medicine. And if you fail financially, they will secretly, deep in their heart, celebrate your failure; that reaction is not their fault either. But it is how they think.

The world is round; it circles around the sun; people will always want their lawyer to be rich and their doctor to be poor—you may not like these things, but there is nothing to be done to change them.

But, I found (as an internist) that unless I started thinking about profit, we couldn't keep the doors open. By only thinking about complicated sick people, I would be unable to pay my staff, buy groceries for my family, and keep the office open to see patients.

I had to learn to think about profit.

Do you doubt me?

Find a cook with a profitable restaurant, staff, and building with prime real estate—easy to do in any town. Now, find a primary care physician with prime real estate and no partners, not an employee of the hospital, but still with prime real estate, who is making it on an insurance-based practice, and opening multiple locations—very difficult to find. Yet, there is a prominent sushi chef in my town who is up to 4 locations and buying up real estate, he gets paid when people eat, and he gets paid well. There are other chefs in town doing something similar. There is no primary care physician in my town on an insurance-based practice doing the same.

So, physicians who learn to prosper must learn to think about profit; but they must keep their profits secret to avoid the disdain of patients and then envy of other physicians.

To think more accurately about profit, it helps to think outside the bubble of medicine; let us do that next.

Real World vs. Medical World Profits

A good hour and a half massage at a fancy hotel is going to cost you $200-$300. It will cost you more than you get paid to spend an hour and a half trying to diagnose a sick person with three organs failing on ten medications. And if you make a mistake, the person dies. And your massage therapist went to school for six months.

It costs more by far to rent a jet ski at the beach than it costs to see your internist for help with a complicated medical problem. I live close to the beach; to rent a jet ski costs more than a level four visit. Just for an hour on a jet ski cost you more than an hour with an internist who's diagnosing and treating a disease that is life-threatening. And if he gets the dose wrong, you die.

But, even considering all the above discussion, the word may still feel wrong— "profit."

Even though, logically, people know you must have extra money after paying your business bills so you can buy groceries and care for your family, it still feels wrong for most doctors and most patients to say the word "profit" when referring to a physician's medical practice.

The word "profit" in almost any context has become tainted. You will even hear politicians talk about "evil" companies making "profit," as if somehow the company could continue to manufacture its products and pay employees, and do research without profit.

If companies are evil for making profit, I promise you, doctors are too.

The Crabs

Where I live, at the coast of the Gulf of Mexico, we label the phenomenon demonstrated by physicians (and by others, maybe almost anyone of any group) with the term "crabs in a bucket."

We call it crabs in the bucket because if you catch crabs in a net for food, you want to boil the crabs while they are still alive. You do not want to eat a crab that was not alive when it was thrown in the pot, not fresh enough.

And so, you catch them, out on a pier with a crab net, and then you throw them into a bucket; but keep them alive until you get home to cook them. Here is the trick: one crab in the bucket will easily crawl out so you may need a lid for the bucket; but if you have more than one crab, you do not need a lid as much because when one crab tries to crawl out of the bucket, the other crabs will grab it with their claws and pull it back down.

They do not want a crab crawling out of the bucket, so they pull it back down to where they all are: "crabs in a bucket."

You can even see threads of the thought of "doctors should be poor" in literature. For an example, think about Charles Dickens.

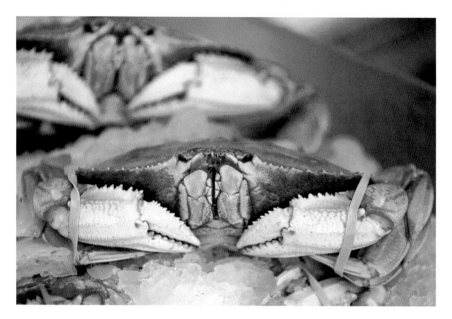

Figure 24. Be very careful of the other crabs; they will try to pull you back into the bucket when you start to crawl out.

Charles Dickens & Doctors

If you read a Dickens novel, *Bleak House*, or *Little Dorrit,* when you read about doctors, you will see that the prevailing attitude of medicine was that it was a calling. You did not go into medicine to make money. If you went into medicine in Dickens' day in London, you either had enough money (from sources other than medicine) to meet your financial needs and could do medicine as a hobby, or you took a vow of poverty. Maybe, that attitude is not so bad. Maybe, that is how it should be. But perhaps there are not enough wealthy people who want to do medicine as a hobby (and risk a lawsuit that takes their wealth) or enough people who want to live out of their car.

So, when you make a profit or consider profit as a physician, you must keep it a secret. Still, I think that to be a good physician, you need to be able to take care of your staff, yourself, and your family, and if you are healing the sick and making people's lives better, you deserve to prosper. To do that, you need to think about profit. Just keep it a secret, please.

Or you will face the wrath of your colleagues and attract the attention of hungry lawyers.

Okay, enough about profit. We needed to talk about the concept of profit, and you need to think about it. Without that discussion, and without your conscious decision to want to make profit, you would see no need for the following discussion of a club—which is a great way to make profits (and help your patients).

Just always remember that for every dollar you make, your patient should receive a value of ten times what you were paid. But, to help you think, always compare the value of your services to real world products and services (not to what insurance would have you think). For example, is what you are doing worth more than a massage, or a night in a good hotel room? If so, then charge appropriately to those who can afford, and give to a number of those who cannot (but not so much that you go broke).

Note: All physicians should do things for free. Frequently. But, as much as possible, you decide what you will do for free; do not let insurance companies decide for you.

Now that we talked about the necessity of profit, I'm going to walk you through how to set up a club. Clubs bring great value to your patients and clubs are a delightful way to make profits.

How to Create Your Own Club

A Look at My BoNT Club

Let's think about some clubs that you may be a part of without realizing. For example, using the button on Amazon.com that says, "click and subscribe," I am a member of a cashew butter club, a toilet paper club, a vitamin club, and more; because for all those things, I pay Amazon to ship to me periodically without me thinking; Amazon bills my card and ships those things to me every month.

Automatic billing with automatic delivery is my definition of a club.

For a multitude of products on Amazon, you can make a one-time purchase, or you can "click and subscribe" and save a percentage because you are now a subscriber to that product—you joined a club that gives you automatic delivery at a discount (because you agreed to automatic billing).

Why I Made Clubs to Survive

In 2003, I was the number two doctor in my state for doing joint injections; moreover, I was skipping cortisone knee injections (which leads to earlier joint destruction) and going straight to Hyalgan for pain relief (which helps prolong the life of the joint). Still, Hyalgan cost more than cortisone—much more. So, BlueCross audited me and fined me some money. After my meeting with the "authorities" at the insurance company, for me at least, it felt unethical to continue the game of an insurance-funded primary care practice. So, with much trepidation, but also much determination, I wrote a letter and gave up my PMD status with the insurance carriers. I went to a cash only practice.

When I went to an all-cash practice in 2003, it was a dramatic thing for me, because I didn't know that when you give up your PMD status with Blue Cross Blue Shield, which rules Alabama, you can't bill anybody who has Blue Cross for *six months*, for anything that is covered by Blue Cross.

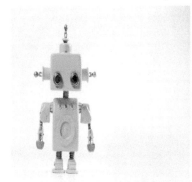

Figure 25. A club requires automatic billing and (if possible) automatic delivery.

So, I eked along on some clinical trials that I had running and lived on that. And then, I started doing for-cash-only medicine (or for free if you were truly poor).

I did not know the word "concierge" medicine. I just asked people pay me to come see me. I was thinking more like 1950s medicine, where you had "hospital insurance" but you paid your doctor. When you think about it, the price of seeing a primary care doctor is less than a fancy haircut in some salons. The idea of having insurance just for a doctor visit did not really come around in the US until the late 1960s. Before then, you had "hospital insurance." But you paid your primary care doctor.

I just thought, "Okay, let me go back to that."

Also, I have been fiddling around building websites since 1998, just to educate people about health and disease (there was no way to pay me on the websites), and I thought, "Well, let me see if I can make some clubs for a steady cash stream." So, I figured out a way to make some simple clubs. It is not that hard.

The first club I made was my "Botox Club."

I started doing Botox before Juvéderm was approved in the US. I do not know if Allergan had its discount club for patients back then, but their club for patients, when I discovered it, did not attract me because people could cash in their points with any physician. Anyway, by the time I discovered their club, I had already made up my own.

The way my club works is that you click a link on a web page, and it bills you $25 a month. Then, after three months, when you come to see me, you have paid me $75, but I give you $100 off your Botox[3] treatment. If you took four months to come to see me, then you've paid me $100, and I give you $135 off.

Now I use Botox and other BoNTs as part of my club. Some people have been in my "Botox Club" for more than a decade. I had people who paid me through COVID; they were still paying me to be in that club.

I've set up vitamin clubs, all sorts of clubs.

A Step-by-Step Process to Make Your Club

(For a video of the following steps, see BoNTClass.com).

Let's walk through a way of setting up your clubs. I realize that for every piece of software that I show you, there are a dozen others that claim to do the same thing. I do my own websites and spend around $50,000 to

---

[3] Now I use a variety of the brand name BoNTs, not just Botox.

$100,000 a year on software; so, you may find something that works better than what I show you. But what I am going to show you was not determined in a haphazard way. I figured it out over 20 years and lots of frustration. So, it may be worth at least looking at my methods before you invest time and money in other software.

You will be able to follow along by reading the following step-by-step plan. If you would rather see it on video as I navigate the internet, then those videos are available at BoNTClass.com But, you will be able to set up your club if you follow the following instructions.

If you do not want to do all the following steps, at least see how easy it is, so you can see that it should not cost you thousands of dollars and require you to wait a month.

If you go to BoNTClass.com, you can see my latest recommendations for who to hire to do the following steps for you (which I update as the software and the companies available to help change).

The Steps (edited from the transcript of the video at BoNTClass.com)

1. Log into your WordPress website

If you are not knowledgeable about building websites, then it will save you loads of time if someone builds your website for you; but once it's built, if you have a WordPress website, logging in is just like logging into

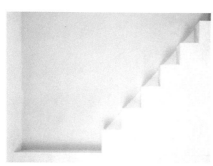

your Facebook page; it works like a blog, where you can just login and write or post photos and videos as if you were writing a Word document.

2. Add a new page or post to your site

After you login, if you want to add a page, just click at the top, "add," then "add a new post."

Then you see something that looks like a Word document.

Figure 26. The steps to building your own club are known and easy. Just follow the steps instead of trying to invent a new staircase.

Making a page is just like typing a Word document. In this example, I'm going to call it "Altar" by typing that word into the title.

Now I have a page on a website to sell the product. That's it, but there is nothing yet on the page. So, next, I will show you how I could set up a way for people to buy our Altar™ cream and subscribe to it (a club).

Most people complicate these things. They start with pictures and lots of formatting decisions. They worry too much about the way it's going to look (and we will make it look reasonably well), but you know what I like to start with first? The button.

Start with the button where they pay you.

Until you have the button that they click to pay you, you may have something that looks pretty, but you do not have anything that is helping your business make money. So, start by making the button where they pay.

Then, build everything else on the page that you need to encourage clicking the button by the person whom your service would help.

3. Make a Pay Button

A Note about How the Parts Work Together

Before you make the button, think about how the button connects to all the parts. The following list may seem self-evident, but it helps make things work better (and make more money) if you think about each part and how they work together in a system.

The Parts of the Online Transaction: (1) Button that the Customer Clicks to Order, (2) The Shopping Cart, (3) Credit Card Processor, (4) Customer to Press the Button, (5) The Customer's Money in His/Her Bank, (6) The Page Where the Button Lives, (7) Your Bank Where You Want the Customer's Money to Go, (8) Emails and Products that Go to the Customer After They Push the Button, (9) The Software (and, also, possibly a person) That Delivers the Product or Service.

Here is how it works together as a system.

The customer lands on a page through word of mouth or because of an email or other communication (postcard, text, social media, etc.).

They read the text or watch a video on the web page and decide they want the product or service.

They then click a button. The button tells the shopping cart what they bought and adjust the inventory to be one less than what you had.

The button also tells your credit card processor to take money out of the customer's bank and put the money in your account. If they just bought a subscription, the shopping cart learns how often to repeatedly take the money from the customer's account and put it into yours. For example, if the customer just bought a monthly subscription, then the shopping cart will take money out of the customer's bank and put it in yours every month without your or the customer needing to do anything to make that happen unless the system breaks (usually by the customer's credit card expiring).

The shopping cart also tells software to send an email communication telling the customer that they bought, and the transaction worked. This communication could also be set up to continue periodically delivering prewritten messages at predetermined time intervals. These communications can come directly from the shopping cart, or they may be triggered by the shopping cart but then be sent by another completely different software application.

The if the product is online information, the shopping cart can deliver a message that links the customer to the online product. If the purchased item is a service, the shopping cart can take the customer (by link or email) to scheduling software to set up a time to receive the service. If the purchased item is a physical product, then the shopping cart can tell a fulfillment person what to ship, provide a shipping label, connect to shipping software (UPS, FedEx, USPS), collect a tracking number, and give the tracking number to the customer.

Note: PayPal can serve as both a as a credit card processor and a bank. But do not use PayPal as a credit card processor if you are selling something that is a prescription drug, or non-prescription CBD products, even if you practice in a state where you can and do have a legal pharmacy in your office. They don't want to get into the pharmacy business, and they will shut your whole account down for just one transaction selling such products. Play it safe and online, only sell non-prescription items; for example, our Altar™ cream is non-prescription. Also, do not make PayPal your only shopping cart processor. Because, if they ding you for something, which they will do occasionally, your only cash register just got shut down—you are out of business. So, do make it one of the ways you collect money, because it will help your sales, but please don't make it the only way you collect money. One irritated customer can complain and, without warning, you are shut down until you clear things up—which can take days or weeks.

My 1ShoppingCart makes PayPal an option when you're checking out; but I can live without PayPal. My shopping cart also processes cards through Authorize.net tied to my bank.

Making the Shopping Cart Button

We already made a page for the button to live on (see above). Now, let's make a pay button that puts people into our Altar™ club--where they pay for and then have shipped to them a bottle of Altar™ cream every month, automatically.

First, you log into 1ShoppingCart. Then you go to "Manage Products," then to "Create a New Product."

Then for this example, I just type "Altar subscription" into the name of the product. Since $97 is the suggested retail for one bottle of Altar, I'm going to bump the price down five dollars and make the subscription price $92 for a one-bottle-per-month subscription.

In review, I just typed in the name of the product, and typed in how much to charge each month.

So, I get to make up the name of my club and telling the shopping cart how much and how often makes it a club. If this was my Xeomin Club, I could just put "Xeomin Club"[i] in the name field and make the price $25.

You get to make this up.

Then, I click to save it.

Easy.

If this sounds simple, it's because it is.

Next, I have to tell the shopping cart how often to bill the new customer—club member.

So, I do two more clicks and type in one number; I click (1) "enable recurring billing," and I type in $92 where it asks for the recurring price (you can make the first price different than the recurring price, but I seldom do), then I click to make it a monthly charge (it could be set up weekly or annually).

That is it!

I don't get bogged down on all the other stuff. Like the first charge is some amount and after some amount of time it does something else fancy. If they happen to subscribe on the 31st and then the next month is February the 28 days, it's OK; the software figures it out and bills everyone who subscribed on the 29-31st on the 28th. You don't have to worry about it. I leave the number of times to bill the person at "no limit." They can tell me if they want to unsubscribe, not a big deal.

And I'm done, so I save it.

Now, what about the button part?

4. Put the Button on Your Web Page

To put the button on your page is very simple. First, while still in the shopping cart on the page where I just made the new product, I find the word "links," and I click on "a link for sharing. "

Then I pick out what I want the button to look like (the software gives you a menu of buttons). I pick the one I like and click on it; then the shopping cart generates the code.

You don't have to know what any of the code means. Very simple, you click on links, then you pick the button you want, and copy the code.

Now, all you have to do is paste the code onto the page you just made (see first of these steps)—and magic!

You now have a button on a page, and when someone clicks and pays, they joined your club!

4. Complete the Page to Compel People to Click the Button You Just Made

Now all you need to do is to put stuff on the page that makes people want to click the button.

Pause and Reflect, Seriously

Here you may want to pause and meditate on something. If your product is truly amazing, you could stop right here. You could just have a button to pay and schedule for your next Vampire Facelift® and your patients would tell other people about your work and people would click the button, if your product or service is amazing. The stuff you put on the page around the button just encourages what should happen if you just have a button.

If you do not have an amazing product or service, forget the shopping cart and your whole website for now and go make your product better. Then come back and work on your website.

All of this falls apart if when the person clicks the button the thing they get from you is not worth much more than what they paid you.

What to Put Next on the Page—the Video

The next thing, after the button, to go on the page, in my opinion, should usually be a video that talks about why the person looking at the page should click your button.

Most of us think in images. We read words, but the words create images. It is difficult to emphasize how important a video is.

What the video says is the magic of sales and marketing, but for now, you may want to just use someone else's video who is selling the same thing. So let's go grab a video.

As an example, for our Altar™ cream, the website for the product is VampireSkinTherapy.com. So, I'm not even going to make a new video. I will simply go to that website and use the video that is on the home page, already made.

Most videos have a share button—and the one on the home page for VampireSkinTherapy.com does.

I only do two clicks, (1) "share," then (2) "embed code."

Now, I just copy the embed code, and paste it onto my webpage. Now, I have a video living on the web page just above the button.

5. Add the click and agree

Now you legally and ethically must add a document that tells the customer that, when they click the button, they are agreeing to pay every month to reorder the product or service

If they call you later and they say (it doesn't really matter what they say), "The moon was wrong," or, "I didn't have my glasses on," or, "I didn't really know what happening," or, "I just need to pay my gas for my car." I don't care what they tell you, if they want their money back, always give it back to them.

But they should not be able to say you tricked them into paying monthly; so by having them click and agree to the monthly payments, you avoid tricking people.

The "click and agree" is just another setting in your shopping cart (under settings), Find that setting, and upload your agreement. If you want to see one, go to VampireFacelift.com/members. Pretend, or actually do, purchase the training there (but you do not have to buy to see the click and agree. Then copy and paste that and have your lawyer approve it or modify it and make it what you use on your website.

It's not that hard to do. There's just getting your attorney to approve your document and then a button that you click.

6. Collect the money & keep the patient

Now you do not have to think about it. After the customer clicks your button, once a month, they will get billed 92 bucks (or whatever your club costs). The shopping cart will make (for you staff) a packing slip that goes in the box that carries to product to the customer, and it makes for a label and a tracking number (that is sent to the customer by the shopping cart).

In other words, in my office, that person is Taylor, and that person's changed over the years, but I have a person (it used to be part of one person's job), but then it turned into a whole job. And sometimes it's been more than one person's job. Depends on how much you're shipping. But this must be someone reliable because if someone pays you and you do not ship, that is mail fraud—which is a felony. So, your shipping person must be reliable, if they pay, you must ship (I prefer the next business day), and if you do not ship promptly (inventory unexpectedly low, hurricane, whatever) then promptly refund (or at least offer a refund).

But all the paperwork and the billing are handled by the software. And what happens is your staff logs into whatever software you're using. I like US Postal Service 2-day mail. And then they copy/paste the address from the shopping cart into the postal service software, and the shipping software generates a tracking number.

And then that tracking number is copy pasted back into your shipping cart--it's just click, click, and they're done. It's easy enough that this is someone that doesn't have to be brilliant, but they must be reliable. My person happens to be very smart too, but they do not have to be super smart, but they must be super reliable.

To Buy Just One & What About Shipping
So now I have a button that starts recurring billing—that makes a club.

Next to the button, I can write "subscribe for $92 a month."

But, I want allow the customer to just buy one bottle of it too. So, I type in, "buy one bottle for $97." It's not per month because they'll just be buying one bottle.

For shipping, I prefer to ensure there's enough profit in the item that I can ship it in the US without having to charge shipping. I'll leave that up to you, but that's how I like doing it.

Words for the Page
Now I have a page with a video, and buttons that allow the customer to buy one item or to subscribe. What about words for the page?

All I have to do is again click the share button on the video. Then, I go to the website, Rev.com.

I click on "Place a New Order," then on "Transcription."

Then I paste the share code into the box and pay.

Now, within a few hours to a day at most, I will get a transcription of the video at the current price of only $1.50 per video minute.

When I get that transcription, I paste that onto the page and now I have a webpage with a video and words and a button to click and subscribe.

Now all you have to do is share the page you made and make sure everyone who clicks your button either loves what they receive or you do not keep their money.

Social Media Makes Me Need a Bath

I don't really like social media so much. I feel dirty when I go on. I do not feel dirty about subject matters, any subject matter, but just the hate and the vitriol and the way people talk to each other on social media in ways they would never talk if they were physically in the same room with other people.

So, I have the website connected to social media such that when I publish the page, a link automatically goes out to social media without me having to look at social media. I recommend you do the same if your subject matter will not get you banned by social media (sometimes they ban articles about sexual medicine).

Email

Primarily, I like to communicate with customers by email. So, for example, after making the Altar™ club, now, whenever someone comes to see me for BoNT, I send them an email with a link to the Altar™ page.

Everybody that's on Retin-A in my office is also on the Altar™ because it keeps them from peeling from the Retin-A. And, of course, everybody gets it after a Vampire Facial®. It really is an amazing product. But people do not like to try and remember to order it; so now I just created a way for people to subscribe to it.

That's how you do a subscription or a club.

But, again, this will not make you much money unless you talk about it. You send emails to your people about it. You have people pull it up on their phones while they're getting their BoNT. You say, "Yeah, if you want to stay on this product, just click and subscribe to it."

Other "Cluster Club" Ideas

Other club ideas: if you have a men's clinic, you can cluster the following: P-Shot® once a year, shockwave treatments, a series of six, and then one a month for the rest of the year. You could add all that up and make some price and then make it a monthly payment and make it a club. It could be the penis club in your office or whatever, Dr. Sally's Penis Club. And I just showed you how to do

Even if you wanted to keep doing insurance, some need to keep taking insurance because that that is how you finance some of the more necessary surgeries that you like to do. You don't want to throw that away. But this is how you can supplement your income and literally make millions—by setting up clubs like this, where people buy and subscribe to products and services.

Examples of Products I sell Individually and as a Club

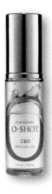

O-Shot® CBD Arousal Oil. O-Shot® providers order wholesale by logging
into the O-Shot® membership site
https://oshot.info/members/wp-login.php
or by calling CMA Headquarters (1-888-920-5311).

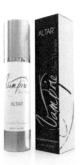

Altar™--A Vampire Skin Therapy™

All CMA members can order wholesale by logging into the membership
sites (VampireFacelift.com/members) and going to "Dashboard"-->then
to "Supplies"

Prewritten emails to promote your BoNT club (to copy-paste into your
software) can be found in the members area of BoNTClass.com

13. HOW TO TURN THE INFO YOU LEARN AT A PARTY INTO A GROWING LIST OF FANS WHO WANT EVERYTHING YOU OFFER

I am going to explain to you a way to turn what you learn at a BoNT party into a growing list of fans who want everything you have to offer. A live presentation of this can be found at BoNTClass.com but you have all the info you need here in print.

What a BoNT Party Really Is

Hopefully, you have studied the previous lessons in this course and know that a *BoNT party is a metaphor for any event where you're in the room with people who are brought into that room by a connector so that you might explain to that group something that will help the members of the group and in return, you get the contact info for the people in the room so that you can continue to grow the relationship after you go home.*

The connector gets something for free: either it is prestige because you're showing up to speak to their group (after all, they were able to attract YOU to speak to their group), or (better) it is a free or discounted service (like BoNT) or product. For example, when I do a BoNT party, the hostess gets free BoNT and the attendees get BoNT at one dollar less than I charge at my office.

That is a review of the party profit model. Now, let us talk in more detail about what happens after the party that makes the model work to grow your practice profits.

What You "Take Home" After the Party and Why

You are there, at the party, and you have people that are wanting something from you in the form of information or services. How do you turn that into a list of people who want everything you can offer them? What is it that you want so that you can make that happen?

Whether I climbed onto a plane to fly (and I have) to New Delhi to speak to a room of people or New Zealand or London or Miami or a half a mile away at the local chapter of the Rotary club, what I want is the names and email addresses (and any other contact info that I can obtain) of the people in the room.

I do the event, they have met me, and some of them may think, "I wouldn't let him babysit my cat."

Great. Not great, but it's great that we figured it out before they showed up at my office and wasted my time and theirs.

But others maybe think, "Oh, maybe he knows something about how to help me with a problem I have."

So that person who becomes interested in me and who likes me and who is interested in what I know may still not show up at my office. They still may not know everything I'm able to do for them (maybe what I spoke about at the event does not apply to them), but because of the event, they know me. So, I take that knowledge and leverage it into a relationship by getting their name and their email address and starting regular communications. And when I do a BoNT party, I get their birthday too because that's what I need for a medical record, and it allows me to offer them something for free on their birthday (usually $50 off anything in my office).

In summary, at the party, I get their name, email addresses, and birthday. I don't usually go for the phone number because it scares people. I might get the number, but the main thing I want is their name, birthday, and email address. And I'm very particular about the email. I want to be sure I can read the email address that they write down on their record card (the card they fill out at the party where I sketch what I did to their face). I want to know, for example, is that an O or a zero, a number "1" or the letter "l", a dash, or an underline? Because the email addresses are sometimes hard to decipher when someone scratches on a piece of paper at a party; you must check them on the spot while you are standing there with the patient. If you do not check the email addresses at the party, while with the patient, at least one in four of the emails you collect will be entered incorrectly and become a waste of your time.

What to Do the Next Day After the Party

Note: *If you do not know how to set up what I'm about to describe, hire someone to set it up for you (UpWork.com) or show up at one of my workshops, and we can talk more about it. But these are not strange things or hard-to-make-happen things.*

Now I'm going to go back home, after the party, and put all the info I gathered into my computer; the name, birthday, and email go into your computer. And now that person's going to receive all your emails because they are on your list.

The Dollar Value of a Name

A plain straight-up email marketer or internet marketer should be making at least $1 per month for every name on their list. That's why you have Kardashians that are billionaires. If you have a hundred million people on your list, if you know what you're doing, you're making a hundred million dollars per month because you should be able to bring something to them to purchase on a routine basis. Even if you're Kim Kardashian and your skill is balancing a champagne glass on your booty or showing cleavage, if you have an audience, you can sell. I'm not knocking her, she's a brilliant woman (would you balance a champagne glass on your booty for $100,000 million a month?). These things bring her attention, and because she has the attention of 100 million people, she can sell them stuff.

If you can sell to 1% of a hundred million people, you just sold a million widgets; sell the widgets for 10 bucks apiece; you just made 10 million bucks. Do you see what I'm saying?

So, you should make a dollar per name per month if you have the attention of people on a list.

As a physician, the dollars per month goes up; you should be making an average of somewhere around $2,000 minimum per year for every name on your list. It doesn't take a big list to start substituting the same income you might make as a primary care physician. And, of course, that number goes up even more if you're a highly skilled surgical specialist. So, the number of people you need to replace a $250,000-a-year insurance-based practice is surprisingly small. To make $250,000 a year as a primary care physician, you probably haver 2,000 to 3,000 patients and answer the phone a lot and maybe even make rounds at the hospital. But you only need an email list of about 300 people, 400 people max, to replace that income.

So that's what you're going to do—build a list of people who want to read your emails and who want everything you sell. When you come back from events, you are going to bring back the emails of people who met you at the event; they go on your list.

Then you care for the people on that list (by teaching them and motivating them) much more than you care for the money you will make from the products and services you sell. Your vow as a physician to care for your patients also applies to the info you send to them by email.

Now that You Have a Growing List of People, What Do You Do with It?

Now that you have a growing list, you are going to send them information and motivation.

You're not going to try to lure them into your office by saying 20% off if you show up in my office tomorrow. Please, no!

Imagine Superman saying, "Twenty percent off if you let me save you today."

I think that's one of the most degrading things a physician can do.

What you are going to do is now make regular, at least every two weeks, emails that give them something: either (1) teach them how to be healthy or beautiful (give how-to info) and/or (2) motivate them to do what they already know how to do (give them volition).

Why email? Isn't that out of date?

You use email (not social media) as your primary communication with your list because email does not get censored unless you're using MailChimp.

Note: *If you are using MailChimp, you should dump it because they've started censoring people—including our providers. MailChimp started off by censoring political views during the COVID times. And then they started censoring our providers based on the services we offer (sexual medicine and PRP both will get your account possibly shut down by MailChimp).*

Also, you cannot run ads on Facebook or Twitter that have anything to do with sexual medicine or PRP. Anything medical puts you at risk of losing your whole account. You can spew hate and vitriol, but if you talk about lovemaking, even in a medical sense, they will shut down your ad account. And I know because mine has been shut down.

So *social media can be frustrating because of censorship, but, so far, no one is censoring email except for MailChimp.*

Currently, favorite provider of email services is ONTRAPORT. Their service has the optimal combination of ease of use combined with expanded options that you will not find in Constant Contact or AWeber, or MailChimp, but it is much easier to use than Infusion Soft or Salesforce.

You can pick up a free e-book about email and how it works in combination with ONTRAPORT on the following web page: CellularMedicineAssociation.org/email. I will keep this page updated with new software that I may find.

The Two Main Subjects of Email, & "Validate the Voyeur"

With your emails, you're either *teaching* the people on your list better ways to relieve their pain, or you are *motivating* them to do what they already know to do. That's it. Those are the only two topics of your emails, except for an occasional update where you let them be a voyeur, and I don't mean balancing the champagne glass on your booty unless that's your thing (you do not need to be outrageous).

By validating the voyeur, I mean let them see your office and who works with you and let them see that you have a family and that you care about your family (including your pets).

They do not care about your hobbies; your *patients will resent your hobbies*. They do not even want you to have hobbies.

They want you to have a family, though. They want you to love your family, and *they want you to travel, but only to learn things about how to be a better doctor and with your family, everything else they will resent*. So, if you have hobbies (which you should), keep them a secret.

You Do Not Have to Dance for Your Money

I know some physicians who do well by being very flashy. And that is one of their gifts, and that is a good thing for them.

Every physician and every nurse can teach what they know.

*To your patients,
what you think
is more important
than news from Mayo.*

They have that talent and become a doctor version of a Kim Kardashian. And some of them are very brilliant physicians and nurses, super brilliant, very amazing clinicians. But if I tried to make a living doing that, attracting people by balancing acts or some sort of dance routine or something to do with being sparkly, I would have to get a job selling shoes. I stick to educational and motivational communications and do not try to be funny or showy.

They do not care about what any other physician has to say compared to what you have to say because you are their doctor. And even if they just met you at a BoNT party, they will develop that depth of trust in you if you earn it by sending them truthful information about medicine. As Hemingway said, write the truest sentence you can think—the truest sentence you can write. That truth has to come from your knowledge and experience in medicine, not from trying to lure people to your office with 20% off because it's freaking Valentine's Day!

Where to Find Today's Truth

That truth comes from your reading of the literature, being the scholar that you are, being the objective, observant, caring, loving, self-sacrificing healer that you are; then sharing what you know with the people on your list at least every two weeks will bring you more people than you have time to see. You can send them messages every day if you have something to say, but at least send an email every two weeks.

Educational & Motivational Format (not pretty)

Your email is not formatted to look like a magazine. You don't try to make it too pretty. It's just helpful information—not *Life* Magazine.

You can write about anything you think may help the people on your list. You can write about the latest procedures you do; but, only in regard to how you can help.

You should also often write about things you do not sell but which help your patients. For example, most of the people who get BoNT and fillers have breasts too. So, let us say that you just read something about how to prevent breast cancer. Your email could be about that too because you care about the people on the list, and give them information about what may help them, even if you do not sell the new thing that may help. You do not just care about the widgets you're selling—mostly you care about the people on your list and your messages reflect that caring.

But the PS in the email you wrote about what you just read about breast cancer can say also say, "Hey, here's where to book your next BoNT appointment." So, the ad for your services lives in the "P.S."

And, when you only communicate in the way I am describing (educational and motivational), that email will get opened by about 30% to 40% of the people on your list, and around 10% will click on your links, and you'll get a very low unsubscribe rate. Your message will not get pulled over in the spam very often, and they may even share your email with their family and friends.

Rinse and Repeat

Then you go to another party or another event, and you bring the names from that event back and they go on your list. And every time you go somewhere, you spread by your email word of (your) mouth, who you are, what you know—your business grows steadily to any size you want.

We could talk for the next week about just how to write emails, and maybe I'll do a workshop on that as well one day. I did that once, but it's been several years. So maybe I'll redo that.

We talk about a lot of this in my hands-on workshops: VampireFacelift.com/members/workshops.

But I just told you everything you need to know to get started and what to do with the information you gather at a party.

The Main Point

You take the list (that you grow through the people you meet at parties) and then turn those on the list into raving fans who want everything that you do because you send to them information that makes their life better and that reminds them of your expertise

14. WHY YOU LOSE IF YOU ONLY DO WHAT YOU PROMISED, & HOW TO GROW YOUR PRACTICE LIKE AMWAY

Here is another little trick that is fun and profitable.

I'm calling them "tricks" because they are not complicated; this is not solving a calculus equation. This is just a simple idea that helps you and your patients.

Know Your Patient Better Every Time They Get BoNT

Care for People You Care for

If I meet a new patient who I do not enjoy, I refer them to my least favorite plastic surgeon. It is a very rare event, less than half a dozen in the two decades (I truly like most people), but when it happens, it is someone who feels like they don't want to pay me, or they want to pay me, but they are never happy with what I do for them (too picky). When either of those

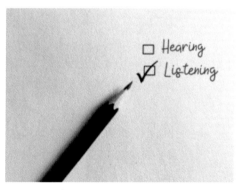

Figure 27. If you really care about your patients, you will listen carefully with every visit with the intent to know them better when they leave than you did when they arrived.

two situations happens, I tell them I'm not having fun. And I send them over to see this guy so they can be unhappy together.

Even if you only do this once every year or two, by permitting yourself *not* to have to take care of everyone who comes to see you, you gain a sense of freedom and joy within your business that makes every day more fun and inspiring. You truly care for everyone you care for.

When I worked in the emergency room, everyone deserved, and everyone received my full care and attention. But, by giving myself permission to choose who I see in my private practice, I am, every day, surrounded only by people whom I like and who like me. It's a beautiful way to spend your day. Unlike say, when you're in the ER, and you're glad to be there because you can be of service, but you must be of service to whoever walks through the door. It's your job. And you must care for them like they're your uncle or aunt or something. You must care for them with the utmost care. Even if it's someone who was just drunk and shot somebody and then ran over three more, you must take care of them, truly. And they are cursing you and puking on your leg while you are trying to take care of them. That is a normal day in the ER and in the inner city, ER, it is what you do, and you love it because you are of help to society and that person has a mama, too, and maybe they just had a bad day. You don't know, but whatever, that is not what you do when you do cosmetic work.

I do not do that anymore.

Always Want to Know More about the Person in Front of You
I must like you, and you must like me, or we do not play together. Because we like each other, it becomes very easy to want to learn, to know more about you.

The goal should be that *with every visit, you know more about your patients when they leave than you did when they arrived at your office.*

With time, we become attached in a friendly and professional way: we care for each other. And because of that, you want to pay me because you want to take care of me because I am taking care of you.

You Become Part of the Most Important Events in Another Person's Life

People often come for BoNT just before the important events in their life: marriages, travel, anniversaries, graduations, class reunions, and birthday celebrations. If you listen and truly care for your patients, you become a part of their most important life events and you start to care for each other emotionally and in tangible ways; you provide services, they gladly pay your fees.

Remember that *it is not really about the BoNT; it is the ceremony of getting the body-temple ready with a kind of anointing for whatever is next in their life.*

That can be beautiful.

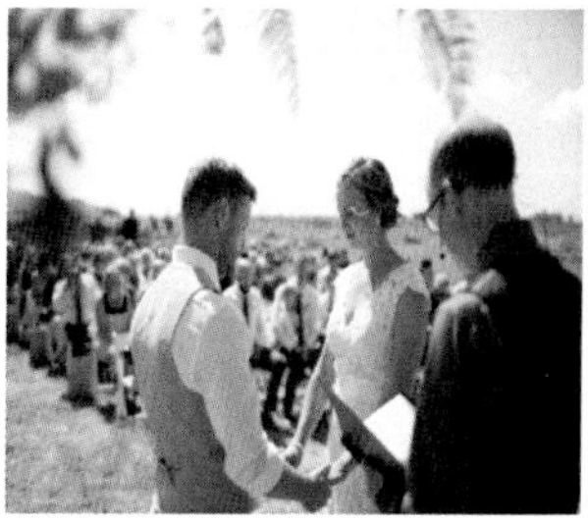

Figure 28. When you provide BoNT, you become a part of the most important ceremonies in the lives of your patients.

Do More Than What They Paid You to Do

As a kid, I was taught always do a little bit more than you are getting paid to do. This is how I was brought up: if I cut your grass, I would pick up the paper too. Or if you hired me to weed the flowers, I would go edge the garden or something, anything so I surprised you by doing more than you paid me to do.

Put another way, if you only do what someone pays you to do, in my opinion, you just *lost* because that is what they expected. So, you only fulfilled your duty. Is that the reputation you want?

You did BoNT for me. I paid you for your BoNT. You are kind to me; *whatever! You only did your duty*. But the moment you do one smidgen of anything more than what I paid you to do, you just put yourself above 99.9% of the people on the planet.

Most people do not even do, in an excellent way, what they are being paid to do—not in a world-class excellent way. And the world is too small to do anything less. But if you do your duty in an excellent way and then do something extra, you are a unicorn rarely seen among men.

If you do not think you can be as good as anybody at what you do, quit doing it. It may narrow what you do but be as good as anyone, or stop doing it, or *do whatever is needed to become as good as anyone who does what you do.*

But you still lose if you only do what you are paid to do; you only did your duty.

So, my goal and my little quick marketing tip is this: *every time, every day in the morning and at night, with every person you see, do a little something more than what they paid you to do after you do (in an excellent way) the thing they paid you to do.*

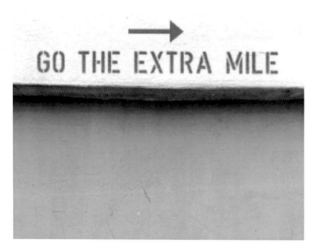

Figure 29. If you only do what people pay you to do, even if you do it in an excellent way, you lose.

It could be simple.

For example, if they got BoNT, well, maybe you give them a little extra unit somewhere you have not treated before to see if they like it, and you do not charge them for the extra.

Or you have a cream that you think they might like, and you give it to them as a sample and say, "Here, I think this may help you, let me know if you like it."

Or you have a book about something that may help them (preferably one that you wrote)—and you give it to them.

Turn Your Office into MLM

The thing you do that is more than what they paid you to do does not need to be huge. It could be a gift certificate (that costs you less than the value of the certificate).

You say, "Thanks for seeing me today; here's a $50 gift certificate to give to someone you love, so they can come to see me."

Gift Certificates Make Your Office Multi-Level Marketing
You can make your business cards into a "gift certificate."

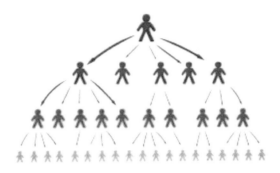

Figure 30. Giving your patients a way to give discount coupons to their friends for your services implements multilevel marketing into your practice.

Take a hand full of cards, eight or ten of them, and write "$50" on the back, and say this to your patient, "Give this to your friends, and anybody you give it to can get 50 bucks off whatever they want in my office. And I'll keep track of it and give you $50 off for every one of these cards that is redeemed."

Stop and Do
I just gave you two huge tips. Please, stop and make note and plane to do both and these two tips alone can grow your practice like crazy: One is to do more than what you are paid to do. The second is to run your office like multi-level marketing by empowering every patient you have with a way to talk about you by giving them money (a card worth $50 in your office) to give away to their friends.

Start Your Own Clubs

As an aside, I do not participate in Allergan's patient rewards club. Why would I want to do that?

If I do, then the patient can cash in their points at another doctor's office. Instead, I hand out the cards that turn my office into multilevel marketing, and I have my own BoNT Club (see Chapter 12).

Module II.

Mixing and Injecting
Techniques to Keep from Hurting or Bruising Your
Patients

15. OFFICE ENVIRONMENT AS A WAY TO LESS PAIN & MORE HEALING

This chapter further discusses how to make relaxing both your BoNT treatments and your whole office. Some of this may sound hokey to you. It may not fit the personality of your office. These are only suggestions or ideas I have found helpful over the past two decades of injecting faces. Take what makes sense to you and disregard the rest.

While teaching the procedures that I designed (Vampire Facelift®, O-Shot®, P-Shot®, Bocox™, and others), I have been blessed to be able to not only have my own office in which to try the following ideas but also to see a variety of practices in the offices of physicians in London, New Zealand, Greece, Spain, and other countries and states within the U.S. And what I have seen, particularly for cosmetic treatments, is the following:

To provide comfortable procedures,
you must provide a comfortable space.

A Cellphone on the Table Poisons Dinner—So, No Sign

If you are at dinner with your family, research shows that a cell phone on the table, even if it is not ringing, even if there's no sound coming from it, even if no one is staring at it or poking the buttons, if there is a cellphone on the table while you're

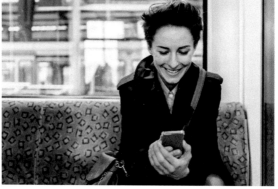

Figure 31. Even if no one is looking at the phone, a phone on the table changes the conversation by introducing the possibility of interruption (even if no interruption occurs).

having dinner, research shows the phone affects con-versation just because there is the *possibility* of interruption.

Even if there is no actual interruption, just the *possibility* of interruption changes the dynamics of human interaction.

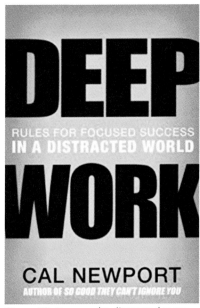

In his book, *Deep Work*, Cal Newport (Ivy League mathematician and computer programmer) teaches people how to avoid the interruptions that break focus. He makes the case that most good things come out of a place of deep focus, but we live in a time where it has become more difficult to focus.

He writes that if you are thinking deeply, doing mathematics, programming your computer, or writing, if you are working on anything that requires focus, then anything that might interrupt you (even if it does not interrupt you but only creates the possibility of interruption), lowers your ability to

Figure 32. You may be distracted more than you think. Read Deep Work to rediscover your best work.

focus. The interruption could be not only your phone but also someone knocking on the door—any possible interruption.

So how does his book relate to what we are talking about regarding BoNT and how to help people relax while you give them shots in the face?

To understand, consider another example.

If I'm alone with my wife and the bedroom door is open, even if there is no one else in the home, it feels less private; I am sure you have felt the same way with your lover. You are alone with your spouse; even if there is no one else in the house, you probably want the door closed, maybe even locked.

You feel safer and more intimate with the door closed and locked— because there is no possibility of anyone coming into the room, even when there is no one else in your home, the locked door feels more private.

Your patients want the same degree of privacy and security when they are doing something intimate—receiving cosmetic or medical treatments in your office.

Even at a BoNT party, I create the perception of distance from the crowd, and the BoNT takes place in a space of contemplation. I intentionally create this miniature temple of contemplation (*con-temple-ation*, contemplation) and conversation, which may be only someone's chair, where they cut hair, but I separate it from the rest of the conversation at the party. And I make that space feel as safe as possible.

You can also create privacy and security in your office. It is part of the reason that my office has no sign.

No sign.

Sometimes people ask me where my office is.

Not too long ago, I was walking on the sidewalk near my office, and a woman approached me and asked, "A lot of my friends and clients see you for BoNT, but I don't know where your office is."

We were only about a block from my office when she asked this question.

I answered, "It's a secret club," and kept walking.

Since she is not my patient, she did not have the right to know.

When my patients go to my office for anything, even just BoNT, maybe they do not want their friends to know or anyone going up and down the street to know that they are visiting me.

There are some businesses where you want loads of drive-by traffic and huge signs. For example, if you are selling hamburgers, you need a big sign, preferably one with golden arches, if you want to make lots of money. But if you're offering a weight loss service, or if you're doing cosmetic work, if you're doing sex-improving procedures, or even if you are doing general medicine, maybe you don't want to be on the street where there's lots of traffic (unless you're running an urgent care center).

Not having a sign makes it feel to your patients there as if an interruption is less likely, and the whole office feels more private and secure. The corollary is that a big sign makes people feel as if the door is metaphorically open and their private medical treatment is at risk of public display.

Deeper Inside the Office

By one study, a primary care physician in the US does not break even financially daily until after seeing patient number twenty-one. To see that many people (and more) quickly enough to make a profit, patients are usually stacked in the waiting room. But, when you come further into my office, there is a sitting area for only one or two people, but there is not a "waiting room"; because it is an all-cash practice, I do not need to see as many people as quickly in order to pay my bills.

My office is close to a bookstore. So, I sometimes ask people to wait next door at the bookstore until it is their time so that they can go straight into my office after my nurse texts to tell them it is their turn. They come straight into the office and into the exam room to be seen without having to worry about seeing anyone other than my nurse and me.

Some of the more well-known people, when they see me, that is how they do it.

So, the first step to privacy is to have no sign (or a very tiny sign on the door) and not a big sitting area where all your patients are sitting in a group and thinking, "Yeah, we are about to see the doctor," almost like sitting in the waiting room at the STD clinic, and everybody there knows your business. It's not quite that embarrassing, but most people (even in the age of selfies and social media) do not want everyone to know their business.

Be at Least as Careful as Starbucks Is About This

Read the book, *Pour Your Heart into It* (by Howard Schultz, the man who started Starbucks); then, go to Starbucks and sit. Whether you like their coffee or not, notice something: they literally have considered *everything*. All the senses, how their cappuccino machines sound when they foam the milk, and all the smells of coffee, the furniture, the temperature, and what is on the walls.

Everything.

For a while, they were selling their own music playlists; you do not hear just anything blaring on the radio in Starbucks. There are no magazines around unless someone bought one. They control the environment— everything you see, smell, taste, and hear. And *people like to sit there. People often buy coffee in Starbucks just so they can sit in Starbucks; the coffee is only a ticket to sit in the store!* You could say it is even a healing place to just sit there.

Would people say that about your office? Would they want to sit there just to feel comfort and peace?

Schultz came from a modest family living in government housing. He built his business by thinking about every part of it, and he is only serving coffee, not practicing medicine. At least, that is what you may first think. He is actually serving a safe and peaceful place to gather.

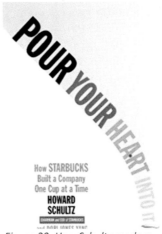

How STARBUCKS
Built a Company
One Cup at a Time
**HOWARD
SCHULTZ**

Now go to your doctor's office; this should be a sacred magic healing place. But you will likely see something stupid blaring on the TV; you will see magazines that sell alcohol and

Figure 33. How Schultz made a coffee shop into a healing place (and made huge profits). Every doctor should read this book.

148

cigarettes; and somebody's yelling for the next patient to come to the back. You may hear the phone ring, and there is a big flashing sign on the interstate telling everybody where you are.

I don't know. Maybe I am wrong. I'm not saying that such a doctor's office is always a bad thing. But that is definitely a different thing. That is different from how Starbucks thinks about selling you an iced mocha cappuccino, a Frappuccino with six shots, and a side of whatever artificial sweetener you add.

When you follow the progression of Starbucks, even though Schultz modeled it after the Italian espresso bars, the Europeans laughed at it in the beginning because there are so many milk products in there. They saw it more like a milk company (with coffee mixed in). It wasn't really an espresso bar. It was a milk bar with flavors of coffee; but whatever, he did not care what they thought, he showed that it worked. And, *it would have never worked had they only served coffee and not a healing experience.*

When you come to my office, why should my office not be as comforting? My office is a healing place. I want you to go there when your relationship is broken or when your genitals quit working.

Why Your Massage Therapist Makes More Dollars per Hour Than You

When you go to get a massage at the Marriott near my office, you pay $385 for a 110-minute massage ($175 for a 50-minute). A level 5 office visit (which is the highest complexity visit involving life-&-death decisions) earns a doctor, for 50 minutes, $183.19 (Medicare maximum reimbursement). Consider those numbers...

Hourly Wages: Massage Therapist vs Primary Care Physician
Massage Therapist—$385/110 minutes *($210/hour)—Training 8 months*

Primary Care Physician—$183.19/50 minutes *($219.83/hour)*—Training 4 years of college + 4 years of medical school + 3 years of residency => *Training 11 years*

But the massage therapist can work outside the hotel, charge even more, and her overhead is one small room or gas money to drive to your home (and no expensive malpractice insurance).

So, if you practice primary care, the massage therapist makes more per hour than you.

The Reason Your Massage Therapist Makes More
Your massage therapist went to an eight-month class. That's all it takes. But because she creates a healing environment, she is paid more per hour than the primary care doctor down the street is paid for planning the care of an 80-year-old woman taking ten medicines and with three organs failing.

And the massage therapist is paid at the time of service. The primary care physician must fill out forms and wait three months for a billing company (who takes 5% of the money) to beg for the doctor's money. And, if the paperwork is done improperly, then at best, the doctor does not get paid; if he makes too many mistakes, he goes to jail for insurance fraud.

So, why does the massage therapist do so well?

The massage therapist creates an atmosphere of healing.

What You Must Learn from Your Massage Therapist if You Want a Successful Cosmetic Practice
Imagine you're getting a massage, where you are in this massage zone, and you are getting your back rubbed, and you are listening to tinker-bell spa music, and then somebody darts in and blares out to the massage therapist, "You're needed on the phone, line 2."

Now imagine they open the door (where you are doing BoNT) and say, "Dr. Jones, you have drug rep, Mary Jo, selling Viagra out there in the waiting room. She wants to give us all a free pen, and she brought lunch and a big chocolate cake. Would you speak with her?"

Imagine that interruption happening if you're getting a massage.

Unthinkable.

But it happens every day at the doctor's office.

Please take note: *one way to make an 8-month class worth more than a grueling 9-year class is simply to pay attention to the environment.*

My Strict Office Rules that Help My Patients Find Peace and Perceive Value

Start with People
The people who work for you matter.

I want an employee in my room, when I see patients, that exudes from every pore *affection and kindness*. You can't teach it; you must find that person because you cannot teach it to them. For what I do, it doesn't even need to be a nurse because I do not need in my assistant the skill set of an RN.

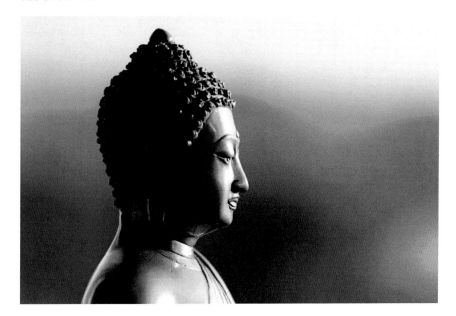

Figure 34. My office should be a place of peace and contemplation; it then becomes a more powerful place of healing.

When I worked in the ER, I needed a woman RN. An RN because I needed her skills to assist me; a woman so that I am never alone with a woman. It appears to me that most women physicians do not use an escort, but I will not be in a room alone with a woman; as a man, it is too risky.

If you are a man, listen closely: *you can never ever be alone with a woman in your office for even one second.*

So, I need a woman employee to help me, and I need a woman who is kind, that exudes estrogen and kindness, that just pours estrogen out of her body onto the floor and makes puddles of kindness, to help counteract my testosterone, to buffer that.

Until I come in the room, my assistant should be as kind to the patient as she would be if the patient were visiting her home, offering coffee and healthy snacks, and pleasant conversation. I like Zone bars because they are healthy. And water. We keep a water machine and Perrier or Pellegrino. So, we have sparkling water of some type, and flat water, coffee, and Zone bars. That's what we have.

The Change that Happens When I Enter the Room

So, my assistant is the kind hostess, the interested conversationalist while the patient waits for me. But things change once I enter the room.

Even with a cosmetic consult, during conversation, you might be on the verge of finding out something important about your patient because you still think about the medicine (even when doing cosmetic work); but your helper does not understand your thought process. So, they burst into your conversation and interrupt you—oftentimes, most often, not even conscious of what you are doing.

If you are good at it, you are taking a skillful history as you appear to be simply having a casual conversation; your unaware helper, who is not able to be quiet when you are in the room, will block your investigations with mindless chatter—time is wasted, and valuable information remains invisible to you.

So, at the very best, people who cannot be quiet (PW-CBQs) will waste your time; more often, they also keep you from discovering something important about your patient, something you needed to know. So, *my staff is trained to be their most tender, loving, conversational, and welcoming self until I enter the room; then, they do not speak unless they are spoken to.* If they are questioned by the patient or by me, they give the shortest possible answer that still feels cordial. Then, they practice complete silence.

When I am in the room, my staff never initiates a new thread of conversation.

PW-CBQs waste your time and interrupt your ability to find answers to questions that you do not even know to ask; pregnant silence can often bring the best information, but PW-CBQs cannot tolerate the silence so they will interrupt silence (silence that may have prompted your patient to reveal the valuable information you most need to know and they most want to tell you) with mindless chatter.

So maybe you just do BoNT, you never even think about medicine; that is still intimate. You still want to know about their life—*you do not BoNT faces, you treat people.*

So, *I want my helper to become invisible when I am in the room.*

If you add to the above problems with PW-CBQs that once you start the treatment, if your patient is talking (because they are chatting with the PW-CBQ), you must stop what you are doing because your patient's face is moving while you are trying to inject; now your PW-CBQ staff is really *wasting your time.*

PW-CBQs Waste Your Time (Two Ways) and Kill the Peace

So, PW-CBQs prevent you from taking a complete history. They give you a moving target, so you can't do your treatment (wasting your time). And they waste time another way by taking the conversation in the wrong direction or in a place that is frivolous for the present purposes, and you cannot finish your work until the PW-CBQ and the patient reach a pause in their chatter.

And the chatter breaks the spell of peace that you are working to create, that is like the peace you find while getting a massage.

So, the person who helps you matters; they should be genetically kind; if you are a male, they should be female; and they should be taught, in my opinion, when to be quiet (anytime you are in the room). And if they cannot be quiet (a PW-CBQ), then you should find them another job in your office or fire them.

You Do Not Need to Follow My Rules

Maybe you don't like to talk, you are not interested in taking a medical history, you just want to do the BoNT, and you want your helper to do all the talking, You don't have to follow all my rules, but these rules help create an environment where my people (I don't mean occasionally; almost every time I see a new patient) are shocked that they get sleepy while getting shots in their face.

No PW-CBQs work in my office. At least not for very long.

Throw Away the Magazines & Display This Instead

So, the person who helps you is part of the environment. I think the most important part. But you also should consider your physical space. As I mentioned, I don't have magazines. I don't have anything in my office that a person could pick up that I did not intentionally put there for their benefit; when they sit in my little waiting area, there is nothing there to read unless I wrote it, or I screened it. Most of it I wrote.

Until you write a few books or have your own brochures, have the brochures about the stuff you do, or if you have a book there for them to thumb through, let it be a book that you have found helpful in regards to health or beauty, not the random subjects of whatever the most recent Cosmo magazine article or ad features (which may be in direct conflict with your treatments and philosophies).

When people bring to me a big stack of magazines and want to donate them to me, I donate them right out the back door to the recycle bin.

Immediately.

Junk Comes in the Front Door and Goes Out the Back Door

When people bring to me, as a gift, junk food (which I define as anything with added sugar), then it can be eaten that day if it's a special occasion (a birthday for example) and it goes home with one of my staff.

When sales reps try to bring me junk food (I don't have to be as forgiving to salespeople as I do to my patients), I tell them to bring me something healthy or don't bring anything. And when my staff wants to have a little party, it can be for that day, they can have cake if it's somebody's birthday or something, then it goes home, or they'll work at keeping each other fat. Because one brings a sugar-filled prize today and tomorrow, she brings her mama's cheesecake recipe, and the next day, somebody brings to you brownies leftover from their child's birthday party.

They take turns keeping each other sluggish and overweight!

So, I recommend that your office become a "safe zone" where *no one is allowed to bring any foods with added sugar.*

That's it. Very simple.

Just that one rule, *"No added sugar foods at work, or you can be fired on the spot,"* will create a healthier and happier environment.

Each person on my staff signs a piece of paper to that effect when they come to work for me.

Until COVID, when they were all working at the office, every staff member who worked for me for the past 2 decades got healthier and skinnier as a side effect of working for me. But with COVID, for the first time in over twenty years, my employees went home and gained weight. Just having a safe zone at work makes everyone healthier.

In my office, they can have fries, hamburgers, whatever. Just that one rule, *no added sugar foods.* They can drink a diet drink; if they want to drink a little poison, that's fine. I do not worry about poison too much. No reason to be paranoid.

155

But the most poisonous poison for most Americans is sugar. So just that one food rule, "No sugar in the office, or you get fired," and you'll have healthier and happier staff.

And they know that rule up front when you hire them. So, if it bothers them, they just work somewhere else. And the smart ones will appreciate a zone where there is no temptation to eat junk. The not smart ones will cave and work somewhere else.

Try this rule if you dare.

But, of course, it means you must follow the same rule.

If You Turn Red, You Cannot Work Where We Talk Sex

All my staff is screened about sex talk. They must be comfortable talking about sex.

And they all sign a piece of paper that says, "We are going to talk about sex in this office, because fixing sex is what we do. And if that bothers you, then don't work here. When we talk about sex, we are not going to call that sexual harassment."

If you do not do sexual procedures (like our O-Shot® or P-Shot® procedures), you may not need this rule regarding sex talk. But if you treat sexual dysfunction, then you need a similar agreement to be signed. Also, as an extra bonus, people comfortable talking about sex usually are comfortable with their own sexuality and are often creative and relaxed and easygoing—all desirable traits in an employee.

Import the Orient (They Thought About This for 4,000 Years)

Video screens are good if used properly. Have one or two, maybe three different little, short one or two-minute videos that are educational, and then one or two videos about something you do.

And maybe intersperse those videos with some spa-type music and with videos of fish swimming, birds flying, and other nature images that relax people.

I don't know if this is true or not, but somewhere I read that, in the East, it is thought to promote prosperity if you have a big stone near the door and wind chimes, and water. So, I have those things by my door. I have a wind chime near the door. I have a stone statue of a woman praying, and I an aquarium. Then, I recently swapped out the aquarium for just a little waterfall; so I don't have to feed fish. I leave town too much, so I'm not here to feed the fish.

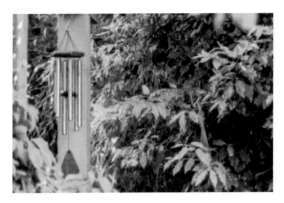

Figure 35. Wind chimes by the door bring peace and prosperity.

I like plants too, but dead plants are not allowed to stay in my office.

For a while, I had a honey beehive move into the wall next to my office door. I think that was a good omen. I did not bother them; they did not bother me. They stayed a little while, and then they moved on. That also was a sign of prosperity. So, I kept it.

All these things come together to create an environment of magic and of healing. You may not think of yourself as a magician, but *if you are a healer, you are a magician*, it seems to me.

As a general internist, before I started offering cosmetic procedures, I had the same philosophy regarding my office environment.

A few times, I had people actually cry in the waiting room and tell me, "This just feels like a healing place."

They cried when they came to see me for the first time because that space had been infused with goodness. Simple things. I don't mean some holy lightning bolt came down; I simply created *an environment absent of poison and full of as much good and magic as I could find.*

At least pay as much attention to your office environment as they do to the environment at Starbucks.

How to Measure You (Because You are Also Part of Your Office Environment)

You are also part of the office environment that your patient visits. Maybe the most important part. So, it's worth giving serious consideration to how you as a person appear.

Here is the short answer...

You will appear as you are.

Here is the all-encompassing rule from which all corollary healing rules can be derived:

You should be the person your patient aspires to be.

You should look healthy, look younger than you are, and natural; and you should truly be happy, sexual, and smart. If there is something on that list that you are not, then it is less likely that people will seek you to help them find the trait that is missing from your list.

You deserve care too!

Music Magic: Never Underestimate It nor Neglect It

I like George Winston's *December* album. If you haven't heard it, listen to it, preferably in the dark with someone you love next to you, in bed.

I think it is the most magical album ever produced. I play it every time I do injections, every time in my office, for over a decade.

Every time.

It puts me in a relaxed state. And if I'm in a relaxed state, the patient feels it.

Never would I let a patient pick out music while I'm injecting their face. What they pick may make them feel better, but it may not make me feel peaceful and happy. They should want me to feel good because if I'm relaxed, they will feel relaxed.

So, I always pick the music.

When I used to do a lot of liposuction, I usually played Prince's *Purple Rain* album because, to me, liposuction was largely mindless work; you must to be aware of what you are doing, but compared to contemplating the face and the shapes and the mouth and injecting fillers where a millimeter off can make someone look stupid, liposuction was more like the hard work of mopping a floor (mostly mindless); it felt that way to me.

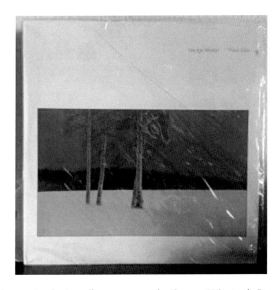

Figure 36. The most relaxing album ever made: George Winston's December Album

So, I played Prince's *Purple Rain* because it energized me, and it was fun. And liposuction then felt more like happy dancing, but BoNT and fillers to me, are more like meditation, and George Winston puts me in that contemplative space.

That album, *December*, may not be the one that does it for you, but at least consider playing the music that both you and the patient listen to for a meditative effect.

Extra Tips for Healing: The Sheets, the Clock, the Thermostat

I also have a clock on the wall that I can see; there's a red second hand

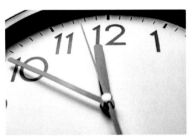

on it. And when we start discussing doing BoNT injections, you will see that the red second hand helps. I use it every day with almost every injection.

That red second hand is a big part of what helps me avoid bruising people. It is the combination of the second hand with George Winston that helps.

Figure 37. I need a red second hand to prevent bruising.

So, there's a clue, but we will discuss this more when we talk about injections.

Temperature

I keep the temperature at 72 degrees Fahrenheit and have the thermostat locked so that my staff is not tempted to change the

temperature based on how they feel that day and on what they wore to work.

Linens, Not Paper

I put linens on the bed, not paper.

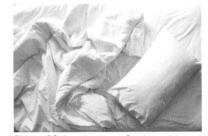

In many of my procedures, the patient will spend anywhere from two grand to six grand, not that much for a plastics guy, but for an

Figure 38. I use cotton sheets, not paper, for covering the treatment bed and the patient.

internist and an injection practice, that is much.

The patient deserves a reward.

The main thing is that if you are dropping cash money that is measured in hundreds or thousands of dollars, you deserve a cotton sheet to cover your body instead of a paper napkin. So, I buy cheap cotton sheets at Walmart, and we run a load once a day or so and use lots of Clorox®.

When I'm doing an O-Shot®, I might even use three or four sheets draped around, under, and over the woman. I want her to feel like an Egyptian princess, someone royal (because *she is* when in my office); and every part of her is warm and covered (except her face); and she feels safe. Compare that state with being covered with a little paper napkin that scratches and tears and feels cold and insecure.

You write on paper; you don't wear it or use it for a sheet—especially if you spend thousands of dollars in my office.

The Walls

Your walls should include the following: (1) diplomas and awards that prove you are smart and educated, (2) medical diagrams and anatomy charts that are instructional and beautiful and celebrate the body-temple, and (3) photos of your family.

The opposite of this would be nothing but your diplomas—too dry and boring.

Or nothing but photos of your family—too much like visiting your grandmother.

Or nothing but the anatomy diagrams—people wonder about your credentials and your office feels too much like your sixth-grade science class.

Or, worse, nothing but plain walls— "Am I in a doctor's office or the psych ward?"

But, if you sprinkle all three on the walls of your office, some of each in in every room, you win.

Beautiful Banners

Also, having roll up, free standing banners that bring attention to the procedures and products (that you offer in your office) can be beautiful and helpful in both education and marketing.

Synergy of Environmental Ingredients

I hope this chapter helped you. I promise you that if you implement all the ideas discussed, your patients will feel it. There develops, when you do all of it, a very powerful synergy that creates a healing and a peaceful environment.

A magic place.

Ignoring just one of the ingredients discussed in this chapter (for example, the wrong music or a helper who bombards you with mindless chatter) will kill the effects of all the rest.

Easy Assignment

Go to Starbucks. Take notes about the environment. Then go to your office and decide if your office deserves and gets the same attention.

Next, go for a $300 massage at a luxury hotel. Is your office as relaxing?

What will you do to bring peace and magic to your office?

Now, it is finally time to learn about the actual BoNT injections. But never underestimate all the rest and focus only on where you stick the needle.

You can be the best injector;
the wrong environment will still kill your business.

---

16. INTRODUCTION TO MIXING BONT

Before discussing where to inject, where to insert the needle, it is imperative to consider how to mix the BoNT in a way that makes it easier for you to do injections that are accurate and painless.

Mixed the wrong way, your BoNT will hurt and cause crazy faces even if you insert your needle in exactly the right place.

Diluent Matters

When you open the BoNT box and pull out the vial, you will see something that looks like a little smudge on the bottom of the bottle. That is 100 units of BoNT. But you cannot inject a smudge, so you must add a diluent. If you add bacteriostatic saline, it hurts less than non-bacteriostatic saline.

So that's what you always use: Bacteriostatic saline (even though the package insert will tell you otherwise).

Next, consider how much to add.

Rifle vs. Shotgun

One of the tricks of doing good BoNT is knowing how to inject the lower face. If it's done inaccurately, you can make someone look like they had a stroke. It's okay. They can still talk and swallow and eat and breathe. Nobody dies, but they look like they had a stroke for a couple of months. So not a good thing. To avoid that, how you mix the BoNT helps tremendously.

First, if you understand guns (which you do if you grow up in Alabama, where I was born), you know that a rifle only shoots one little bullet that is only about ½ inch to one inch long for most sporting guns (not military). But a shotgun has multiple pellets, so if you are even 30 yards away, the pellets might spread into a pattern 3 feet in diameter. If you mix your BoNT in a high volume, and you have one unit in your syringe, you are shooting a shotgun; it can spread and inadvertently hit muscles you did not intend to hit. But if you reconstitute the BoNT in a small volume (the same amount of BoNT but in a smaller volume), you can put your needle exactly where you want, and the volume will be small enough that the BoNT will stay there (without spreading to muscles you do not want to relax).

How to Mix BoNT

Cosmetic BoNT comes in a one-hundred-unit vial.[4]

If you add 1 cc of Bacteriostatic saline, that gives 1 unit of BoNT per 0.01 cc of liquid.

An insulin syringe is marked such that one unit of insulin is in 0.01 cc of liquid. So, mixed in this way, 1 unit of on an insulin syringe would also be 1 unit of BoNT.

Use the 30-unit insulin syringes (BD brand, 31 gauge).

A 50-unit syringe makes it more difficult to draw up only 1 or 2 units of BoNT accurately—so do not use a syringe larger than a 30-unit insulin syringe (0.3 cc).

Now you have a magic-wand, rifle-of-beauty, not a crazy-face-making shotgun.

---

[4] For Dysport, use the same dilutions and inject the same amounts, but the number of units will be three times as much and it will be exactly the same in effectiveness.

17. MIXING BONT FOR MORE ACCURACY & LESS PAIN

Let's think more about mixing BoNT in such a way that you do not hurt people.

When you first take the BoNT bottle out of its box, it looks like there is nothing in it, only a smudge at the bottom of the bottle; that smudge is BoNT.

Use a 1 cc syringe with an 18-gauge needle to pull up 1 ml of bacteriostatic saline (more accurate than measuring the 1 ml with a 10-cc syringe). Pull up about 0.02-0.05 extra because some volume will be lost in the transfer.

Then stick the 18-gauge needle into the rubber stopper of the BoNT vial. Because the BoNT is vacuum-packed, most of the liquid should be pulled into the vial. If the vacuum is lost on the vial, and the liquid is not pulled into the vial, then something is wrong, and you should discard the vial and contact Allergan. You may need to push the plunger to empty the last few drops out of the syringe.

The Math of Dilution—Use a Small Volume

When you look at an insulin syringe, on one side, you will see a scale of "units." On the other side, you will see a scale of "milliliters." With an insulin syringe, you will see that 30 units of insulin is equal to 0.3 milliliters of liquid; so, *one unit in an insulin syringe is equal to 0.01 milliliters of liquid.*

Summary

If you have 100 units of cosmetic BoNT in a vial and you add one milliliter of bacteriostatic saline, that makes a dilution where there is one unit of BoNT in 0.01 milliliters of bacteriostatic saline.

So, adding 1 milliliter of bacteriostatic saline makes it easy—*1 unit on an insulin syringe is equal to 1 unit of BoNT.*

The package-insert instructions that come with Botox recommend adding over 2 ml of non-bacteriostatic saline to the Botox. But, if you add that much, it makes you less accurate since the BoNT is more likely to inadvertently affect muscles that you did not intend to inject (especially in the lower face).

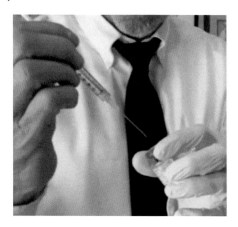

Figure 39. Adding 1 cc of bacteriostatic saline to 100 units of BoNT using a one cc syringe.

After you add the fluid, you can't really see the liquid well unless you look through the gap in the label. There is not very much in there.

Part of the way you make BoNT injections not hurt is by mixing the smaller volume. The other way you make it not hurt is by using tiny 31-gauge needles. The 31-gauge needles hurt significantly less than even a 30-gauge needle. Do not use 30-gauge needles. I think the 31-gauge *BD brand* hurts the least of all.

The Needle Touches Nothing Until It Touches the Patient

The other way to make BoNT hurt less is to make sure that the needle touches nothing until it touches your patient's face.

After you mix the BoNT, take the cap off using a bottle opener. Then remove the rubber stopper.

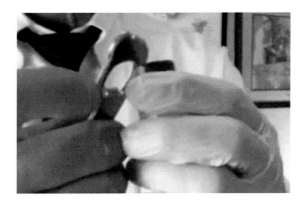

Figure 40. Beer-bottle opener removes the metal cap so that you can remove the rubber stopper to avoid dulling the needle when you extract the BoNT.

Now, you can extract the BoNT without touching the needle to anything other than the liquid.

Use the Needle No More than Three or Four Times

As an experiment, take one of your insulin syringes with the 31-gauge needle, then stick yourself on the back of your forearm using the same needle four times in a row.

By the time you get to the fourth time of poking your arm, you'll say, "Oh wow!"

The fourth injection, using the same needle, hurts noticeably more than the first.

So, to lessen the pain for your patients, use a separate syringe for each muscle group: one for each corrugator, one for the procerus, one for each side when you treat crow's feet, etc.

Never use a needle more than three or four times. That's another way you keep from hurting your patients.

Summary

In summary, by using (1) a small volume for dilution, (2) using *bacteriostatic* saline as the diluent, (3) not touching anything with the needle until it touches the patient, and (4) using a tiny 31-gauge needle to inject, you greatly decrease the pain your patient experiences with your treatments.

Next, let's talk more about how to extract the material from the bottle. If done improperly, your injections will be more painful and less accurate. So, please do not underestimate the importance of the next chapter.

18. EXTRACTING THE LAST DROP WITHOUT DULLING THE NEEDLE

Remember my recommendation that (when you pull BoNT out of the bottle) you never touch the needle to the glass, or else you will dull the needle and hurt your patient. But not touching the bottle with the needle presents a problem when you have only a small amount of liquid left in the bottle: to extract the fluid, you must very carefully pull the liquid from very close to the bottom of the bottle.

A small volume of BoNT is nearly impossible to remove without dulling the needle; so how do you extract those last few drops?

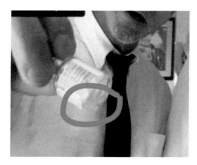

Figure 41. The last drops of BoNT in the vial are impossible to extract without dulling your needle.

The answer is that when you have only a few drops left in a vial, stop, leave those last few drops where they are, and mix another a fresh new vial.

Now, take the bottle that doesn't have much in it, take a needle that you intend to discard, and pull up all that is remaining. Pull out every last drop. Scrape away with the needle (you don't care if you dull this needle because you are going to discard it).

After you have every drop of the old vial in the syringe, then discard the now empty bottle, take the new bottle that you just mixed, and add the remnant from the last BoNT bottle.

Now you are ready to go. And your new bottle has 100 units plus what was transferred from the last one.

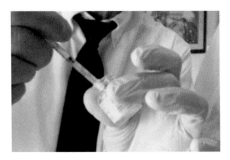

Figure 42. Adding the remnant from the almost-empty bottle to the newly mixed 100-unit bottle.

Now, throw away the syringe you used to scrape the bottom of the last bottle to withdraw those last drops.

RESULT: *It becomes easy to draw BoNT out of the new bottle without dulling the needle, and you did not waste the last drops in the almost empty bottle.*

I go through this process every time I open a new bottle: I scrape the last remnants of the last bottle and add to the newly mixed bottle.

Why go to so much trouble to transfer that remnant?

It wastes my time to try to extract the last remnant of BoNT without dulling the needle when the bottle is close to empty. So, once I get near the bottom (around 10 to 20 units remaining), I'll go ahead and mix a new bottle and transfer the remnant.

19. THE "ONE THING" YOU MAY BE DOING THAT *DOUBLES* THE PAIN

When You Hold the Syringe, Think Smoking

Most of the nerve pain fibers are on the surface of the dermis. After teaching a few thousand doctors for the past 12 years, I have seen that the most common way that people unnecessarily torment their patients with pain when injecting BoNT is by taking too long to pass the needle through the dermis, where most of the pain fibers reside.

Passing quickly through the skin with the needle hurts much less than passing slowly.

If you are going to move quickly, what can you do to keep from surprising the person?

First, hold the needle like a cigarette. That gives you the best control. Now you are ready to inject.

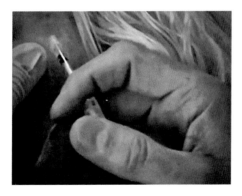

Figure 43. For best control, hold the syringe between the pointer and middle fingers, with the thumb near the plunger and the fifth finger lightly touching the skin of the patient.

Next, if you quickly insert the needle, with no warning, the patient will jump with surprise and perceive the injection as hurting more, even if the pain is minimal.

Also, if you alert the patient by saying something like, "Are you ready?" or with a countdown, "1, 2, 3" –then saying such things adds to the patient's anxiety and takes too much time.

So, instead, with each injection, lightly touch the skin with the needle (for less than a second) at the place where you are about to inject. This light touch does not hurt, but it notifies.

Then, after you touch the skin lightly, go in very quickly with the needle; then inject.

After injecting, quickly pull out the needle. The pull-out is a separate, distinct step, or you risk injecting BoNT on the way out and giving the patient a hose-down with the BoNT (outside the skin onto the surface). That's a very expensive way to bathe the face.

There is no reason to go slowly as you pull out the needle. There is nothing to be careful about when removing the needle.

For the least amount of pain, the rhythm goes as follows:

1. Touch the needle to the skin with very light pressure, letting them know you're going in.

2. Quickly push the needle into the skin, stopping at the hub, unless it is one of the areas (like the crow's feet) where you only advance the needle until the lumen is subcutaneous.

3. Inject, pushing the plunger to empty the syringe or to the intended marking for a partial emptying of the syringe.

4. Quickly pull out the needle.

The whole 4-step process takes 1 to 2 seconds per injection.

It takes a little practice; there is a little knack and a rhythm to it. But it is not complicated surgery.

It's a shot! That's all.

There is no reason to overthink it. It's just a shot. But you make a shot worth many thousands of dollars (over the years that a loyal BoNT patient will visit you) by making the shot not hurt or bruise and by knowing where to put the needle.

BoNT is a procedure concierge,
requiring both elegance and flare.

---

20. A MARKETING METHOD WITH SOUL

Same-Day Appointments or Lose the Patient

Offer same-day BoNT appointments, or you will lose people.

If your patient has an important event coming soon, BoNT *is an emergency.*

The BoNT Emergency
It usually goes something like this: Mary wakes up and she's getting ready for work.

Then she thinks, "Oh, Wow! My daughter's wedding is in 2 weeks. If I do not get my BoNT today, it will not have time for it to start working, and I'm not

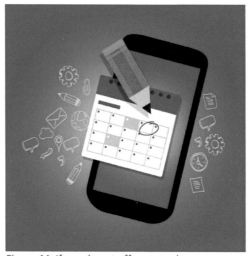

Figure 44. If you do not offer same-day appointments for your BoNT patients, you will lose many patients.

going to look good in the pictures! I need an appointment today!"

You Always Have Time for One More BoNT Patient
After a little practice, a BoNT visit with someone who is already a patient can be done easily in five or ten minutes (really); so, you can always work a BoNT visit into your schedule. This assumes you can see someone and keep conversation to near zero. Normally a BoNT visit involves more conversation and discovery than what can be done in five minutes, but if you work someone into your schedule at the last minute, they understand you are too busy for a normal visit and will be happy just to get the BoNT, even if they only get a few minutes with you.

Snacks Get You Out of Jail

Research shows that if you are in prison, and your case comes up for review by the parole board, you are more likely to get out of jail on parole if they review your case immediately after lunch than if they review your case when hungry just before lunch.

People are happier when not hungry and when not in caffeine withdrawal. So, offer your patients fresh coffee, water, snacks, and whatever else matches your philosophy; if that is beignets and cake, LSD, mushrooms, and a shot of Jack Daniels, then I guess that is good for your office. But, if you are a primary care physician and think and teach your patients about overall health, especially if you are running a weight-loss clinic in your office, then *offer your BoNT patients only healthy drinks and snacks*, whatever you recommend as part of your eating plans—maybe Zone bars and fresh fruit, and the meal replacements you recommend.

Consider having a nice *cappuccino machine in your office* and offer a scaled-down version of Starbucks. Caffeine makes people happy if that is their drug of choice. The cappuccino machine goes far in creating the VIP feel to your office.

A Question That Gauges Patient Treatment

When your patient arrives at your office, she should feel like she is arriving for a concierge service, as if she were a VIP at the Bellagio in Las Vegas or the Hotel Pierre in New York.

Another way to gauge how your patients are treated at your office is to ask yourself, "If this person came to my home, what would I do?"

You would not ask a guest in your home, on their arrival, to sit in a separate room for thirty minutes until you have time to see them.

After visiting with your friend in your home, you wouldn't tell them goodbye and let them find their way out to the door. Instead, you would walk them to the door, maybe even to their car, and tell them how you enjoyed seeing them.

So, I do not finish a BoNT treatment and then just say, "Goodbye." Instead, I walk them to the door of the exam room and often to the door of my office and express my gratitude for their visit.

A BoNT Patient Who Died

When you provide cosmetic treatments, you are not poking faces with a needle; you are helping people with their relationships and their self-esteem; you are helping them take care of their Body Temple. The procedure of injecting BoNT will eventually come to you organically, almost without thought. Use your remaining brain power to *practice taking a genuine interest* in your patients and exploring who they are (not just in where to inject the BoNT).

Say, to yourself, as someone leaves, "Do I know more about this person now than I did when they arrived?"

Then make a short note about what you learned about their life (as well as how you injected their BoNT) in their chart; then, when they see you for their next appointment, you remember, "Oh, they were going on vacation the last time I saw them, I wonder how that went."

So you ask them about their vacation.

Are they getting along with their spouse? How old is their grandbaby now? If you are truly interested in your patient, curiosity about such things comes naturally to you, but it still helps to remind yourself to take interest in your patients and to make notes about their life, not just about their faces.

Knowing my patients is a major part of what makes cosmetic medicine fun for me.

But, sometimes, like all branches of medicine, even cosmetic medicine can bring sorrow. For example, a young woman came to see me at a BoNT party and received treatment.

Then, *she kept coming to see me for BoNT every three months—for over a decade!*

During that decade, she evolved into a tender, caring, most delightful, and loving elementary school teacher (and aged to be in her late thirties). Over more than ten years, she brought to me (for BoNT) her sister and her mother. And for more than a decade, we talked every year about the children in her classes. She taught the third grade.

Then, she got breast cancer and recovered.

I treated her hair with PRP, for free, to help her regrow it after her chemotherapy. She had spent money on BoNT for over ten years. So, I helped her grow her hair back faster after she finished chemo, not to get a morality badge, simply because I wanted to do something, any little thing, to help.

She loved her new hair, which grew back thick and shiny over the next year.

Then, a few months after a visit where she showed me her new hair, while at my office to get BoNT, she told me that she was going to see a doctor the next day for something odd that she could feel in her abdomen.

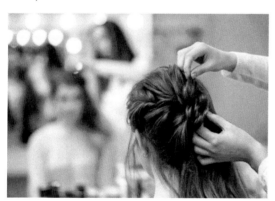

Figure 45. Caring for the body temple involves not only medicine but also magic.

She was worried.

I BoNT-ed her and asked her to let me know what the doctor said.

She texted me a couple of days later, "They think it may be cancer, again."

Less than a month later, not yet forty years old, she was gone—colon cancer.

I grieved.

More than I expected.

All she ever got from me was BoNT, and I treated her hair.

That was it.

But *we had a decade of conversations.*

I did not treat her cancer. I was *not* an important part of her medical treatment, ever, if you consider my role from the internal-medicine textbook viewpoint. But I was *important to her* because I cared about her and did her BoNT and helped her grow her hair so she felt pretty.

She grew her hair back thick.

Then she died.

And I miss her.

That is a long way of saying it, but the point of that story is the following:

The best way to market is to care for the people you care for.

If you are new to cosmetic work, you will be surprised by the fun of taking care of people who are happy almost every time they visit. Unlike, for example, in the emergency room, where you do valuable services, but your patients are usually afraid and angry at you (but not really at you because they are afraid).

But, with cosmetic work, your patients smile.

Summary of a Marketing Method with Soul

Your patient is a guest.
Care.
Know them better,
Repeat.

---

21. NEEDLE SECRETS
TO AVOID PAIN & BRUISING

More about How to Extract BoNT from the Vial

Over the years, those receiving BoNT from you will pay you thousands of dollars.

You should not hurt them.

Receiving BoNT should be like a treatment at a concierge spa—a relaxing interlude, not a trip to a torture chamber.

Part of the way you make BoNT relaxing is to make it pain-free. Dull needles hurt much more than sharp ones. So, I will describe a few more tips about getting BoNT out of the vial in a way that is both accurate and keeps the needle sharp.

Make it Smooth.
When I pick up a new syringe, before I fill it, I move the plunger up and down 3 or 4 times so that the movement will not be sticky or jerky when I do the injection. A sticky plunger will cause me to inject less accurately.

The Cap
If I am prefilling syringes for a BoNT party, then I save the cap to the syringe and recap the syringe after I fill it. So, when I attend the party, I may have twenty syringes prefilled with five units each, all in a plastic cup labeled with the number "5," and maybe sixty syringes prefilled with eight units, recapped and in a cup labeled "8." (See Module I for more about preparing for a party.)

But if I am in my office filling syringes at the bedside, I do not recap the syringe. I discard the cap and put the syringe onto the holding board.

Bubbles Make You Inaccurate

Note: The following will be much clearer if you read with a syringe and vial in your hands.

I use the following seven steps to quickly fill a syringe with exactly the amount of BoNT that I want and to keep bubbles out of the syringe since bubbles cause an inaccurate injection. You can watch a video of the process at BoNTClass.com, but the following tells you all you need to know:

1. After picking up the syringe, I move the plunger back and forth a few times to make it less sticky.
2. I pick up the vial with my left hand (my non-dominant hand) and hold the vial with my middle finger and thumb and the barrel of the needle with my index finger and thumb. This grip turns the vial and the syringe into one unit.
3. The label of the vial blocks my view of the top level of the fluid, so I look through the gap in the label to see where to direct the needle into the fluid without touching the vial with the needle.

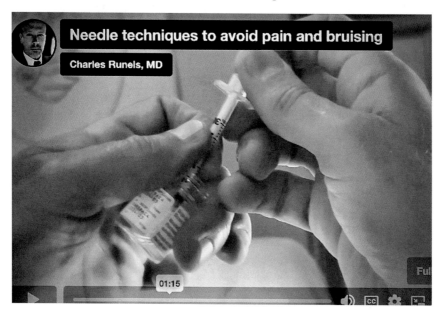

Figure 46. The way I hold the syringe & the vial for a quick & accurate extraction of the BoNT from the vial. (A screenshot from a video on BoNTClass.com)

4. I pull the plunger up (with my right hand) just enough to pull fluid into the syringe, then I push the plunger back down, completely emptying the syringe and squirting the BoNT back into the vial

(with the needle lumen still submerged). *This removes the bubble from the syringe.*

5. With the needle still submerged, I pull the plunger back up until I have a few more units in the syringe than what I have planned for this syringe.

6. I pull the needle lumen out of the fluid and (with the needle still inside the vial but now hovering over the fluid) slowly push the plunger back down until I have exactly the amount of BoNT that I want to inject.

7. I pull the needle out of the vial and place it in the proper place on my BoNT board or in a pile of syringes (that will be recapped and put into a plastic cup to take to a BoNT party) on a clean gauze

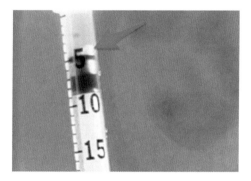

Figure 47. Close view of the approximately 0.01 ml bubble (in a 30-unit insulin syringe) that happens every time you draw up BoNT. You remove the bubble by pushing the fluid back out of the syringe with the needle submerged; then drawing the fluid back in.

For example, if I'm going to do a seven-unit injection: first, I get rid of the bubble, then I pull up the plunger to fill the syringe past where I want to go (to around 10 or more), and then I push it back down until I have exactly the amount intended—seven units.

Then I pull the syringe out of the vial.

A Tiny Injection Demands a Small Syringe & No Bubble

Some BoNT injections are only one or two units; if I'm doing a two-unit injection, a one-unit bubble included in the measurement would cause an error equal to half the intended dose—not acceptable.

181

As a reminder, always use a 30-unit (BD Brand insulin syringe with a 31-gauge needle) because you cannot accurately measure one unit or two units with a 50-unit syringe. You will do many treatments with only one, two, or three units.

Important: *If at any time, I even lightly touch the needle to the wall of the bottle, then I push all the liquid back out into the vial, and I discard that dulled needle/syringe. Even lightly touching the needle to the glass dulls the needle enough to make your BoNT treatment hurt. The 30-unit syringes cost about 3 cents apiece; it is worth 3 cents to avoid hurting people. After practice, you will seldom touch the needle to the wall of the bottle.*

In the beginning, you may waste many syringes while you learn. But, even if you threw away ten syringes per treatment because you kept bumping the glass with the needle, it is worth 30 cents (10 x 0.03) to keep from hurting your patient.

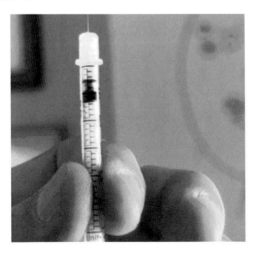

Figure 48. Demonstration of the tiny volume of 2 units of BoNT using the dilution of 1 cc per 100 units of BoNT. This dilution allows for increased accuracy (needed when injecting the lower face).

Lighthouse

To improve accuracy, pull up the liquid, and then with the needle still submerged, push the plunger all the way back down—that removes the bubble. Then pull the plunger back up, and the syringe contains liquid without a bubble.

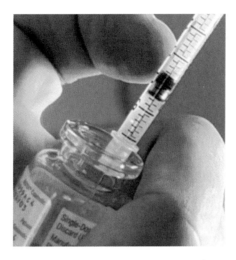

Figure 49. Slightly more than 7 units of BoNT in a 30-unit insulin syringe (using a 1-cc-to-100-units dilution)

Watch how to extract the BoNT quickly and easily on the videos at BoNTClass.com

22. THE "HOLDING BOARD" FOR SAVING TIME & AVOIDING PAIN

In the last chapter, you learned how to pull BoNT out of the vial in a way that does not dull the needle and that provides an accurate amount. With a busy BoNT practice, you fill thousands of syringes, so having a way of filling the syringe accurately and quickly is necessary.

In the next module, you will learn injection points for twelve muscle groups that allow you to achieve gorgeous results. By discarding a syringe after treating each muscle group, the needle is only used one to three times—meaning the syringe is discarded after the needle is dull. If you pull up all the BoNT into one big 50 or 100-unit syringe and use the same needle to treat the whole face, the pain is much increased, and you will lose patients.

So, for each person that you treat, you will usually use six to sixteen syringes. For that many prefilled syringes, you need a way to keep the syringes clean and orderly. That solution is the BoNT Holding Board.

Making & Loading the "Holding Board"

The holding board is made by Gorilla gluing the rubber tops of ten BoNT vials to a fiberglass cutting board (like you would use in the kitchen). These tops then serve as holders for the syringes to both keep the syringes in order, and to allow you to move around your office with the syringes on a tray that keeps them from rolling off.

When you place a syringe into the board, you will notice that the syringe is held away from the surface of the board. So, the syringe stays clean and sharp because nothing is touching the needle until it touches the patient's face.

Loading

After evaluating the patient and making a treatment plan, I fill the syringes for each muscle group and place each of them into the holders on the board.

I always load the board in the same order (you will understand this more after you study the injections). This keeps me from forgetting to treat an area, and it allows me to know immediately which syringe is intended for which muscle group.

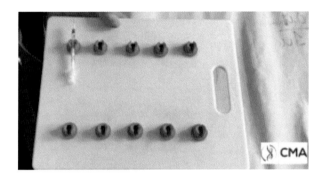

Figure 50. BoNT holding board loaded with one syringe.

For example, I always first fill the syringe to treat the procerus. I then place that syringe into the groove of the first holder.

Then, I fill the syringe for the patient's right corrugator and place that one in the groove of the second holder. Since I am facing the patient, the right corrugator is on my left—so I am working from my left to right.

Next, I fill the syringe for the left corrugator and place that one into the next holder.

Continuing in that manner, from the left to right and from the top to the bottom, I usually load the board as follows:

TOP, left to right: (1) procerus, (2) right corrugator, (3) left corrugator, (4) brow lift (includes the BoNT for both sides), (5) right crow's feet.

BOTTOM, left to right: (1) left crow's feet, (2) frontalis, then the extras that may be needed depending on the person's face, like Bruxism, gummy smile, bunny lines, etc.

Now that you know how to find new BoNT patients with the BoNT party and how to draw the BoNT out of the vial and organize your syringes, it is time to learn how much to put in the syringes and where to inject the BoNT.

Module III.

Twelve Injection Points & the Exact Dosages to
Create Gorgeous Results
These 12 Are All You Need to Know

23. FOUR GUIDING PRINCIPLES OF PROVIDING GREAT BONT

Guiding Principle #1: Follow a Consistent Sequence

In the next section, I will show you twelve injection points that allow you to do great BoNT, allowing you to create gorgeous results for your patients. I will go through each of the twelve in the order that I normally inject them.

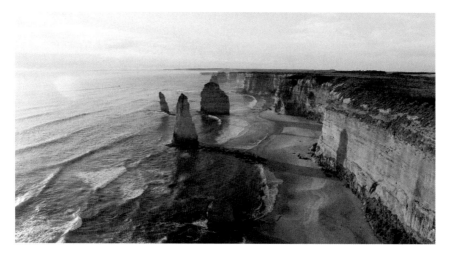

Figure 51. The "12 Apostles" in Australia represent the 12 injection points (even though there may not be exactly 12 of either).

You do not need to follow the same order that I follow. You can proceed in any order you please. But always inject in a specific, predetermined order—for efficiency and so you do not forget to treat an area.

Then you can inject on autopilot, allowing you more brain freedom to think about the patient's face and about what you should be learning from the conversation.

I always treat the procerus first because it seems to hurt the least. And everyone gets the procerus treated. Then, I treat the corrugators, followed by a brow lift, crow's feet, and the frontalis (assuming the patient opted to receive all of these).

Guiding Principle #2: Facial Muscles Attach Skin to Bone

Most of the voluntary muscles connect *bone to bone*; for example, the bicep connects the scapula to the radius; contraction of the bicep causes movement across the elbow. But, with the facial muscles, the muscles connect *skin to bone, so contraction causes movement of the skin—the bone does not move.* You know this difference between facial muscles and the other voluntary muscles, but it helps you do better BoNT to pause and consider the difference.

So, when you contract your corrugators, for example, the two corrugators attach to the skull between your eyes and to the skin just above each of the brows. Contraction causes the skin of the brow to move closer to the center of the face—making an angry or worried expression.

Guiding Principle #3: Muscles are Belts that Make Pleats

Each muscle works like a belt; when the belt contracts, it shortens the material adjacent to the belt, causing pleats that are oriented perpendicular to the belt.

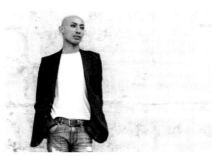

Figure 52. Belts go horizontally and pleats go vertically.

Visualize the belt on your slacks. If you tighten the belt, the material beneath the belt shortens and pleats appear up and down, crossing the belt.

The belt goes horizontally, the pleats go vertically.

If you loosen the belt, the pleats are pulled out.

189

That is what BoNT does; it loosens belts (muscles) so that pleats (wrinkles) are pulled out.

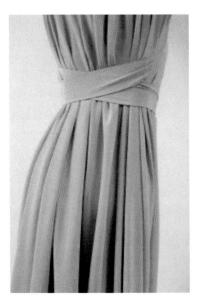

Figure 53. The pleats (wrinkles) run perpendicular to the belt (muscles).

Guiding Principle #4: Before Injecting, Watch the Face Move

Since facial muscles attach the skull (on one end) to the skin (on the other end), to find the exact location to inject, visualize the exact location of the muscle, and to "see" the muscle, you look for the insertion site—where the distal end of the muscle attaches to the skin.

As an example, consider the frown lines or the glabella area. This area is the most common for people to want treated and includes three muscles: (1) procerus, (2) the left corrugator, and (3) the right corrugator.

To visualize these three muscles, if I ask the patient to "frown," they often do crazy things with their face but still do not contract the procerus or the corrugators—which is what I want them to do. But if I tell ask the patient to "knit your brows together," they will usually contract all three muscles of the glabella.

When the corrugators contract, a dimple appears where the corrugators attach to the skin; the skin becomes "corrugated" (shortened) medial to the dimple; the skin is pulled toward the midline (like a curtain).

With contraction of the corrugators, the skin becomes smooth lateral to the dimple (where the skin is pulled tight).

On different people, due to variations in anatomy, you will see the dimple (skin attachment of the corrugators) appear anywhere within a circle of at least two inches in diameter just above the brow.

But even though you will see variations, when you see the dimple, you can easily *understand* where the corrugators lie beneath the skin. This understanding of the person's face allows you to "see" beneath the skin and so know where to inject.

A Common Mistake that Can Cause Either a Lack of Effect or a "Crazy" Effect from BoNT

A surprising number of physicians inject all faces in the same location without watching the face move to understand *that individual, unique face*.

When I meet someone who says to me, "Botox doesn't work on me," usually I find that the person has a corrugator that is either longer or shorter or somehow configured in a way that varies significantly from what is found with most people; so, someone has probably been injecting that person without watching the face move and therefore has missed the target muscles with the needle.

For example, a very wealthy woman (who had visited several physicians in another town) came to one of my BoNT parties and she told me, "Botox *never* works for me, I'm just here to visit my friends."

I said, "Let me look at you."

She sat down in front of me and I asked her to knit her brows together; the insertion site of her corrugators lay very close to the midline. So, she had a tiny little corrugator that was half the length seen for most people.

Her previous BoNT doctors likely missed the corrugator by injecting lateral to the insertion site.

So, I said to her, "I will do your BoNT for free today. In two weeks, when it starts to work, call my cell phone with your credit card."

I gave her my cell phone and injected her BoNT. She called to pay me two weeks later.

WARNING: If you estimate where to inject by the location of the eyes and brows without watching the face move, you will often miss the ideal injection point, causing either a lack of effect or a crazy result that makes the patient look as if she had a stroke.

But do not worry; I will make it very easy for you to understand every face and all twelve injection points on every face.

Example of Using the Principles

In summary, the best way to treat frown lines is as follows: Ask the patient to "knit your brow together."

Pleats will appear along the part of the skin that is contracted by the corrugators; the muscle contraction will pull the skin tight lateral to the insertion site.

Starting laterally and moving medially, when you see where the smooth ends and the wrinkles start, you will see a dimple; that dimple is the lateral insertion site of the corrugator. The medial insertion site will be visualized as midway between the eyes (more about this later when we learn each injection point).

The point is that for all twelve injection sites, there is a simple way to find and "see" each muscle by watching the face move.

As an example, look at Alex's face (my wife). Without the blue arrow, could you find her insertion site?

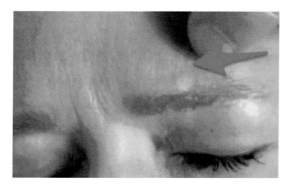

Figure 54. The skin appears "corrugated" medial to the insertion site (at the tip of the arrow) and smooth lateral to the insertion site.

In the photo, you see vertical wrinkles (corrugations) medial to the insertion site and smooth, tight skin lateral to the insertion site. The insertion site appears as a dimple.

The procerus, usually more visible in men, pulls down and makes a "dash," or horizontal line.

When the corrugators relax, that pulls the 11s out.

When the procerus relaxes, that pulls the dash out.

Lighthouse

Belts tightened,
make pleats—wrinkles;
Belts relaxed,
pleats pull out—smooth.

When you understand (by knowing the anatomy and by watching the face move) exactly where every belt (muscle) is and exactly what moves when each belt relaxes or tightens, then (and only then) you can provide amazing BoNT that is custom made for each individual face.

24. FACE CONSULT: CLEAR THINKING & ACCURATE PROMISES

Sometimes, while at a social event, someone (after discovering my profession) will say to me, "How would you treat my face?"

When that happens, because I seldom interact with someone socially and simultaneously contemplate what I might do with their face, I must stop what I am thinking and doing. Usually, if I am interacting with

someone socially, I focus on the person—who they are, not how they appear—not because I'm a soul-searching, perceptive prophet, but simply because who they are interests me more than their wrinkles. So, I am usually focused on them as a person, and when they ask me to contemplate their appearance, I stop and do what I call *"swapping brains."*

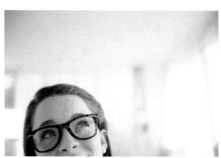

Figure 55. It helps to stop and swap brains when you think about faces.

Learning to consciously swap brains on demand will make you a better BoNT injector. Here's how...

How to Swap Brains (and Why You Must)

You have three brains: your left brain, your right brain, and your lizard brain (your instinctive or midbrain).

When someone says to me, "How would you treat my face?"

Then, I pause and methodically use each of my three brains to think about the four characteristics of the appearance of anything (not just faces): (1) size, (2) shape, (3) color, & (4) texture.

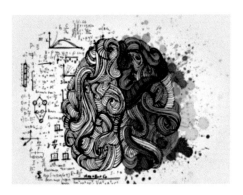

Figure 56. All parts of the brain are used when you think about faces (left, right, and lizard).

First, I go left brain and think about size.

What about symmetry, size, and proportions—what are the measurements, the numbers?

To understand more about how to think about these measurements, repeatedly study the topographic maps on the following website: BeautyAnalysis.com

I cannot emphasize enough how much Dr. Marquart's ideas (the author of BeautyAnalysis.com) have helped me over the past 2 decades. *Print his topographic maps of both the attractive male and female faces and study the measurements*; think about them when you look at faces in movies, in magazines, and when you are with your patients.

I use his maps to direct my left brain about measurements. For example, is the cheek wider than the jaw? What is the ratio of the width of the upper lip at the midline compared with the lower lip? How does this person's e-line appear?

You will understand the e-line and those ratios when you study Dr. Marquart's website (and it is free): BeautyAnalysis.com

Those are some of the left-brain measurements.

Then, I go Right Brain and think about shape.

After going left brain, then I go right brain and think about shapes (using Dr. Marquart's maps). Where does the face look convex, and where is it concave? Does the cheek swoop down toward the corner of the mouth or does the cheek swoop toward something else? What about the jaw line—is it straight, or is there a "jowl"?

Studying Dr. Marquart's maps will help you understand shape. But, of course, you gain your own experience as well; if you decide you will become an expert in shape, then study your patient's faces and those in magazines and at the movies.

With time, you will develop your own nuances and preferences. Then, like a designer of clothes, *from your preferences, you will witness an evolution (without strain or forced effort) of your own style.* Your experience and ideas of beauty will translate into your patient's face.

Then, I think about Color and Texture.
The easiest thing to see immediately when you look at a face is color and texture. Does the texture look smooth or wrinkled? If wrinkled, then where do I see wrinkles? For each wrinkle or set of wrinkles, is the etiology only aging skin, or have repeated muscle contractions and relaxations caused the (dynamic) line?

Do I see scars? What caused them? Has there been trauma, disease (zoster, pox, poor nutrition), or acne? Do I see sun damage? Do I see basal cell carcinoma, melasma, or hypopigmentation? These are all color-texture changes (not shape or size).

By color, I do not simply mean the amount of melanin. For every ethnicity, you can see an underlying color of red for good circulation or gray for those who are elderly, who smoke, or for another reason, suffer poor health.

Finally, I lose my thinking brain and go lizard brain.
After observing the person's face using my left brain and my right brain, and noticing color and texture, then I go to my "lizard brain," and think, "Does this person feel like they are older than their birth certificate? Or do they feel younger?"

"Do they feel attractive, or do they feel tired and older than what their birth certificate says?"

When I say "Lizard brain," I am talking about that part of you that *feels* (more than looks) to understand if someone is attractive or not, to what degree, and in what ways.

Although the maps help with the lizard evaluation, the full equation cannot be defined; you feel it more than you see it. This is the part of your brain that does not think, the part that gives you desire or repulsion. When you look at someone and become sexually attracted or feel the need to assist because of their old age, or when you feel afraid, you are not doing mathematical equations; you are using your lizard brain.

Since I live near the Gulf of Mexico, where we enjoy the company of huge "lizards" called "alligators" in our ponds and streams (and sometimes in the backyard), I can watch lizard behavior on a grand scale. An alligator or a lizard does not contemplate much of anything that I can see other than hanging out and waiting for the opportunity to eat. Though some will argue that alligators will avoid people, the truth is that (given the opportunity) they will not hesitate to eat you or your dog. They do not do the math; they do not contemplate the species or any ethical dilemmas; they only seem to know if they are hungry and if the thing in front of them seems edible and available to eat without too much of a fight; if it is, then they will. Their brain is pure instinct.

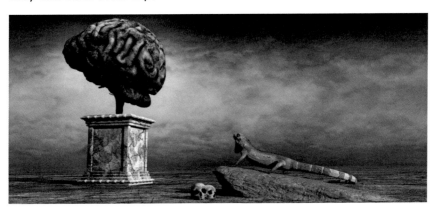

Figure 57. Always use your "lizard brain" when you study the faces you inject.

Education seems to beat the instinct out of people. The more educated the person, the more difficulty (it seems to me) that the person will have in accessing their lizard brain. Professional con men (I have worked in

197

prison) will tell you that the educated are the easiest to dupe; the uneducated more easily detect a lie, sometimes not by reasoning (left brain) but because they "smell the lie." The con man may be very intelligent, but he also keeps a well-developed lizard brain.

As an educated professional, you may have taught yourself to keep your lizard brain locked away where it became atrophied. One way to access the lizard part of your brain when seeing a patient is to note your first impression when you walk into the room. A second way is to briefly leave the room, then walk back into the room and simply feel your first impression of the age and the attractiveness of the person.

That first impression tells you how old, young, or attractive the person *feels to your lizard brain*. This leaving and coming back into the room also gives you a way to check your work; sometimes (after staring at someone's face for 30 minutes while treating them with BoNT or fillers), you will not be able to see as well with your lizard brain; you get stuck in left-brain mode. Just as it helps you to proofread your writing, if you let it sit and come back to it the next day, you will understand what you have done and what you may still need to do with your injections if you stop, leave the room, and then walk back into the room while noticing what you feel with your lizard brain.

Then, using your other two brains (left and right), try to understand why your lizard brain just felt that. Now, you know what you need to do next or if it is time to stop injecting because all is as good as you can make it.

Now we have discussed the three brains with which you see: the left brain, right brain, and lizard brain. And we have discussed the four characteristics of the appearance of anything: size, shape, color, and texture. Next, let's consider patient-doctor discussions.

Your Patients Are Not Looking for Compliments

If someone comes into my office and sits down, they are not there for compliments. They will not discard compliments if I offer them, and I do like pointing out what is attractive about a person's face before I offer my ideas about how to improve their appearance. But compliments are not why they came to see me.

When patients visit me for cosmetic work, they want expert advice about what to do to accomplish two things: (1) the healthiest, easiest strategies to help them stay *natural* to the way they were built (made by their creator), while simultaneously finding (2) a way for them to look *younger*. Looking younger can be almost synonymous with looking more attractive—but not quite.

To accomplish those two things (younger and natural), I need to be able to see what is attractive, young, and natural to their face, and pointing this out would be the complementary part. But I also need to be able to see the parts of their face that reveal aging, worry, or declining health. I cannot improve a person's face if I cannot recognize the characteristics of their face that, if pointed out in a social gathering, would be considered an insult.

Example of a Patient Conversation

As an example, I might say to a new patient something like the following: "Your mouth looks young up top. You have a beautiful cupid's bow with prominent columns and a youthful shape. But the corners of your mouth are downturned, and the lower lip is rolling in (or "inverting") such that I cannot see the color laterally. Your cheeks are nice and wide (wider than your masseter's, which is good since you are female), but I see flatness anteriorly and some depression of the tear troughs."

The preceding is only an example; the conversation, obviously, varies with every patient. As I am saying these things, I point out my observations (using the tip of a capped insulin syringe) directly on her face (with her looking into a hand-held mirror) or by pointing to her photograph on my phone.

The main idea is that the person should hear from me what I find to be youthful and attractive about her face, but that is not why she came to see me; she came to see me for an expert opinion about what parts of her face show aging and what can I do to reverse that aging without making her look weird.

Why You Should Study Faces in Movies

Because the roles in movie plots involve caricatures, you can observe what is it about the face of the character who plays each part that gives them the characteristics of the role. What about the angry person that makes them look angry? What makes the evil person look evil? What makes the caring mother look like a caring mother or the seductress look seductive? What do they do with make-up to make a person look older or younger? The role defines the face, and the face defines the role— making it easy for you to study the characteristics of faces that portray all manner of messages.

For example, watch *Benjamin Buttons* with Brad Pitt. What did they do with make-up to make him appear older or younger in that movie? What about his face makes him appear attractive, trustworthy, and kind? That movie is an extreme example because he demonstrates everything from a very old man to an infant.

But many movies show a progression of age; therefore, you have an opportunity to see on a big screen what they do with the face to make it appear younger or older.

When these ideas about the appearance of youth and of aging become embedded in your brain, then you understand what to do with your patients to give them a younger appearance without doing things that make them appear strange.

What Every Patient Wants

"Younger" and *"natural"*—that is what they want.

You can find this rule embedded in every part of this course, but it is worth repeating:

> *Younger and natural—that is the goal.*

If she is 80 years old or even 40 years old, she does not expect you to make her look 18 (young). But she expects you to help her look young*er* when she walks out of your office (or at least a short time after she walks out) than she looked when she walked into your office—while doing nothing to make her look odd or unnatural.

That is the game you play, and if you win, the person will be your fan for life and will send to you everyone they know.

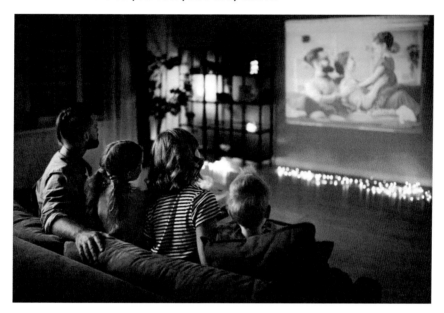

Figure 58. By thinking about the faces when you watch movies, you become a better injector by understanding the traits of old, young, angry, kind, evil, and 10,000 other things.

My Favorite Aesthetic-Consult Question

To accomplish that purpose (younger and natural), as part of the consult, I must tell them what might be made better (and what I cannot do).

One of my favorite questions to help find the best strategies is to *hand my patient a mirror* and a capped insulin syringe and say, "If this (referring to the insulin syringe) were a *magic wand*, what would you want to make better?"

I usually hand them a BoNT syringe (a 30-unit, BD-brand insulin syringe) because it's a better pointer than a finger, which is much thicker than the tip of an insulin syringe, making it more difficult for them to point exactly to what they want me to improve. I refer to it as a magic wand because in my hands (and in yours), it is.

Notice that *I do not ask, "What bothers you?"* because that sounds like I am implying that she needs psychotherapy.

Also, I do not ask, "What do you not like?"

That's not a good question because I assume that she is a grown-up woman who likes everything about herself, but she may want something to be made better. I do not want to imply she does not like anything about herself; I want her to like herself when she comes to my office and like herself when she leaves my office.

I simply want to make her face look younger while keeping it looking natural—nothing more or less than that.

The patient will often say to me, "What do you think?"

Even though I have ideas when the person walks into the room, I resist answering that question until I elicit their opinion about their face. Only after they tell me what they would want to "make better" do I then take out my camera (an iPhone) and I take pictures and I look at those pictures, and then I answer their question, "What do I think?"

I look at the photos before offering an opinion (not just their actual face) because I will see in 2D, in their photos on my phone, many things that I do not see if I look only at their real, 3-D face. With the phone, when I move the photo around and expand it and contract it and look at different views, then I better understand their face.

Do not look to see;
look to understand.

Also, if I am looking only at their face, there could be some awkwardness while I stare at their face for a prolonged time, whereas if I am looking at their photograph on my phone, I do not create that awkwardness.

As a minimum, I contemplate appearance until I understand at least the following about:

1. What is causing each wrinkle? Is it from a muscle? Then which muscle? Or is this wrinkle from skin aging?
2. Where do I see volume loss?
3. Are there scars? What caused them?
4. Are there pigment changes? Why?

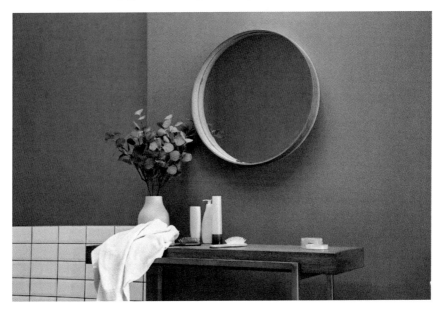

Figure 59. I can only do a facial aesthetic consult if I have a mirror, a small hand-held mirror that stays within reach of my treatment bed. I also keep a mirror on the wall for the patient to look into after the treatment (as they leave the room). The treatment bed has an overhead light, so I can see shapes. The mirror on the wall is in a place with a soft diffuse light. If they like my treatment when looking into the mirror with the harsh overhead light, they will love what they see in the mirror with the soft light.

You will know more to consider after you complete this course. It is not a difficult process after you know what to practice. But, always, *understand before you inject.*

I reach that understanding while sitting and thinking about their face and looking at their photos on my phone, not while walking around them and staring, which could make us both feel uncomfortable.

If You Are Trying to See Better, Use Less Light

Use an *overhead* light while taking photos and while doing injections. In my office, it is a light made to go over a kitchen table, with a dimmer switch. The only other light coming into the room where I inject is a diffuse light from one window covered by stained glass.

I do better work with an almost dim overhead light (and no other direct light) so that I can see shapes and shadows. *If you cannot see shadows on the face, it is very difficult to see shapes.*

If I were doing glamour photography, I would use at least three lights projecting from three different directions to take away shadows. If you have too much light, your "before-treatment" photos make it difficult for you to see what you need to do. So, do the opposite of what is done in glamour photography. Instead, use one light positioned over the head of the patient and directed toward the floor.

An important part of the consultation process is to set appropriate expectations. Not everything can be helped with an injection of any kind. Sometimes, you need surgery or creams. When you can use your injections to help someone look younger and natural, you may still lose them if you over-promise or if you do not make it clearly known the time frame of the progression of your treatments.

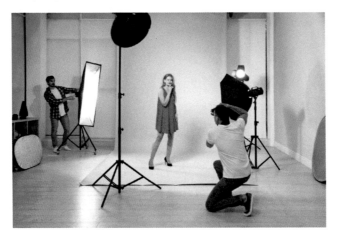

Figure 60. Bright lights from multiple directions take away shadows; without shadows, it becomes more difficult to see the shapes and lines that you want to erase (which is exactly why the glamour photographer uses multiple lights).

To help set those expectations, plan a few little canned speeches to give your patient. I'll give you those speeches in the next chapter.

Note: Watch videos of canned speeches at BoNTClass.com

25. "LITTLE SPEECHES" THAT HELP YOU IMPROVE YOUR TECHNIQUE & MAKE MORE MONEY

The "little speeches" in this chapter are only *one to three sentences long. Each is memorized and used when the time is appropriate.* The purpose of the little speeches is to *set realistic expectations and to avoid unnecessary calls* of worry.

For example, if you treat someone with BoNT and do not inform them that it takes two weeks for it to take full effect, you will likely get a call two to three days after the injection with the patient complaining that your treatment did not work.

The "It Didn't Work" Speech

When you inject BoNT, always tell the patient (especially first-time patients), "BoNT[5] starts to work in two days, the full effect is two weeks, and it lasts two to three months—unless you do it every three months for a year, and then it can start to last longer."

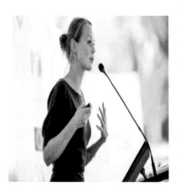

Figure 61. Canned speeches make life better for my patients and me.

Even after giving that little speech, an occasional patient will still call you after only a few days and say, "It isn't working."

Usually, they are referring to only one of the injection points. But sometimes, there can be an inhomogeneous onset of action. So, if you treat someone with BoNT and it is only two *days* or

---

[5] Substitute the brand name you are injecting.

even a week later, and your patient says, "It didn't work," then you can answer with the following little speech:

"The full effect is not until two weeks after the injection, so give it two weeks before we decide. If I reinject that one spot now, and there is a delayed reaction in that same area from the first injection, then the *additional BoNT I give today to try to make things straight could make things crooked*."

If between two and four weeks, the patient still has an area not working, then you can reinject that one area, but usually not before.

My Little "Go-Home" Speech that Can Help You Become a Better Injector and Keep You from Losing Patients

Here's a possible variation of the go-home speech for the first-time BoNT patient:

"Come back to see me between two to four weeks. Even if you think it's great. I'm going to be pickier than you are. I may add to it. I may change your recipe for next time because I think you may need less. I won't charge you to add anything to an area that I've already treated. If there is something new to treat that you want, I will charge you for that. But, if I only touch up what I have already treated, I won't charge you. That way, I will be able to better understand your face. I'll just add the touch-up to make your perfect recipe for the next time and will do it all at once."

I often use the word "recipe." You want to be the person who knows their face better than anyone and who knows their "perfect recipe" for BoNT.

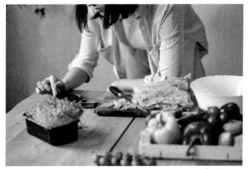

Also, by scheduling the two to four-week follow-up appointment when

Figure 62. Every person deserves that you find their perfect recipe.

treating someone for the first time, if the person is not happy with the results, you can discover and fix the problem instead of them simply going elsewhere for their next visit (thinking that you do not know what you are doing).

Finding the perfect recipe for their face brings up the principle of "how to become excellent."

How to Become Excellent at Anything

Why would you want to provide anything for patients except in an excellent way? So, How do you become good (maybe even *excellent*) at anything?

Not just BoNT—anything.

The following is a simple, 4-step way to become excellent at anything:

Step One
First, you read about your chosen subject; and you go to classes until you know almost everything. Then you keep going, even after you are bored, looking for anything you do not yet know, and you think about the subject.

Step Two
Second, even while doing Step One, you do it. Then you do it again. You practice. You practice a lot. You practice more than anyone you know.

Step Three
Third, as you practice, you look at your results and get feedback—preferably from another person who is already excellent, and (with BoNT), you get feedback from the person you treated.

Step Four
Then you repeat steps one through three; you repeat them over and over and over—assume that you know enough today to do your work but that you will always want to know more. And if you want to know more, never forget that your patient can be your best teacher.

Becoming the Expert for Each Patient

Keeping in mind the idea of "how to become an expert," consider the following: if you wait until everyone's BoNT has worn off before seeing them again, you do not obtain first-hand feedback about what you have done, so you are not able to improve.

Only by seeing the person between two to four weeks after the injection do you see the full results of your injections. You cannot do this with every patient (many will not come back until it is time for their next treatment) but try to do it with as many first-time patients as possible.

If the patient is too busy to come back to see me between two to four weeks, I tell them, "If you are not able to visit in two to four weeks, then at least text me a non-smiling selfie using an overhead light. Then I can see the results and see how to improve the treatment on your next visit."

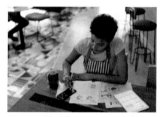

Figure 63. All my patients have my cell phone. But I encourage text instead of calling when possible. They can text selfies as an option for follow-up.

All my cosmetic patients have my cellphone number, and they never abuse it.

If they text a selfie and all looks great (which happens most of the time), then I save that selfie in their Dropbox folder and text them back that they look gorgeous and that I look forward to seeing them on their next visit.

If I see something on the selfie that could be better, I might ask them to come back to the office, or I may only make a note to alter the treatment on the next visit.

Most of the time, they are proud of the results, and they send a selfie to show me how well it is working and to say thank you; we are all happy. But, without the option for you to see and for them to tell you what they think, your results will not improve as much as they could, and you may never even know that your patient was not happy—they just quit coming back.

Since I only treat the forehead on the second visit (if the person is new to me), those first-time patients who want the forehead treated will usually make the second visit. But most of the others will just see me on the next visit to tell me that things worked beautifully and to repeat the same recipe.

The "Free Offer" Speech I Make after Every BoNT Treatment

Even on repeat treatments, almost every time, after every treatment, I say to my BoNT patients, "After two weeks (before four weeks), if it isn't perfect, just let me know, and I will touch it up for free."

Be very specific about two to four weeks. Otherwise, they will sometimes come back at two months and want you to touch it up when, really, their BoNT is wearing off, and it is time for another treatment (not a touch-up).

I sometimes say, "Between two to four weeks, if you don't love it, let me know; you must love it. If there's something that isn't perfect about it, come back, and I'll touch up anything I've already done for free. If you want another area treated, I charge you. But, if something I treated is not perfect between two and four weeks, I will touch it up for free."

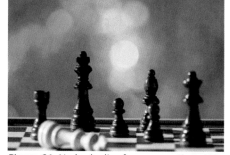

Nobody Dies

Let's say that they come back at 3 weeks, and you (on the first treatment) put 10 units into each corrugator, and you see

Figure 64. No body dies from cosmetic BoNT. But still do the consent and do not treat those with myasthenia gravis or who may be pregnant or if they feel too demanding.

that they really needed more (because they can still make the "11" sign); so, you must add another 5 or 10 units to each side—it's okay, nobody died.

If you *underdose* BoNT for wrinkles, it is not like under-dosing someone with triple antibiotics when they are septic in the ICU (they die if you get it wrong). If you under-dose with BoNT, their wrinkle does not go away; that's it.

And if you *overdose*, nothing bad happens; but perhaps you spent more of their money than necessary and perhaps increased their propensity to develop antibodies to BoNT.

But, still, nobody dies, ever, from cosmetic BoNT.

You never lose sleep.

Even though nobody died, you still want to know when your treatment is not as perfect as possible so that you can fix it. The next little speech helps you know.

The "If-You-Can-Do-This" Speech to Help You Improve

Another little speech I often give is the following: "*If you can do this at all* [said while knitting my brows together, which I must do by using my fingers since I BoNT my own corrugators] *between two and four weeks, I want to know so I can add more to your frown. I do not want you to be able to frown at all.*"

After you give this speech, if your patient comes back at two weeks and can still frown, you add more BoNT to the area. If they need an extra 5 units on the follow-up, 2-week visit, and you initially gave them 10, then, next time, you give them 15 on each side. You just add it to their recipe.

Not a big deal, but it helps you become an expert by giving the person permission to come back to see you, and it helps you find the perfect recipe for every patient (and that keeps them loyal to you no matter what doctor nearby offers a Groupon discount).

The "Reassurance" Speech

Your patients will almost always find the following speech to be endearing.

When someone comes back for a touch-up, they will often apologize for "bothering" you. They may feel as if they are acting picky and therefore feel guilty and self-conscious.

When this happens, you must *thank* them for coming back to see you and tell them, "Only by coming back am I able to learn more about your face. It only takes a few seconds to make things perfect and I am glad to do it. I would never want you walking around crooked or with a frown."

Without *rewarding* them with praise for allowing you make things right, they may simply find another doctor because you either left them

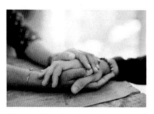

Figure 65. Comfort the patient with the idea that they are doing you a favor when they ask you to make it better.

unhappy with your treatment results or you made them feel guilty for asking you to make things right.

It only takes only a few dollars' worth of BoNT and a few seconds of your time to make someone happy with a touch-up and therefore retain a patient that will give you thousands of dollars over a lifetime. So, be truly grateful when they give you the chance to make your work as perfect as you can. *If they try to pay you for the touchup, refuse to take their money.*

Often, when they come back and ask you to touch up an area, they will ask you to treat something new or will buy something else from you (one of your creams, a filler treatment, almost anything) because they are grateful you did the touchup and want to reciprocate; when they do, take that money (but never for the touchup).

The Forever Challenge

Keep practicing, keep learning, and never think you know enough—you know enough to do your work today, that is all. Always assume that while you are proud of the wagon wheel you are making, someone else, down the street from you, is making a rocket ship about which you do not yet know.

So, learn everything that is in this book. Practice like crazy—even my little speeches. Practice like a fiend while you keep looking for the information that may hide in your blind spot by reading and going to more classes.

Then throw this book away and write your own book. Write something so wonderful that this book becomes irrelevant.

Somewhere, I will smile and congratulate you.

26. BEFORE & AFTERS, AN OVERVIEW, & A FRONTALIS WARNING

You must take pictures *before* you inject.

Always.

Otherwise, if your patient is asymmetrical before you treat her (almost everyone is), she might blame you for causing her to be crooked even

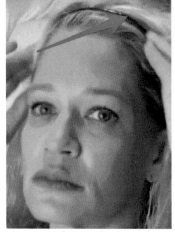

though she was so before you started. This happens more than you might expect, so *always take the before photo—not only to show what you did but to prove what you did not.*

A Prize for the Patient

Before taking the photo, for every patient, I give her a throwaway hairband. We buy them by the bag full, and I let the patient take hers home if she wants.

Figure 66. Those with enough hair to block the forehead put on a disposable head band before I begin taking photos or injecting.

She puts on the headband before I take her picture.

I always take at least three views. First, I take a photo from straight ahead, then from tangentially on each side. For consistency (to make it easier to compare the before and afters), I prefer to align the medial corner of the eye with the bridge of the nose. Some injectors align the tip of the nose with the cheek when they take their tangential views; that is also acceptable. Just be consistent.

I take a profile view, too, if I am interested in her e-line. The e-line becomes more important when injecting fillers (you can see more about that in my book about the Vampire Facelift® procedure). But, with the injection of BoNT alone, the e-line and the profile view can still be helpful.

The main idea is that your before-and-afters should be taken from the same angle every time.

A Frontalis Pearl that Saves Two Units of BoNT

For the frontalis, when your patients raise their brows, in the very center, there may be an absence of lines (making the forehead smooth in the center); but the lines manifest all the way up to the hairline on both sides. In some people, there is no smooth center.

In the photo, you see a continuation of the horizontal lines all the way to the hairline on the patient's right, but there is smoothness near the hairline in the center and even some asymmetry with the lines stopping further from the hairline on the patient's left. The smooth areas show you where the frontalis is absent.

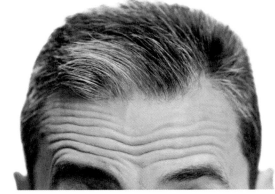

Figure 67. Example of a split frontalis showing a lack of muscle superomedial. Also, there is less muscle on the patient's left superolateral.

If I put BoNT in the smooth areas, nothing bad happens; but I would be causing no effects and therefore wasting the BoNT.

Usually, if there is a split frontalis, there will only be smoothness in the center, and you will see the horizontal lines on both sides all the way up to the hairline.

Short-Hand Notation for BoNT

Looking for a quick way to document the number of units injected and

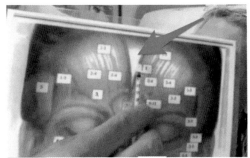

Figure 68. Absence of frontalis in the superomedial forehead.

the location of each injection, I tried a variety of software programs and devices. I have still found none that are both as quick and as accurate as simply using a pen and paper. If you find software that you like better than pen and paper, then use it. But you should be able to document your face injections in less than ten seconds; more than that is a waste of your life.

In the following sketch, the red numbers indicate where I injected and how much. The circled numbers (written in black) indicate the sequence that I injected. I do not usually document the sequence in the patient's chart (the black numbers).

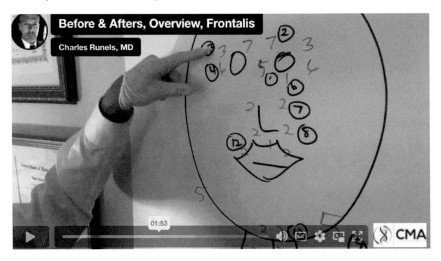

Figure 69. Screenshot (from BoNTClass.com) showing how I document injections with a simple diagram. I usually only write the red numbers (the number of units). The black numbers show the usual sequential order that I follow when injecting.

You will understand my shorthand documentation more after studying each of the twelve injection points in this course.

If you must use software, the fastest accurate method that I have found is to take the photos with an iPad; then, using iPhoto, you can write directly onto the photo (on the screen) both the number of units you used for each injection. But I still think paper and pen are much faster.

I usually draw a simple oval, add a circle for each eye, a capital "L" for the nose, and then draw a mouth. It looks childish but simple works better. This is not art class; it's a medical record.

When I am with a *new* patient or at a BoNT party, I make the diagram before I inject and then use the diagram as a tool to discuss the plan and the price with the patient. With a repeat patient, after I inject, I write the number of units I used on the face diagram.

A "Disclaimer Speech" that Brings Them Back

If your patient has never had BoNT (or if only inconsistently), then even when she relaxes her face and even if you take your fingers and pull the 11's flat by stretching the skin between her brows, you will still (in most people over 30) be able to see two lines at the location of the folds.

If you do not give your patients the following speech, even though your BoNT worked, and they cannot move their corrugators, they will still see the residual lines (making the "11") and think your BoNT failed, so they will never come back to see you.

To avoid that misunderstanding, first, hand the patient a mirror. Then ask her to knit her brows together to make the number 11s.

Then, ask her to relax her face, and take your fingers and pull tight the skin between her brows, trying to make the 11s go away—and demonstrating that they do not.

Even though the corrugators and the over-laying skin will be stretched tightly by this maneuver, you will often still see a line at each of the folds because the skin has remodeled due to the repeated frown.

After pointing out the two lines (the patient is looking at her face in the mirror) that are still there, you give the following little speech:

"Even if I pull your skin tight, you still have the 11 lines. So, when your BoNT[6] starts working, you will still have these lines. If you cannot frown (knit your brows together), then the BoNT is working. If you want the lines to go away, then get your BoNT every three months, and you will never knit your brows together; so, the skin will remodel and become smooth again. This usually takes six months to a year. But, if we let the BoNT wear off, the corrugators recreate the folds, and the lines will never go away."

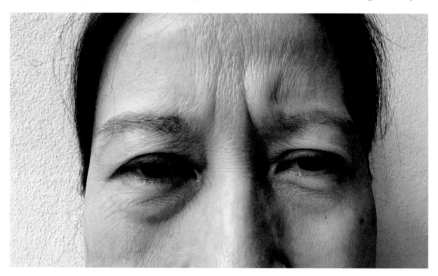

Figure 70. The vertical creases caused by the corrugators: the 11s.

The first time they receive BoNT, it will wear off around the second month. That's officially (by the package insert) how long BoNT lasts—about two months.

So, the rest of the speech goes like this:

"Get your BoNT every three months for the first year, even if it seems to wear off at two months. Then, after a year, it will start to last the full three months or even longer—four or five months. Also, after a year of

---

[6] Replace "BoNT" with the brand name of the material you are injecting.

receiving BoNT every three months, you can often see the same effects with a lower number of units."

What Makes BoNT Valuable?

BoNT is safe, and the injections are easy to do.

These little ideas about explaining, and follow-up, and documentation, and understanding your patients (not just their faces) give value to your injections even if your understanding of the facial anatomy is no deeper than the injectors down the street from your office. The anatomy of the facial muscles is simple (at least as required to do BoNT). For comparison, one might argue that the female pelvic muscles are less well-understood and more complicated in function.

You learn the facial anatomy, but you distinguish your practice by learning the unique anatomy of each individual.

Time to Inject

The preceding part of this course considered how to find and talk with your patients. Now, we are ready to consider the easy part—how to do the actual injections—twelve injection points, only twelve, that will empower you to provide gorgeous BoNT treatments.

27. INJECTION POINT #1: FROWN LINES, THE DASH & THE NUMBER 11'S

First, a Word About Gloves

Before we think about the procerus and the corrugators, think briefly about your hands. You can wear two gloves. I only wear one.

With my non-gloved hand, my dominant hand, I hold the syringe that holds the BoNT. I also touch things on my Mayo stand, touch bottles, my BoNT board, etc. I want that hand to stay clean (no blood on it).

But with my non-dominant hand, I always hold a gauze with which I blot oozing drops of blood when I do an injection. And I hold pressure after every injection with that gauze. Also, the patient feels like the procedure is cleaner because I only touch their face with the gloved hand. Even though the glove is non-sterile, it is still new and fresh out of the box—which feels cleaner to them when I touch their face (especially around the mouth).

In summary:
*My *dominant* hand (ungloved) holds the syringe and never touches blood.

*My *non-dominant* hand (gloved) holds the gauze and touches the person's face (blots blood and holds pressure) and never touches anything else in the room

I developed this one-glove habit while working in emergency rooms for twelve years. Often, the ER would grow so busy that I would have no one available to assist because all the nurses had their own tasks. While working alone, if I had a sterile field, the gloved hand would stay sterile, and the non-gloved hand could touch items in the room to assist the gloved hand.

If the one-glove idea seems odd or confusing, skip it and wear a glove on both hands. I am telling you *everything* I do to keep things clean and efficient: this one-glove habit saves time and is safer because I am not tempted to touch things in the room with a hand contaminated with blood.

So, counterintuitively, one glove instead of two increases safety while saving money (fewer gloves); I think, if you try it, you will never go back to both hands gloved when injecting BoNT.

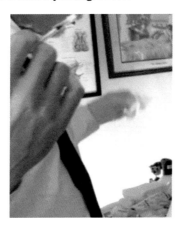

Figure 71. Gloved non-dominant hand (holding gauze); non-gloved dominant hand holding syringe.

Skip Betadine & Alcohol

With BoNT, there is no need to cleanse the face before doing injections. You can even inject through makeup. With fillers, that is different—you must cleanse the face because fillers are injectable implants.

But, with BoNT, you do not need to cleanse the face.

Go Into Your Peaceful Space

When I do injections, as mentioned previously, I always play George Winston's *December* album.

Every time.

For almost two decades.

By always playing the same music, when that music plays, it instantly puts me in a peaceful place, and I am focused on only the person in front of me.

When I started, it was a George Winston CD. Now, before I inject, I get George and his Steinway going by saying to Alexa (who sits on the shelf near my treatment table), "Alexa [pause until she's listening], play George Winston, December album."

Alexa answers, "Here's some music by George Winston on Amazon Music."

Then I say, "Alexa [pause], volume three."

Volume three on the Alexa is loud enough to calm me but soft enough to not interfere with conversation.

Then, with my prefilled syringes loaded onto my BoNT board (see Module 1), I take a breath and listen to George for a second or two while I restudy the patient's face for orientation. Then, I inject.

Maybe that seems like too much winding up for a BoNT injection. But my injections take on a higher level of excellence and the patients seem happier when I follow the described process.

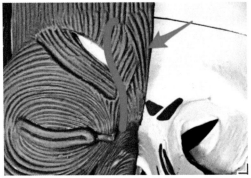

Figure 72. Procerus connects to the bone (inferior) to the skin (superior). It weaves into the occipitofrontalis, making it challenging to distinguish the two muscles in the inferomedial forehead.

Glabella = (Procerus + Corrugators)

Think of the "frown lines" as the combination of lines formed by the two corrugators (left and right) and the one procerus.

Procerus

The procerus attaches the *skin* of the inferomedial forehead (the top of the procerus) to the fascia

222

overlying the superior surface of the nasal *bones* and the superior parts of the upper lateral nasal *cartilages* (the bottom of the procerus).

1a. Injecting the Procerus (Erasing the Dash)

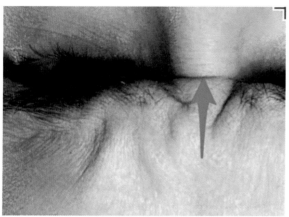

The procerus pulls the skin (and the brows) down between the eyes causing a dash wrinkle between the eyes. The person looks angry, sad, or worried. You will learn more about this group of wrinkles (called the "Omega" complex) in Chapter 40 about treating

Figure 73. The "dash" or "-" caused by the procerus muscle is usually more prominent in men.

depression with BoNT.

See the Two Invisible Lines Before You Inject

Unlike with the corrugators, to find the spot to insert the needle to inject procerus, you do not need to see the face move. Simply *imagine*

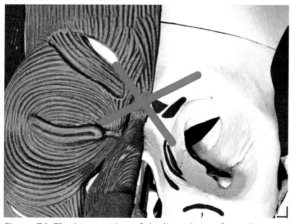

an X that goes from the end each brow to the medial corner of the opposite eye.

Stop and Meditate About Something Wonderful

Before thinking more about injecting the procerus, consider what I just described: "The landmarks for

Figure 74. The intersection of the lines drawn from the medial end of each brow to the medial corner of each eye.

injecting the procerus are the corners of *the eyes* and the medial end of each *brow*."

Could you ask for easier-to-find landmarks?

BoNT, compared to (for example) doing a spinal tap on a screaming child, is so very easy. And, as you progress through this course and learn about the other eleven injection points, the techniques do *not* grow more difficult.

You never lose sleep doing BoNT.

Inject the BoNT

After you visualize the two lines and where they intersect, use your non-dominant gloved hand to *gently* pinch the skin away from the skull; this pinch makes the pain from the injection near zero. Inject the procerus at the intersection of the two lines (between your thumb and forefinger).

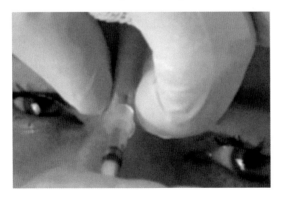

Figure 75. Procerus injection at the intersection of imaginary lines connecting the medial corner of each eye and the medial end of the opposing brow.

The syringe for this injection should only contain the amount of BoNT you plan to use for the procerus—usually around 12 units for a first-time female and five units for a woman who has received BoNT repeatedly. For a male, the numbers are usually 15 (first time) and ten units (repeat). Fill a syringe with only the BoNT needed for the procerus injection, then discard the syringe after the injection. That is correct; you only use this syringe once.

The needle, for this injection, goes all the way to the hub; the hub of the syringe touches the skin but is not pushed so far that it indents the skin.

I hold the syringe as I would hold a cigarette, not as I would hold a dart.

Watch for Bleeding Before Moving to the Next Injection Point

After the syringe has been emptied, I quickly pull the needle out of the skin (there is no advantage to pulling the needle out slowly) and hold pressure using the gauze in my left (nondominant) hand. I keep holding pressure, *very lightly as if comforting a child*, until I do not see a dot of oozing blood when I take the gauze away. If I do see a dot of active bleeding when I take the gauze away, then put the gauze back in place and keep holding pressure.

To Avoid Bruises, Follow the "Full-Minute" Rule

Usually, almost with every injection, after only a few seconds, you will see no bleeding when you take the gauze away. But, occasionally, usually one or two injection points per patient encounter, you will see brisker bleeding. This brisk bleeding indicates you have punctured a

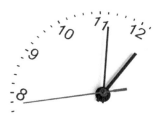

larger arteriole (instead of the capillaries encountered with most injections).

Do not worry.

When you puncture an arteriole, if you put your gauze back in place, hold gentle pressure, and *wait a full minute*, you will usually avoid making a bruise.

If they still develop a bruise, "Oh well, not good, but nobody dies."

I never promise that I will not cause a bruise. But, almost every time, my

Figure 76. If you see brisk bleeding, holding pressure for a full minute decreases the chances of a bruise. A second hand on the wall and George Winston's December album help you wait the full minute.

patients have zero bruising after a BoNT treatment, and that consistency grows my business.

I do not care if they had a handful of aspirin and drank three glasses of wine while driving to see me; the full-minute wait after hitting an arteriole will still allow me bruise-free treatments for almost every patient.

Waiting a full minute, however, can be maddening when the office is busy. And because of my impatience, if I estimate a minute, I may rush, wait less than a minute, and cause a bruise. So, I keep a clock on the wall near my treatment bed and the clock has a second hand. If I see brisk bleeding that heralds a potential bruise, I watch that second hand and hold pressure for a full minute. But, without that second hand and George Winston to keep me patient, I would make many more bruises.

Sometimes, I will even close my eyes, listen to the *December* album for a few seconds, take a little vacation, then open my eyes and watch the end of the minute on the clock so that I make the full minute. Then the patient goes home bruise-free and tells all their friends they got sleepy while getting shots in their face and saw no bruises afterward.

Magic!

Leonardo da Vinci said, "I want to do miracles."

It is OK for you to want the same.

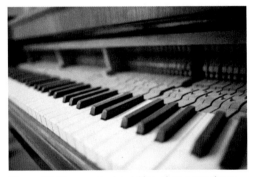

Figure 77. The music should be whatever relaxes the injector.

A Note on Music

I never let the patient choose the music in my treatment room.

The music is for me. If I am relaxed and peaceful and methodical and accurate and not hurting the patient, then the patient will be peaceful too. For that to happen, I need music that relaxes me.

Very often, maybe even most of the time, my first-time patients will comment, *"Is it odd that I am getting sleepy [while you are giving me shots in the face]?"*

And I will say, "It happens all the time. This is your time to relax and treat yourself."

Remember, to save time, my staff is not allowed to chatter when I do BoNT (read Module 1). If they do, they waste my time, but *they also defeat my efforts to bring the patient to a relaxed state.*

Chatter saves us from our thoughts.
There are times when almost everyone prefers silence: imagine a chatty massage therapist while you are getting a massage—not relaxing. The same principle applies to BoNT.

You may find that being chatty helps relax your patients. I suppose chatter could be better for some than complete silence; complete silence makes most people uncomfortable. A big part of the reason your patients and your staff want to chatter is that they are uncomfortable with their own thoughts—which come barging into their consciousness when there is silence. But peaceful music without chatter soothes the discomfort of silence and relaxes most patients more than incessant talking.

If the patient feels chatty, however, I let them go for a while because I truly want to know about their life. But, *if they talk, I stop doing injections, and I converse with them* for a few minutes. I quit trying to inject. I forget about BoNT and focus on what they are saying.

Never chase a chatting face.

Eventually, when I feel there is a potential pause in the conversation, I discourage further conversation by saying, "OK. Let's just think about your face."

Then, in my head, I go back to the music and to their face; nothing else matters. Nothing.

1b. Injecting Left & Right Corrugators (Erasing the 11)

After first injecting the procerus (which I think hurts the least of all the injection points), then I inject the left and right corrugators.

To find the corrugators, I must see the face move; so, I say to the patient, *"Knit your brows together."*

When they do, a dimple will appear at the most lateral end of each corrugator. This dimple marks where the "corrugated" skin stops and the smoother skin lateral to the insertion site begins.

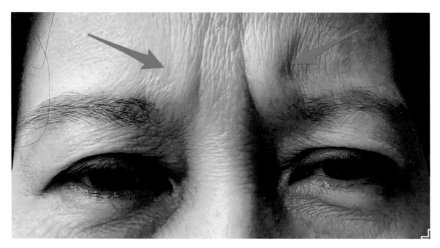

Figure 78. Arrows mark the insertion sites of both left and right corrugators. The site varies from face to face and sometimes from side to side.

When I see the dimple, I put my index fingertip into the indentation (on the side I am about to inject) to feel the insertion site. This palpation of the insertion site is not necessary, but it helps me see beneath the skin and to be more accurate with the injection.

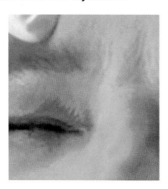

Figure 79. Fingertip palpating the insertion-site dimple.

Then I visualize the corrugator going from where my finger marks the dimple to a place between the eyes—the same intersection of the "x" we imagined when we injected the procerus.

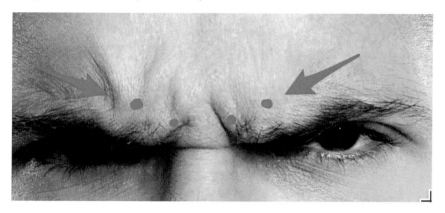

Figure 80. The arrows mark the insertion sites for both the left and right corrugators. After seeing and palpating each corrugator insertion site, I ask the patient to relax her face. Then, after the face relaxes, I inject the corrugator at the dots.

After finding the insertion site and visualizing the corrugator, I say to the patient, "Relax your face."

Then I inject near the lateral part of the corrugator about one-third of the total amount I intend to inject into that corrugator.

You could probably inject it all in one place, so do not worry too much about injecting exactly one-third. But I do think the treatment works better if you split it into two injections.

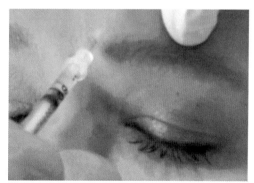

Figure 81. Injecting the more medial of the two injection sites for the left corrugator.

Then, I inject the rest of the syringe intended for that corrugator into the more medial part of the muscle.

After injecting, after every injection, I hold gentle pressure until I see no further bleeding.

229

You can watch a video of me injecting both the left and right corrugators at BoNTClass.com

Gentle Massage After Injection in Two Places

With the glabella (glabella = procerus + corrugators), your injections will show better results (more complete relaxation of the muscle complex) if you gently massage between the eyes immediately after injecting. I also massage gently after injecting the frontalis. I do not massage the other injection points. For all the others, I only hold gentle pressure.

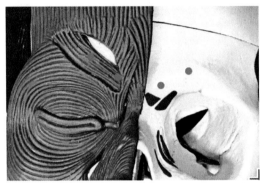

Figure 82. Blue dots mark the injection points for the corrugators.

The reason I do not massage the other injection points is that I want the BoNT to stay only in the exact place that I injected—not to spread. For example, if you massage the area after injecting to lift the brow, you could cause ptosis of the eyelids. But with the glabella region

and the frontalis, I think you do see better results and relax the patient more if you massage after the injection.

Always, with both massage and with simple pressure, I think about comforting the patient after the injection; I never think about "poking the hole" where the needle entered. Instead, *the attitude is one of holding softly with the flat of my hand (with a gauze between my hand and the patient's skin) as if comforting a child.*

A Fast & Accurate Record

The following diagram shows you how I would document the injection of seven units into each corrugator and five units into the procerus.

The simplicity of making a sketch in a chart or on an index card and then snapping a photo of the sketch documents your injections as well and is much faster than any software I have found.

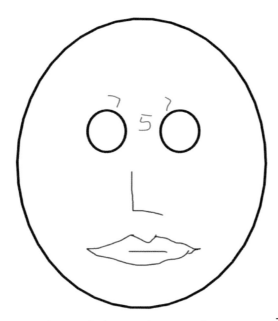

Figure 83. A simple diagram documents the injection amounts without slowing me down with unneeded software.

An alternative method is to snap a photo of the person's face with an iPad and then use iPhoto to sketch numbers onto the photo to indicate where and how much you injected. I am showing you the simple and quick, and accurate method that works for me. I have tried an embarrassing number of alternatives. For only one of those alternatives, I paid over $10,000 for the software and then went back to making sketches with a pen on paper.

If you need an electronic record, the photo of the sketch turns it into an electronic record.

28. INJECTION POINT #2: BROW LIFT

It is easy to understand how to expertly lift the brows (which most women and some men want) if you understand the cumulative tension on the brow—the vectors pulling up and the vectors pulling down.

The Muscles & Vectors that Control the Brow

Only one muscle lifts the brows, the frontalis; that is the only one.

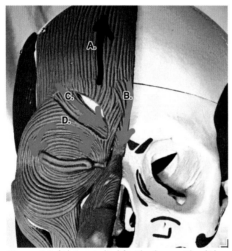

Figure 84. (A) Frontalis lifts the brow. The (B) Procerus, (C) Corrugator, & (D) Orbicularis oculi lower the brow.

Five muscles pull the two brows down: (1) the left and right corrugators, (2) the procerus, and (3) the left and right orbicularis oculi.

You cannot tighten muscles with BoNT, you can only relax muscles. So, to lift the brows, you relax the pull-down muscles (corrugators, procerus, orbicularis oculi) more than you relax the one pull-up muscle (frontalis).

Think of lifting the brow like a physics-vector problem (or a tug of war). In that case, the brow rests at the place where the tension (vector) from the frontalis equals the cumulative tension (addition of the vectors) of the procerus, the corrugators, and the orbicularis oculi muscles.

Said in a third way: *if I relax all the pull-down muscles and I don't relax the one muscle that's pulling up, then the pull-up muscle wins the tug of war, and lifts the brow.*

How to "Tailor-Make" Brows

With some people older than 50, and some as young as twenty, if you fully (or even partially) relax the frontalis and all the pull-down muscles simultaneously, the net effect can be to drop the brow.

When the brow drops (in both men and women), it is not attractive; the brow becomes heavy, and the patient looks like a Neanderthal. Because I don't really have a good way to predict what will happen if I treat the pull-ups and the pull-downs simultaneously, on the first visit, I only treat the pull-downs and do not treat the one pull-up (frontalis).

When you do not treat the frontalis on the first visit, but you do fully relax all the pull-down muscles, you cause the maximum lift of the brow because you left the pull-up muscle (frontalis) maximally strong and unopposed.

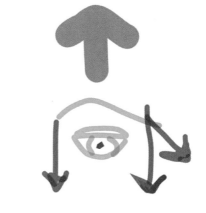

Figure 85. Before treatment, in the relaxed state, the brow will rest where the force from the pull up (frontalis) equals the pull downs. If the pull up happens to be much stronger than the pull downs, then if you fully relax all of them, the brow will drop. It is nearly impossible to predict what will happen if you fully relax them all; hence, the best results will be seen if you fully relax the pull downs (achieve maximal lift), and then tailor make the treatment of the pull up on a second visit two to four weeks after the first visit.

I just explained the brow-vector idea four different ways. I did so because it is an important point: *if you break the rule and treat the pull-downs and the pull-ups both on the first visit, if the brow drops, that person will not come back to see you and maybe not ever get BoNT again from anyone, never ever.*

For one mistake, the person may opt out of what may be the best treatment for their migraines, their bruxism, their depression, and/or for the maintenance of their facial youthfulness—all because they were inappropriately treated the first time.

Never treat the frontalis on the first visit.

On the other hand, if you leave the frontalis untreated (on the first visit), when they come back, between weeks two and four post-first treatment, now if they droop after you treat the frontalis, they will still come to see you again. They will just ask that you not treat their forehead (frontalis) anymore—because they saw how great they looked with a maximum lift before you drooped them.

Many women have never seen their brows with a maximum lift because they always had the frontalis treated and never experienced this tailor-made, stepwise approach. When they see how high you can lift the brow, they sometimes choose to wear bangs or just put up with the frontalis lines so the brows can stay high.

If they only want to treat the forehead
Some people will visit you and only want to treat the lines on their forehead. Since I cannot do that without risking dropping the brow, when someone asks me to only treat their forehead, I explain the brow vectors to them (using a photo of the facial muscles so they can visualize the muscles). It can be a tedious explanation that takes a full minute. But the explanation is necessary if you want patient cooperation; it goes something like this:

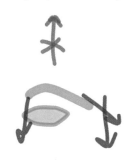

Figure 86. If you relax the frontalis (treat the forehead) without relaxing the pull-down muscles, then all the vectors pull down and you almost always create a neanderthal look.

"If I relax the only muscle holding your brow up, and do not relax the muscles that pull down, your brow will drop. So, let's relax all the muscles that are pulling the brow down, come back in two to four weeks, and then I will tailor-make how I relax your frontalis based on how high and on where your brow is lifted (and see if we can do that without drooping you)."

Almost everyone appreciates this tailor-made method of adjusting their BoNT treatment.

When they come back for the second visit, to tailor make their forehead treatment, for many of my patients, I inject to achieve only a partial relaxing of the frontalis to allow movement (and a natural look) and to avoid drooping them.

Where to Inject to Lift the Brow

You lift the brow with two separate injections.

The *first injection goes right through the eyebrow*; the needle passes through the brow. So, you have a line already drawn for you to help you find the spot. But where along the course of the brow do you put the needle?

When you relax the orbicularis oculi in the best place and keep the frontalis strong in the best places, the frontalis wins the tug of war and lifts the brow into the shape of a gull's wing.

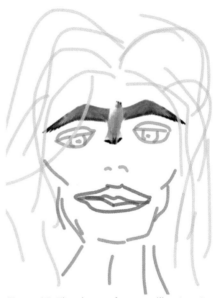

Figure 87. The shape of a seagull's wings in flight reflects the shape of a woman's brows.

The way I find the exact place along the course of the eyebrow to insert the needle is to find the "corner of the head." The actual name is the "lateral process of the zygoma", but I like calling it "the corner of your head."

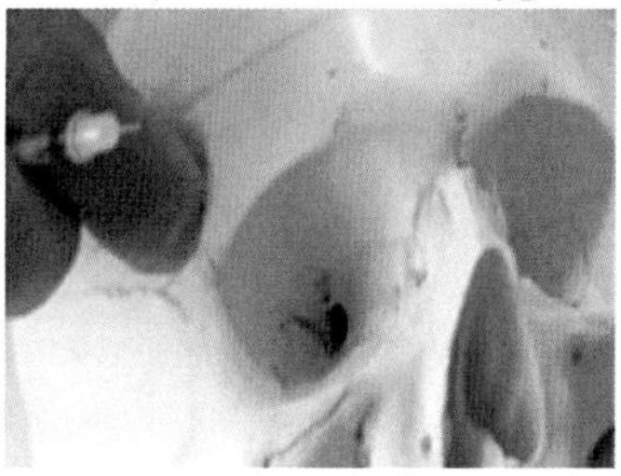

Figure 88. Finding the "corner of the head" or the lateral process of the zygoma.

If you look at the skull, you can see the edge of bone between the space where the temporalis muscle lies and just above the orbit, that edge travels vertically and crosses the brow (which goes horizontally)—intersecting the brow exactly where you should inject the orbicularis oculi.

235

To find that edge, if you slide your finger back and forth (always very gently), horizontally, just above the eyebrow, you will feel an edge; that edge is the "corner of your head."

When you find the edge, if you put your thumb and forefinger against that edge (lateral to it), and then gently pinch the brow from top to bottom, you can now inject the BoNT between your fingers into the brow, and you will create the perfect gull's wing shape. (You can watch me demonstrate finding the exact spot at BoNTClass.com.)

In the photo, I am holding the brow with my fingers, and my fingers are abutting the edge (indicated by the vertical blue line). Then I simply pass the needle between my fingers and inject the BoNT into the brow (at the spot marked by the arrow point).

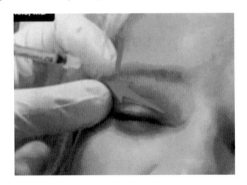

Figure 89. The injection point (marked by the arrow) is between my fingers which are holding the brow while simultaneously abutting the lateral process of the zygoma (indicated by the blue line).

So, first I find the edge, then grab the brow lateral to it. And then I inject three to five units of BoNT between my fingers right through the brow (wherever she has drawn it or plucked it); the needle goes directly through the center of the brow into the muscle below.

I use one syringe exclusively for the brow lift.

For most women, I will inject three units in each side; so, I start with a syringe (30 unit, BD-brand, insulin syringe) that has a total of six units (3 for each side).

After I inject three units into each brow, I discard that syringe.

236

Can't Touch This

This injection into the brow is the one most likely to cause ptosis. Tell the patient, "Avoid touching your face here [pointing to where you just injected] for the next four hours or you may cause your eyelid to droop."

As far as I know, I have drooped only three eyelids in almost twenty years. But, when I do, then I give that patient the next BoNT treatment completely free. *I always try to make up with people so that they feel like they came out better because something went wrong.* Following my plan, you are unlikely to droop anyone. But, if you do, I recommend you follow the same policy to make up with the patient.

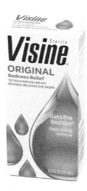

Figure 90. The tetrahydrozoline in Visine® is a sympathomimetic amine that will open the lid and counteract at least some of the droop from a BoNT-associated ptosis.

When they droop (and if you do BoNT long enough, you will droop a few people), then a simple and effective way to treat the droop is to tell them to use Visine (the original formula with the red letters) every three hours when they are in a public place and want to lift the lid back to near normal. They will need to use the drops every three hours as needed for up to two to three months (until the BoNT wears off).

Usually, when people droop the brows, it is not from a true ptosis as we just described; when people complain of a droop, it is usually because the frontalis was over treated and both brows drooped giving a heavy look; but the orbicularis oculi was not affected (not a true ptosis). If it is a true ptosis, usually only one lid will be affected, and the frontalis may still be treated correctly (the lid droops, not the brow).

Documentation of the Brow Lift

I use a very simple diagram to document the brow lift.

In this case, I would have started with one syringe with a total of six units and injected three on each side; then I would discard that syringe.

Occasionally, I will use 5 units on each side, or I will use slightly more on one side than the other to correct asymmetry.

What's Next?

We just covered the first injection to lift the brow. Treating crow's feet is the second injection that will lift the brow. We will discuss that in the next chapter.

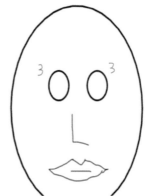

Figure 91. Documenting three units on each side to lift the brow.

Further Help

You can watch movies of me doing a brow lift at BoNTClass.com.

29. INJECTION POINT #3: SOFTENING CROW'S FEET

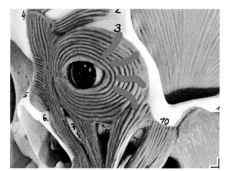

Figure 92. When the orbicularis oculi shorten, they make pleats that are the crow's feet.

If you visualize the orbicularis oculi like a belt encircling the eye, you can see that if you tighten the belt, you will see pleats that are the crow's feet.

Smile Lines vs. Eye Lines

Without showing your first-time patients the following demonstration, they will think that your crow's feet injections did not work.

First, you hand your patient a mirror and ask them to look in the mirror and wink one eye without closing the other.

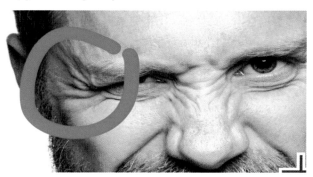

Figure 93. The orbicularis oculi cause crow's feet.

Then, while pointing to the crow's feet, you say to the patient, "Those are the lines that happen from closing your eye—your crow's feet. I can 'soften' those lines [never say you can make something go completely away]."

Then, say to the patient, "Now, keep both eyes open and smile very big.

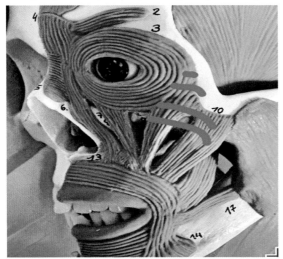

Those lines are from the smile muscles, and I will not be able to make those go away when I treat the crow's feet."

Continuing, you say, "If I BoNT your smile muscles, you will look like you had a stroke."

The smile muscles make some of the same lines as those made by the orbicularis oculi. By demonstrating this to your patient using the mirror, on their own face, you give them realistic expectations and avoid the phone call where they tell you that your BoNT did not work.

Figure 94. "Smile muscles" make lines that overlap with crow's feet.

Where to Put the Needle

To find where to put the injections to soften crow's feet, first palpate, *very gently*, the orbital rim.

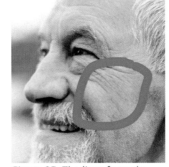

Figure 95. The lines from the "smile muscles" overlap with the crow's feet and do not go away when you treat orbicularis oculi.

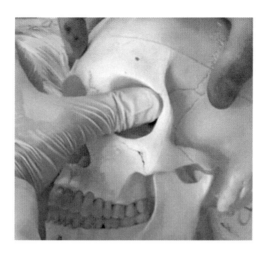

Figure 96. Palpating the orbital rim very gently. Then the injections are placed about 1/2 to 1 cm lateral to the orbital rim.

After gently palpating the orbital rim, I usually put three dots of two units each. The blebs are separated by about ½ cm and placed about ½ cm from the orbital rim and injected sub-q from a tangential orientation.

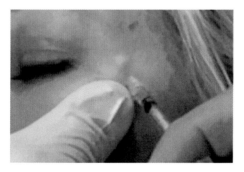

Figure 97. Injecting crow's feet: shallow and tangential orientation of the needle about ½ cm from the orbital rim.

The skin and the muscle here are extremely thin; so, the injection works better done sub-q. I am not trying to go deep into the muscle.

Also, after finding the orbital rim by gently palpating the rim with the tip of my left thumb (I am right-handed) and visualizing the injection points, then I move my left thumb to a place inferior to where I intend to inject so that I can stabilize the skin.

241

More About the Amount

If someone is over 30 years old, then each injection is two units.

If I treat a 20-year-old to prevent lines, I might, instead, only inject one unit in each of the three injection points. That gives a total of three units on each side.

If I am treating someone with deep lines (over 50 years old), I might inject three units in each injection point, for a total of nine units on each side.

Whatever the amount I plan to inject on each side, I start with one syringe for each side. For example, with most women, I will inject a total of six units per side, so I start with two syringes, each containing six units. Starting with a syringe per muscle group keeps me organized. But, more importantly, it helps me avoid hurting the patient. After about three injections, the syringes become significantly duller and more hurtful.

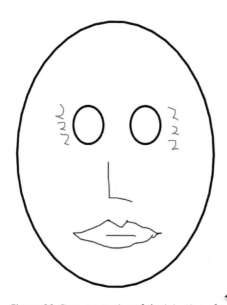

Figure 98. Documentation of the injection of six units on each side to treat crow's feet. to decrease pain, use two separate syringes (one for each side), each with six units.

If you succumb to temptation and wrap the injections all the way around, with more than three injection points and some of them below the eye, you may change the shape of the eye. But also, you may smooth out the skin inferolateral to the eye; but smooth it out so much that there can be a curtain effect causing new vertical lines that appear beneath the medial eye because you pulled the skin beneath the lateral eye so tightly that it appears the way curtains open and fold. So, I usually do that semi-circle of 3 injection points, two, two, and two, with most women because most women I'm treating are not 20, and they're not 80, but if I have deep lines, I might go three, three, and three.

Avoid the "Crow's Feet Catch"

If you see a vein lateral to the eye (as you often will), avoid it. But if you happen to catch it with your needle, no big deal. This is where your second hand comes in handy.

The mantra is *"If you need a band-aid, you're making a bruise."*

So, if I see brisk bleeding after injecting and inadvertently puncturing a superficial vein, I hold pressure. And *if I hold pressure immediately for a full minute, I will likely avoid a bruise.* This is why I always have gauze in my left hand when I am injecting with my right hand. Even the short time it takes to reach over and grab a gauze is enough time to cause a bruise.

You can see a video of me injecting crow's feet at BoNTClass.com

"Don't Touch This"

With all the BoNT I do, they can touch the injection point afterwards except for the crow's feet and the brow lift. In theory, if they rub where you treated crow's feet or for the brow lift, they can cause ptosis. So, I tell them to wait four hours before they touch near their eyes.

I will look at the clock, calculate a time 4 hours from my injection time, and tell them to wait until then before touching around their eyes.

For example, if it's 2:30 pm when I do their BoNT treatment, I would say, "Do whatever you want, have sex with your husband, go exercise, whatever, but don't touch this [pointing to where I injected] around your eyes until after 6:30."

What's Next
That's how you treat crow's feet. Next, we will discuss how to smooth the forehead.

30. INJECTION POINT #4:
THE FOREHEAD SMOOTHER

When I watch other teachers, I see more variation in how the forehead is injected than I do with any other part of the face. *With that much variation, perhaps it means that many different techniques work well.* I will show you how I think about the frontalis; take what has worked for me for two decades, learn it, study what others say, then create something new that you like better.

The danger of doing something for decades is that you start to believe everything you say. For everything I put in this course, there is something better that is yet to be found.

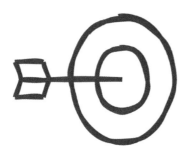

Find it!

But first, learn what has worked. *How do you know if you found something new and better until after you fully understand the existing?*

Where to Inject Frontalis

As with most facial muscles, *you cannot inject the frontalis accurately for the most beautiful results without watching the face move.* So, to inject the frontalis,

Figure 99. Changing the injection location by only a few millimeters can be the difference between a gorgeous result and a crazy face. But do not worry: the landmarks are easy.

first ask the patient to lift his brows as high as possible.

Then, look carefully, take a photo with the brows lifted and another photo at rest; then sit and study the photo.

Use the distribution of the horizontal lines to understand the distribution of the frontalis muscle.

With the frontalis, the muscle extends to approximately one half to one centimeter superior to the most superior line (wrinkle).

Remember: *Lines do not show you muscle; lines help you understand muscle.*

> *Do not inject lines.*
> *Inject muscles to treat lines.*

The other principle to remember when injecting the frontalis is that *the frontalis is the only muscle holding the brow up.* At least five other muscles pull the brow toward the floor. So, treating the frontalis with BoNT is like cutting the suspenders that hold the brows up (and there is no backup belt).

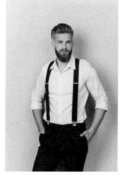

Figure 100. The frontalis acts as the only suspenders holding up the brows.

The Over Forty Frontalis Fix

Remember (from the previous chapters in this book} that I prefer to tailor-make the frontalis injections by treating the frontalis on a second visit between two to four weeks after treating the rest of the face.

Tell the patient, "Come back between two and four weeks," because if you tell them, "Come back *after* two weeks" (when BoNT reaches its most effectiveness), the patient may come back to see you at *eight* weeks when their BoNT will be starting to wear off; by then, they need a second treatment, not a touch-up of the first. Best is to make the appointment for two to four weeks before the patient leaves the office after the first treatment.

I also tell my first-time-to-get-BoNT patients, "The package insert says BoNT wears off at two months, but if you get BoNT every three months for a year, you will possibly be able to go down on the dosage or spread the treatments out to every four or five months."

When the patient comes back between two and four weeks, see how high her brows are when at rest. Sometimes, the brows may be high enough that she loves it and does not want to risk drooping them with a second treatment.

Sometimes her brows are not up so high, even before you treat the frontalis. In that case, especially in the woman over forty, warn her that

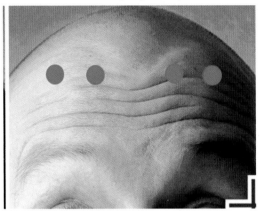

Figure 101. To preserve movement and to avoid dropping the brow, with a split frontalis in the person over forty, I often inject only two units at each of the blue dots (and do not inject the split in the center).

you may droop her brows if you treat her forehead.

Usually, I still proceed with treatment, but if she droops, she will still come back to see me and ask that we do not treat her forehead in the future. But, if I had treated the forehead on the first visit, and she drooped, I would have lost her as a patient forever.

So, usually we do treat the frontalis on the second visit. Then, after this first and second visit, on following visits (every three months for the first year), I will always treat the frontalis and the rest of the face all in one visit.

Split Frontalis
Here's the *usual distribution (from left to right) that I use for the woman or man over forty years old with a split frontalis: 2 units, 2 units, skip the split, 2 units, 2 units.*

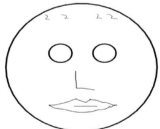

Figure 102. Documentation of treatment of the frontalis with a total of eight units with a split frontalis.

The rule is to *treat the forehead high on the forehead with the lowest effective dose to avoid drooping the brow* and to allow some natural expressions of happiness and surprise.

So, for the frontalis, *"Go high and low."*

246

Softening the Non-Split Frontalis

For the person without a split frontalis, I usually inject five points, instead of four, with two units each (since I need an additional two units to inject the center, where there is no split).

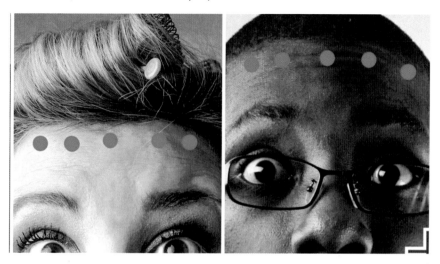

Figure 103. For a person over forty with a non-split frontalis, I usually inject five points with two units each (at the blue dots) to preserve some movement.

The Forehead Younger than Forty

For the person younger than forty, or the person over forty who shows a very high lift of the brow on the second visit, I will often use two or three rows of injections, with each injection point containing two units of BoNT.

The forehead is very forgiving; do not over think it. There are, however, three traps to avoid.

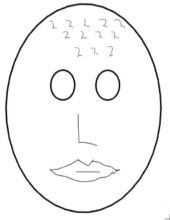

Figure 104. Documentation of a more aggressive, three-row, treatment of a non-split frontalis.

Three Frontalis Treatment Traps & How to Avoid Them

There are *three traps* that can trick you when treating the frontalis: all three lead to losing patients—forever. They are (1) the Neanderthal Trap, (2) the Spock Trap, and (3) the Touchy-About-Touch-Ups trap.

1. "Neanderthal Trap"

The most common trap that catches almost every new injector happens

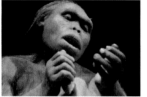

Figure 105. *Both the person with an over-treated frontalis and the Neanderthal man will demonstrate a heavy and drooped brow.*

in one of two ways (both create the Neanderthal look).

"Only Treat My Forehead"

The first way you may be tricked into making a Neanderthal happens when the patient says, "I only want the lines on my forehead treated—nothing else."

If you agree and only treat the frontalis to smooth their forehead but do not relax the muscles that pull the brow down (procerus, corrugators, orbicularis oculi), their forehead will smooth but you risk drooping their brow; they will walk around their home and their office for three months looking like a Neanderthal, and never return to your office.

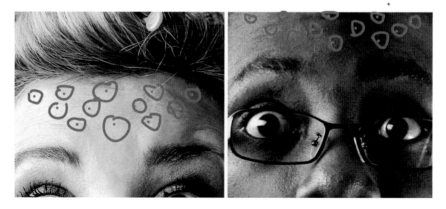

Figure 82. *One way to inject a strong or young forehead on the second visit: The top row has five injections of two units each; the second row has four injections of two units each; the third row has three injections of two units each.*

248

So, instead of agreeing to only threat the forehead, you take out your diagram of the facial muscles and explain, "The frontalis is the only muscle holding up the brow, so if you want to relax that muscle to smooth the brow, then we should also relax all the pull-down muscles to avoid drooping you."

If the patient insists that they only want their brow smoothed, then, at the least, also relax the procerus and both corrugators on the first visit; then see them back between two and four weeks and tailor-make where you treat the frontalis.

"Just Treat It All Today"
The second way you may be tricked into making a neanderthal will happen when your patient says, "My previous doctor just treated my forehead and the rest of my face all in one visit. Why do I need to make two trips?"

Then, you will be tempted to treat everything on the first visit. But there is a good chance that you will not do your best work (and perhaps droop the patient's brow) if you take this approach.

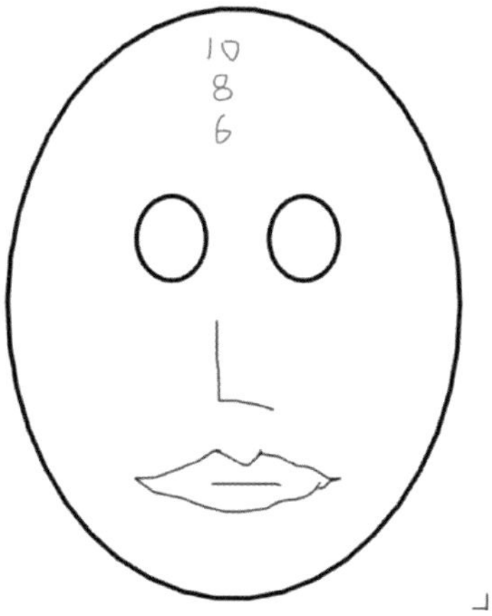

So, you answer the patient's request, "If you wish, I can treat both your forehead and the rest of your face all in one visit, but that does risk drooping you, but if I split your

Figure 106. An even shorter, short-hand notation for a three-row treatment of the frontalis.

treatment into two visits and treat your frontalis on the second visit, then I can tailor-make how I treat your frontalis and create a better shape."

Almost always, answering patients in this way will cause them to appreciate your efforts to make things as beautiful as possible by taking a more meticulous approach to understanding their face.

249

The Secret to Become Your Patient's Best Injector Ever

When they return for the second visit, you charge them to treat the as-yet untreated forehead, and you indeed tailor-make a gorgeous recipe for their frontalis; but you also do something else much more important than treating the forehead, and this "something else" is the little secret that helps you become the best injector they ever had: by giving them a reason to come back for the second visit before everything wears off, you get to see the results of what you did to the their entire face; (*before it wears off*), *you get to learn to be a better injector* by offering to "touch up" anything that is not perfect.

For example, if they still can contract the corrugators (weaker, but they still move), then you may decide to add another four units to each side. Or maybe you treated the triangularis, and only one side seems to have taken effect, so you add three units to one side even though your patient may not have even noticed.

I even tell my patients, "I will probably be pickier than you, and I will not charge you to touch up anything I think is not perfect."

The point is that you get to evaluate what you did and touch it up to make it better—*the ability to see your work before it wears off gives you a way of understanding that patient's individual face and a way to improve your overall injection skills*. That is the secret learning method that helps you become an excellent injector. The doctor who only sees the patient back after everything wears off will not learn in this way.

Summary of the Second Visit

When they come back for the second visit, you charge them for what you add to the frontalis, but you never charge them to touch up something you already treated. Instead, you thank them for teaching you how to better inject their face.

2. The "Spock Trap"

To avoid the second trap, tell them on their first visit that if they "Spock Out" at two weeks or even at two days (their brow jumps up so high that they look like Spock), you want to know about it immediately.

With that statement, you are implying more than what you said: you are warning them that if you do a great job with relaxing the pull-down muscles, there is a chance that instead of a perfect gull's wing shape, the brow could jump too high and that you are recognizing this as a possibility and if it happens it does not mean that you made a mistake. It just means that you did a great job of relaxing their frown.

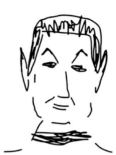

Figure 107. When an attempted gull's wing goes too high, the person looks "Spocked Out."

Other ways people describe the Spock Out is that they look "surprised all the time," or they "look like a clown," or "like the Joker."

If you do not warn your first-time patients that this could happen, then they may think you made a mistake and never come back. Instead, if you warn them and they then "Spock Out," they perceive that you have simply treated all the pull-downs and found that they have a strong frontalis; so now you know that you can treat their forehead aggressively without drooping them.

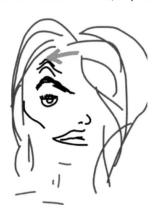

Figure 108. If someone "Spocks Out," simply add 2 units of BoNT at the peak of the "A" formed by the frontalis wrinkles. The brow and the wrinkles will relax to a gorgeous shape.

The "Spock Out" Second Visit
If they come back to you Spocked Out and they want to keep the brows high but lose the Spock look, the fix is very simple: put two units at the peak of the capital "A" (formed by the wrinkles). Those two units will drop the peak of the "A," and they will enjoy a natural look with a beautifully lifted brow.

You could also probably treat the whole frontalis in this person with two (maybe three) rows of BoNT with little risk of drooping them.

3. The "Touchy about Touchups" Trap

Even after you have injected someone's face for years, there will be times that, for some unknown reason, one small area on the forehead does not seem to work well.

The trap is that when the person calls or texts to tell you that something did not work as well as usual, you then express reluctance to see them—you just lost your patient.

The other way this trap gets you is if when you do see them, you charge them to touch up what did not turn out so perfect—*the patient will perceive that you charged them to fix your mistake, so you just lost them.*

To avoid the "touchy-about-touchups" trap (expressing frustration or charging your patient to touch up what you already charged them to do), when they complain about something not being perfect, you say to them (with a genuine smile), *"Thank you for letting me know. Come see me today at [time]. It will only take two minutes to touch things up. I do not want you walking around crooked."*

After you say that, they will come to see you, thank you for seeing them, and offer to pay you for the touch-up.

Do not take their money.

They will love you for standing behind your work.

They have made a second trip back (inconvenient and costly to them) to see you for something they already paid you to do, so consider the few extra units in the touch-up the price of your continuing education and *be grateful for the lesson and for the chance to keep your patient happy.*

You still made profit, and the patient will be devoted to you for life.

A Tip About Those Who Have Had a Surgical Facelift

Even if they are 90 years old, you will not likely droop them if they have undergone a recent surgical facelift. They will be lifted tightly enough that you can usually treat their frontalis aggressively with two or three rows of BoNT, and their brows will not droop.

31. INJECTION POINT #5: EYE OPENER

Why Open the Eye?

There are three reasons for opening the eye with BoNT: (1) asymmetry (one eye is wider than the other), (2) both eyes are more narrow than desired, and (3) the eyes are satisfactorily open when at rest but close more than wanted with smiling.

Asymmetry

In a group of four or five people, you can usually find at least one person with asymmetrical eyes—with one eye wider from top to bottom than the other.

Some people are unaware of the asymmetry. Some know but do not care. But often, there is enough asymmetry that the woman is aware of and would like to correct the asymmetry but does not know there is that possibility.

So, when someone is in your office for BoNT, always notice if there is an asymmetry of the eyes.

Then, if there is, offer to correct it by pointing it out in the mirror (or in a photo on your phone) and saying, "If you want, I can make your eyes even with only one unit of BoNT."

She will almost always want the correction. Moreover, this is a very simple correction; but she will become a regular client because you know this trick and offered it and no one else did.

Both Eyes Less Open than Desired

Sometimes, due to genetics, the woman wants both eyes opened a few millimeters when at rest. This occurs in every race but can be common with women of Asian descent. You can keep the beautiful Asian shape and show more of the color of her eye by using the eye-opening injection equally on both the left and the right.

Her eyes Close More than Desired When She Smiles

The third situation in which the eye-opening technique can help is when the woman finds her eyes to be satisfactory when at rest but notices (usually in her photos) that her eyes are almost closed when she smiles.

This complaint is almost never volunteered. You pick it up by taking photos in your office of her face at rest and while smiling.

Then, if in the photos you notice that her eyes nearly close when she smiles, you show her the photos of her smile and say, "Because you smile with your whole face, your eyes nearly close, and it becomes difficult to see the color of your eyes. If you want to adjust your eyes so that they can be better seen when you smile, I can do that with only two units of BoNT (one unit for each side)."

This adjustment of the eye-opening width while smiling seems to be something most wanted by professional models or by women in their twenties. Others may say yes, but those are the two main groups who love it.

Give This to Make Your Patients Happy and Your Profits Grow

When I have a new patient, if I see asymmetry in their eyes, I often will not even bring it up on their first visit. If I do bring it up, I show them the asymmetry but tell them we can treat it on the next visit if they want, but I want to learn their face and add more ideas later.

Here's one of my best marketing tips (that also helps you create better results):

Say less than you know,
Do less than you can,
And patients will always
Believe your plan.

What you do, you do with excellence, but you save some treatments for a future visit, or else people feel like you did all you could to take as much money as you could; then they have less reason to come back because they think you have nothing left to offer.

But, if you point out the ideas you might want to try in the future, even if it is only a tiny idea like treating one eye, they feel more as if you are taking a stepwise, strategic approach (which you are) instead of trying to take every penny you can from them (which you are not).

Then, when they come back for the second or third visit, I might say to them, "I have thought during your previous visits that you may really like it if I correct the asymmetry of your eyes (or whatever other additional treatment you want to offer). Let me give you the treatment for free today (they still pay me for their usual treatment). If you like this new idea, then you can pay for it as part of your next treatment. If you do not like it, then we will leave it off your next treatment—no big deal."

For something that you think might help but that the patient did not really know or ask for, this try-free approach makes it easier for them to say "yes."

Of course, I never offer anything unless I feel the patient will love it. But, by giving it to them the first time, I take away resistance they may have to something new. Then, when they love it, they are grateful and more attached to me because I found a new way to improve their appearance and gave it to them. If they do not like it, they do not feel like I pushed them to do something unhelpful just so I could take more money.

Most people have a strong sense of reciprocity and will repay you with devotion (never paying attention to the Groupon deals in someone else's office) if you routinely give them more than they expect.

Ectropion & A Warning About Treating Eyes

For an older person with weaker muscles, sometimes there can be an ectropion of the lids with a turning outward severe enough to require surgical correction. Of course, you would never BoNT the lids of someone with an ectropion; the warning is that the older person may not have an ectropion, but when you treat their lower lid with BoNT, you can cause an ectropion resulting in a chronically dry eye due to difficulty blinking.

The Snap Test (Learn It, then Forget It)

The usual proposed way to avoid causing an ectropion with your BoNT treatments is to do the "Snap Test."

How to Do the Snap Test

To do the Snap Test, pull gently down on the lower lid for a few seconds; then, you release the pulldown and see how long it takes for the lower lid to "snap" back into place. If there is a delay in the lid snapping back to the resting position, then you do not treat the lower lid with BoNT (you never treat the upper lid, that would cause ptosis).

How to Grade the Snap Test
Here's how you grade the Snap Test:

Grade 0-IV (0 = normal, IV = severe laxity):

 *Grade 0 – a normal lid that returns to position immediately on release

 *Grade I – it takes 2-3 sec for the lid to return

 *Grade II - 4-5 sec

 *Grade III - >5 sec but does return to normal position with blinking

 *Grade IV - never returns to position and continues to hang down in frank ectropion after the snap-back test

Now Forget It

Learn that test if you want. Some people use it as a guide, so I am showing it to you.

But *I never do the Snap Test.*

I showed you the test, so you know about it when you go to your next hands-on class, and so you do not think I am ignorant about its existence and think, "Why did he not teach the snap test?"

But my rule is that I do not treat your lower lids if you are old enough to need a snap test (usually patients over 70 years old). But no matter how old the patient, if they have such poor enough muscle tone that I think to do the snap test, I skip the test and do not do the treatment. Why risk making someone unable to blink for months?

256

There is never a reason to be a cowboy when doing BoNT.

Exactly Where to Put the Needle

It is important to put the needle in exactly the right place when you do this injection. But it is easy to do and causes almost no pain.

First, ask the patient to look straight ahead (you may need to hold up your finger to give them a focal point).

Then, with the eyes looking straight ahead, you will see the iris in the center and the sclera, both medial and lateral to the iris.

With the patient's eyes looking straight ahead, find the spot one or two millimeters below the lower lash line that is in line with the lateral edge of the iris: this is where you inject. But, if you try to inject with their eyes looking straight ahead, they will blink.

So, after you identify the spot where you will inject, then ask the patient to look up (keeps them from blinking when they see the needle coming) and inject.

When you inject, barely go in with your needle (only just beyond the lumen of the needle) and make a sub-q bleb (two millimeters below the lash line and in line with the lateral edge of the iris).

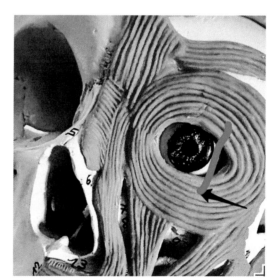

Figure 109. The orbicularis oculi are injected in line with the lateral edge of the iris about 1-2mm below the lash line using a lateral-tangential approach.

Not only do you avoid the patient blinking when injecting with the lateral approach, but it is also not as scary for the patient (as is coming straight

257

at her eye). With a lateral approach, she knows that if I get bumped, I won't poke her eye. If I approach from the front, even if her logic tells her otherwise, her lizard brain worries that I am about to stick a needle in her eye.

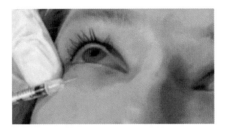

Figure 110. To widen the eye in the resting or smiling position, inject in line with the lateral edge of the iris; use a tangential approach while the patient looks up; only the lumen of the needle is inserted to create a small bleb (done properly, there will be no pain or bruising).

You never want your patient to worry while you are treating them. You want them to go into a parasympathetic state of relaxation.

So, I slip the needle in from the side; there is no pain to that. It is a little pesky, but there is no pain to it.

Important: to Keep from Injecting Too Much

You *cannot* measure one or two units accurately with a fifty or a one-hundred-unit syringe. So, always use a 30-unit insulin syringe (BD Brand) with a 31-gauge needle.

Do this injection (and all injections of only one or two units) with a syringe that starts with only the intended amount in it. That is the only purpose of the syringe and after using it, you discard the syringe.

You carefully draw up the BoNT to something more than one unit, then empty it to only one unit. Then, you simply and easily empty the entire syringe when you inject the orbicularis oculi. This strategy keeps you from inadvertently injecting more than you intended (which would be easy to do if you tried to inject only one unit out of a syringe that contained five or ten units).

You can see now why the BoNT board (see the first two modules of this course) helps you stay organized. When preparing for a complete facial treatment, you often fill ten or twelve different syringes. Without the board, the syringes are easily shuffled into disorder by just a bump of your mayo stand—wasting your time.

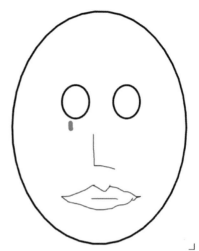

Figure 111. Documenting injecting one unit of BoNT into the patient's right orbicularis oculi.

32. INJECTION POINT #6:
BUNNY LINES ERASER

Bunny lines can be seen when people "scrunch" their noses.

These lines appear as dynamic wrinkles, most prominently in someone who has been getting BoNT for several years; when the person squints

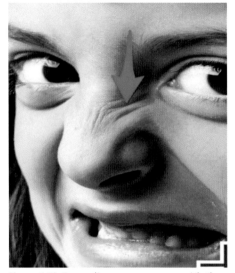

in the sun, they cannot use the corrugators, so instead, they use the nasalis to narrow the eyes, and that makes bunny lines.

Facial Muscles Allow You to Read Minds

One of the fascinations of the facial muscles is that they are contracted at varying degrees in relation to emotions. So, the facial muscles allow us to see emotions in real time. To see photos of the nasalis in action, on a stock photo

Figure 112. Bunny lines, appear even with the face at rest in someone who has gotten BoNT for several years.

database, you search for the term "disgust." The nasalis will also contract when someone is laughing and when angry.

Finding the Nasalis Injection Point

Find the nasalis of your patient by contracting your own nasalis while you say to the patient, "*Scrunch up your nose.*"

Often, when they "scrunch" their nose, they will also contract the corrugators and procerus; when they do, it is OK; you can still see what you need to see: the nasalis pulling up the skin to make a bridge going from nose to cheek.

260

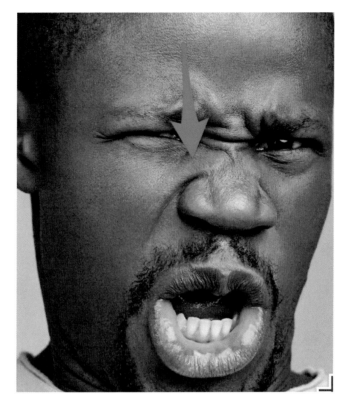

Figure 113. Showing disgust with contraction of the corrugators, procerus, and nasalis.

Your injection goes into that bridge about one-half centimeter from the center of the nose.

![Injection point for nasalis]

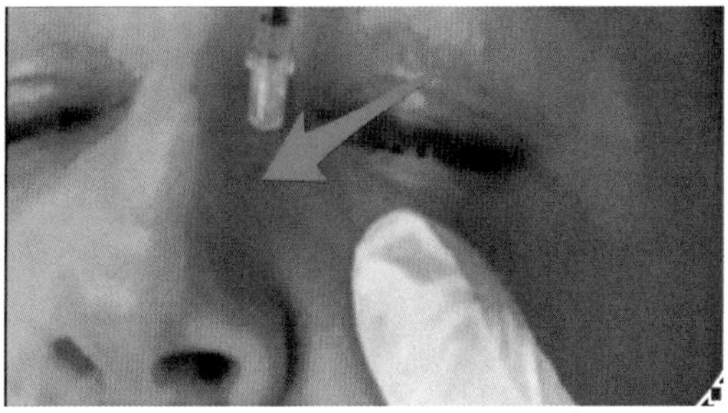

Figure 114. Injection point for nasalis is 1/2 cm from the center of the nose at the location of the bridge made with nasalis contracted. Find the injection point with the muscle contracted. Then ask the patient to relax the muscle before doing the injection.

In a previous lesson, when I opened the eye with BoNT, I used a syringe with only one unit so that I did not inadvertently inject too much (which could easily accidentally happen if I had more than one unit in the syringe).

The nasalis is treated similarly; pull up two units into two separate syringes (for a total of four units).

261

After you find the injection point with her nose scrunched, before you inject, ask her to relax her nose.

BoNT-Technique Order
1. Ask the patient to contract the muscle.
2. Watch, understand, and decide.
*3. Ask the patient to **relax the muscle.***
*4. **Inject.***

The nasalis treatment is not a deep injection. Insert only about one-half of the needle (but if you accidentally insert the whole needle, you will do no harm).

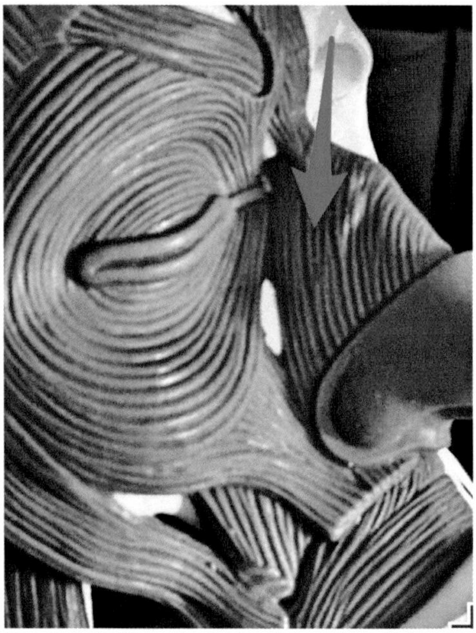

Further Help

You can see a movie of me injecting the nasalis at BoNTClass.com (for less than what you will be paid by one BoNT patient).

Figure 115. The orientation & location of the needle when treating the nasalis. Use two separate syringes, each with two units.

33. INJECTION POINT #7: GUMMY SMILE ERASER

What is a Gummy Smile?

I will usually see a gummy smile in one person out of a gathering of twenty.

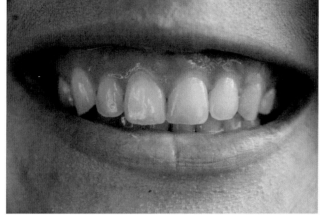

Figure 116. The gummy smile can be endearing, and some would rather not treat it. If the person is bothered by their gummy smile, they are usually most displeased about their smile in photos.

I don't know why, but it usually correlates with blondes and redheads, but not always. I see it in every ethnic group.

When the upper lip rises higher (with smiling) than usual, you see more of the upper gums than usual; hence the name, a "gummy smile."

Example of Gummy Smile You Should Not Treat

Kat Timpf is a comedian, libertarian journalist, and Cable News personality.

She has taken off her glasses on camera and admitted that the glasses are for show; she does not need them to better see. You can look at her photos and discern the same by noticing that there is no refraction of the lenses—there is a smooth line of her brows and lashes between what you see through the lenses and what you see outside the lenses.

So, why does she wear the glasses?

Answer: They make her look vulnerable—not perfect.

She also has a gummy smile.

People do not usually fall in love with perfect people. By wearing glasses and keeping her gummy smile, she is more lovable even when she is brilliant and gorgeous.

Put another way, she would not be as funny or likeable without the

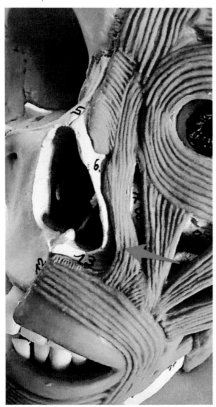

gummy smile; her intellect and beauty would risk making her too perfect, more enviable, and not as loveable to some of her audience.

So, some people should keep their gummy smile and others want it treated.

How do you decide whom to treat? That's next...

The Question to Ask to Discover if You Should Treat a Gummy Smile

Most people do *not* want to keep their gummy smile; they dislike it but do not know that you can easily treat it. As a possible fix, they have usually been offered only expensive, painful surgeries by a dentist or

Figure 117. Where to insert the needle when treating levator labii.

an oral surgeon (not out of malice, but because only about half of the states in the U.S. allow dentists to inject BoNT). The dentist may not know there is an easier treatment than surgery.

To find out if someone wants their gummy smile treated, I ask them the following question after they are already on my BoNT treatment bed: "I notice that when you smile, I can see your upper gums. That can bother some people when they look at their photos because it looks like their smile is too big. If you want me adjust your smile, I can do so with only four units of BoNT."

Almost always, but not always, they will answer, "Really!?! Yes, please, let's do it!"

After you treat a gummy smile with BoNT, you often help a teenager, or an older woman feel more confident when she is having her photograph made. That may not be curing cancer, but that is still a good day's work.

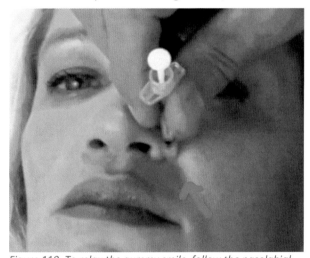

Where to Put the Needle & How to Inject

The *levator labii* is the primary muscle that lifts the corners of the mouth. *It passes by an easy-to-find landmark—the nose.*

Figure 118. To relax the gummy smile, follow the nasolabial fold until it reaches the nose. Then, with the syringe touching the nose, insert the needle. Aim the needle neither left, right, up, or down; aim straight at the back of the patient's head. Inject 2 units on each side for a total of 4 units.

And, you actually have a line drawn to show you where to insert the needle to relax the levator labii. Follow the nasal labial fold starting at the mouth and going up until it meets the nose.

Lightly touch the spot (where the nasolabial fold meets the nose) to avoid surprising your patient; then, aim the needle straight toward back of the patient's head; quickly go in with the needle (stopping at the hub); inject quickly and pull out quickly.

There is no advantage to pulling the needle out slowly.

Use two units for each side. As with the eye, use a separate syringe for each side.

Doing this injection will often aggravate your patient. Since your needle is close to their nose, it is like a fly landing on their nose. Though not painful, something about goofing with their nose makes them angrier than (for example) goofing with their elbow.

Who knows why; it just does.

But nobody ever dies with BoNT.

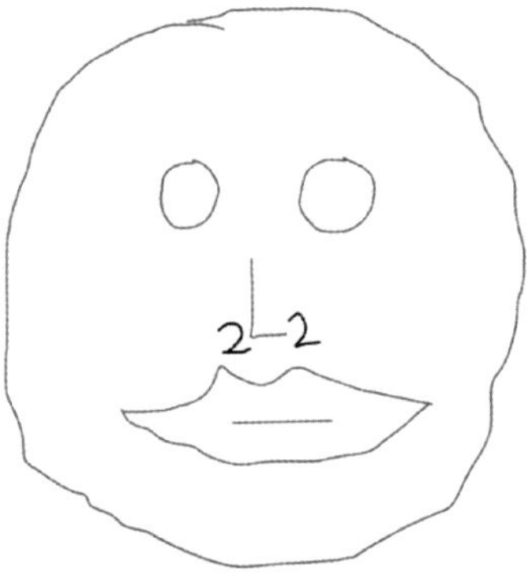

Figure 119. A simple sketch in chart to document two units on each side to treat gummy smile.

Warning (to Avoid Making Your Patient Look as If She Had a Stroke)

This is one of those injections where if you dilute the BoNT as they suggest in the package insert (using more than twice the volume to reconstitute than what I recommend), then two units will spread twice as far when you relax the levator labii and perhaps inadvertently relax a muscle not intended—causing a crooked smile.

The patient then looks as if she had a stroke.

But by doing my recommended dilution of only one milliliter of bacteriostatic saline per one hundred units of Cosmetic BoNT, you are shooting with a rifle (instead of a shotgun), precisely into a small space.

How Valuable is This Simple Little Trick?

I just showed you how to treat a gummy smile.

So, what?

It is so simple. Can that really be a big deal?

266

I have enjoyed the honor of a noticeable number of people trusting me with for almost two decades *for all their cosmetic work* (and bringing their families), mostly because I am the one person who offered this simple little treatment for their gummy smile. But, *because I treated their gummy smile, they avoided painful expensive surgeries.* And for that, they are grateful and loyal and perceive me as an expert.

Do not underestimate the value of offering this service. Like many ideas in medicine, the reward to the patient is much greater than the skill required by you to offer the technique.

The value to patients
does not correlate
to your difficulty
to prepare the plate.

Further Help

To watch a video of me treating a gummy smile, go to BoNTClass.com. Also, see the section at the end of this course, called "Further Help."

34. INJECTION POINT #8:
FROWN ERASER

Sculpture or Engineering?

Injecting fillers involves thinking about shapes and using your right brain, but BoNT mostly involves engineering, your left brain.

When you consider where to put hyaluronic acid fillers, you think, "How much should I inject and where to cause the desired change in shape."

Considering shape is a right-brain art question.

When you look at the face to inject BoNT, you think, "If I relax this belt (facial muscle), how does it change the expression of the face; which 'pleats' does it pull out?"

That is a left-brain, engineering question involving "ropes" and "pulleys."

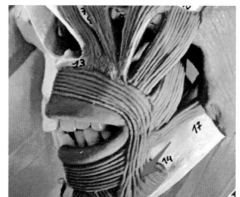

The Triangularis Connections

As an example of thinking in terms of left-brain engineering, consider the depressor anguli oris

Figure 120. Depressor anguli oris (triangularis) muscle.

(DAO). I prefer the synonym "triangularis."
It starts at the corner of the mouth (where it attaches to the skin), then it comes down, broadens to make a triangular shape, and attaches to the mandible (bone).

When the DAO contracts, it pulls the corner of the mouth toward the mandible, causing a sad or angry expression. If, in the resting state, the DAO overpowers the levator labi and other "smile" muscles, then the resting expression of the face looks angry or sad (some call "resting b**ch face").

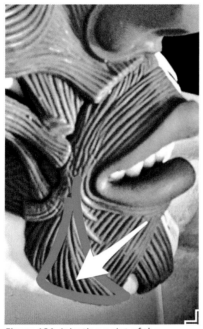

Figure 121. Injection point of the depressor anguli oris.

Who Wants Their Frown Fixed?

If you put filler in the lower face, for any reason, then BoNT in the lower face can help the fillers last longer (decreased movement increases the longevity of fillers).

So, I treat the DAOs for two reasons: (1) when someone shows resting downturned corners of the mouth or (2) to increase the longevity of hyaluronic acid (HA) fillers after injecting HA below the corners of the mouth or around the chin.

Some people inject the DAOs near the corners of the mouth. But the margin of error is small near the corner; if you inject near the corner and the BoNT spreads even a few millimeters in the wrong direction, you could inadvertently relax one of the adjacent smile muscles and cause the smile to be asymmetric—the patient then looks as if she's had a stroke for the next two to three months.

Since the whole muscle is relaxed if you inject any part of it, a more reliable strategy is to inject the DAO near the mandible where the muscle is broad and there are fewer adjacent muscles.

If you watch the videos on our <u>Vampire Facelift® membership</u> website (<u>https://vampirefacelift.com/members</u>) you will see how I use fillers to prop up the corners of the mouth. When I do that prop up with fillers, I tell the woman to go ahead and add BoNT in the DAO so that *the two strategies (BoNT and fillers) work in synergy* to lift the corners.

Where to Put the Needle

Here's how you measure where to put your needle when you inject the DAOs: First, put your needle right where the nasolabial fold meets the nose.

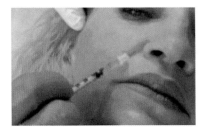

Figure 122. The starting point for measuring to inject the DAO's.

Then wrap your needle across the corner of the mouth and down onto the mandible. Where the barrel of your syringe crosses the mandible is where you do the injection.

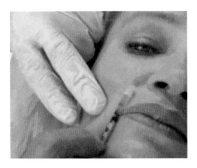

Figure 123. Wrapping the syringe around to find the place where you will insert the needle.

Another way to find the injection point is to ask them to turn down the corners of their mouth (frown). You will see where the muscle is pulling at the insertion site when they do.

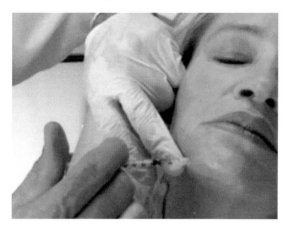

Figure 124. Injecting the broad base of the DAO.

I find this second method (asking them to frown) to be more confusing; it involves seeing something more subtle than the nose, the nasolabial fold, and the corner of the mouth. So, I prefer the first method where I put the needle where the nasolabial fold touches the nose and then wrap the syringe across the corner of the mouth and down to the mandible: *where the barrel of the syringe crosses the mandible is where you inject.*

Aim the syringe horizontally (see the figure), with the needle aimed towards the mandible and then inject five units into the muscle; this one is deep. Touch the mandible with the needle, then inject.

I usually put five units on each side for a total of 10 units. Use one syringe that starts with 10 units and inject ½ on each side.

Other Ways

As with everything that I am showing you, there are many ways to do this injection. I'm showing you what I think is the most reliable method with the least chance of causing an unexpected and unwanted outcome.

Some doctors are fearful of injecting the lower face at all. I think, perhaps, their fear of unpredictable results is either because they are using a dilution that causes their BoNT to spread and relax surrounding muscles (using more than one cc to reconstitute a 100-unit vial), or they are using a different technique that makes the results less reliable and less accurate. So, if you are a beginner, do as I have shown you for a while; then, if you want to create a better way, go for it. Please write to me (or write your own book) and teach me your better way after you find it. I will be eager to learn.

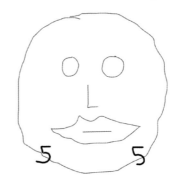

Figure 125. A simple diagram for chart documenting five units in each triangularis.

Be glad for you what you know.
But know:
Everything you know
becomes a mirror show.

What to Say & Do to Keep Your Patients from Leaving after a Triangularis Treatment

People seem to either love the results when you inject their DAOs, or they think it does not help at all. It is a pass-fail system, much more so than the other injection points. I am not sure why.

What to Say to Keep Them from Leaving

To prepare the patient (and avoid discouragement), before I do the triangularis injection, I say the following: "You're either going to love this, or you're going to think it does not help. If you love it, we'll keep doing it; if you do not love it, we won't do it again. Do you want to give it a try?"

By forewarning them of the two possibilities and giving them the option to try the injection or not, they are less likely to be upset if they see no benefit. In contrast, you can always relax the corrugators, but relaxing the DAOs is less reliable, so use my little speech, and your patient will not be upset if they see no benefit.

It is worth the try, though. People who love it (more than ½ of those you treat) will want it every time you treat them.

What to Do to Keep Them from Leaving

If the person calls you two days after you treated their triangularis and says, "My smile is crooked," then ask them to text a photo of their mouth at rest and another while smiling.

If their smile is crooked (one corner higher than the other), the side that is lower than the other is the side where the DAO was not affected by the BoNT. Bring them back to the office and inject the lower side (measure in the same way but go slightly more medial with the injection).

Always makeup in a way
that makes your patient say,
"Your mistake made a better day."

Do this touchup for free; they are not responsible for the asymmetry. They will forgive the trouble to come back to see you if you get them in quickly and treat them. If you charge them to fix the asymmetry, they will never come back.

When you touch up their crooked smile, you might suggest that you omit the DAO on their next treatment and give them one of your facial creams or ten percent off their next visit.

273

Never leave anyone feeling damaged, even by the inconvenience of the return visit. Make up by giving something to them that they value more than the trouble resulting from what they view as your mistake.

35. INJECTION POINT #9: ORANGE PEEL CHIN

"Crinkle, Please"

An orange peel chin, also known as "peau d'orange," is a condition where the skin on the chin appears dimpled or uneven, like the texture of an orange peel. The condition can be caused by the accumulation of fat deposits beneath the skin, resulting from genetics, weight gain, or hormonal changes. It can also be caused by repetitive contraction of the mentalis muscle.

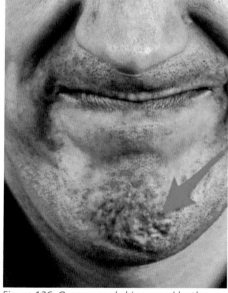

Figure 126. Orange-peel chin caused by the mentalis muscle.

You can see the activity of your patient's mentalis muscle by saying to them, "Crinkle your chin please."

Whom Should You Treat?

Some carry tension in their lower face and crinkle their chin as a frequent expression; this habit can make them look worried and age their appearance. This frequent-chin-crinkling person seems to benefit most from treating the mentalis; but one who usually enjoys a relaxed chin would not likely benefit.

If I try to show the habitual chin crinkler what I intend to treat by holding a mirror, for some reason (that I do not understand), he will almost always relax his mentalis when I hand him the mirror. Therefore, it is difficult to use a mirror to show the patient their contraction of the mentalis.

So, instead of showing their mentalis contractions to them in the mirror, I take a picture of their chin while they are contracting it (they see me take the photo but do not know why).

An Orange Peel chin
Will not a lover win.

Then, I show them their mentalis in action in the photo (on my iPhone) and say, *"Contracting your chin like this seems to be something that you often do. You are one of many who carry tension in their chin. This is called 'orange-peel chin.'* If you want, I can help your face relax and help you look younger by treating your chin with only four units of BoNT."

They most often answer with something like, "Uggghhh! Yes, please!"

Where to Put the Needle

After you scare the person with a photo of their contracted mentalis, you will need to know where to put the needle. As a rule, stay close to but not directly in the center of the chin. If you inject too laterally, you inadvertently effect muscles involved in smiling and make their mouth crooked.

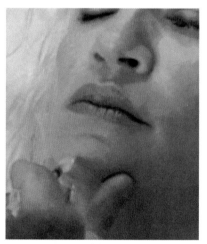

Figure 127. One of the two injection points for the mentalis (inject both sides of the center of the chin).

Here's how I do it:

First, I ask them to crinkle their chin so I can see the distribution of the mentalis.

276

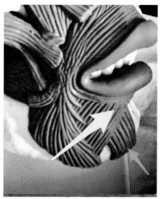

Figure 128. The large yellow arrow points to where the mentalis attaches to bone. The green arrow points to where the muscle attaches to skin.

Then, I ask them to relax their chin, and I imagine a dot right in the center of the chin.

Then, I inject at about ½ cm on either side of the dot (two separate injections) and within the area where I previously saw dimples.

I usually inject four units, two on each side.

For this one, I use one syringe loaded with the entire four units and inject one-half of the syringe on each side. If one side receives slightly more than the other, it will not create the same asymmetry that happens if you are slightly off when injecting the levator labii.

A Tip for Injecting Mentalis

The next time you want to relax for three hours, watch Kirk Douglas in his 1960s movie *Spartacus*. Notice the dimple in the center of his chin.

See it.

Then imagine it when you inject the mentalis; put two units on either side of the imagined dimple. It's a great landmark (and I think *Spartacus* with Kirk Douglas may be the best movie ever made).

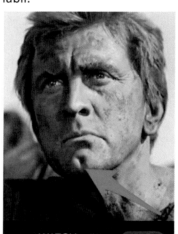

Figure 129. Imagine Kirk Douglas' chin in Spartacus and inject 2 units just on either side (but not into) the dimple.

Why Do You Need a Mentalis Muscle Anyway?!

I can easily see why I need most of the muscles of my face: the temporalis to chew, the orbicularis oculi to keep my eyes moist and to protect them, for example. But why do I need a mentalis muscle?

The mentalis muscle helps with movement of the lower lip and the protrusion of the lower jaw. It connects to bone at the incisive fossa on the anterior aspect of the mandible and inserts into the skin of the chin.

Since it is involved in wrinkling skin on the chin and protruding the lower lip, it is sometimes referred to as the "pouting muscle." It is also used when speaking certain sounds, such as "m" and "b."

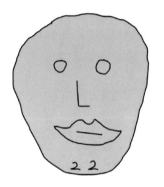

Figure 130. Simple documentation diagram of injecting the mentalis with two units of BoNT on each side.

Mentalis Warning

Because it is involved with speech, I avoid treating the mentalis in professional speakers, singers, attorneys, and actors—people who make their career with their speech and may suffer from a change in their enunciation.

Note: the mentalis treatment is much less likely to change speech than is injecting the orbicularis oris muscle (injection point # 12 in this course), which should never be injected in professional speakers and singers.

I have never had anyone other than professional speakers (singers, newscasters, etc.) complain of their speech changing after injecting either the mentalis or the orbicularis oris.

Most who habitually crinkle their chin love the mentalis treatment.

Further Help
You can watch me inject the mentalis on the videos at BoNTClass.com

36. INJECTION POINT #10: WEBBED NECK

Platysma Bands

There are two techniques you can do to improve the neck. The first to consider is platysma bands. We cover the next technique, "necklace lines," in the next chapter "Injection Point #11."

What Are Platysma Bands?

The platysma extends from the fascia of the pectoralis major and the deltoid to the level of the corner of the mouth.

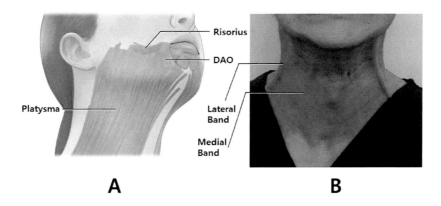

Figure 131. The lateral and medial bands of the platysma are created by its edges; two edges for the left and two for the right platysma--making four bands. Photo courtesy of Yi et al. (2022); © Yi et al. (2022).

Its extent across the center of the neck varies but usually spares the center especially in the lower half.

The pull of the platysma can contribute to *pulling the corners of the mouth downturned* and *worsen the contour of jowls.*

The platysma's anterior and posterior lateral edges create "bands."

The Treatment of Platysma Bands: Two Methods

For almost two decades, I have used a conservative treatment of platysma bands that uses only twenty units in total. This conservative

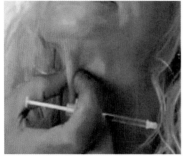

Figure 132. Grabbing a platysma band while the patient says, "Eeeeeee." Screen shot from a video on BoNTClass.com.

method works great for most, but not all. So, I am going to also show you a more aggressive, more expensive, but sure-to-accomplish-maximal-relaxation strategy that uses forty units in total.

With both techniques, to see the platysma bands, you ask the patient to say, "Eeeeeeeeeeee."

While they say that, you will see the platysma bands jut out from the neck.

Where to Put the Needle: "Save Strategy"

For a conservative, save-your-patient's-money approach that accomplishes the most with the least amount of BoNT, watch your patient's neck when she says, "Eeeeeeeee."

Then, as she says "eeee," grab one of the bands *in its most prominent place of protrusion* using the thumb and forefinger of your non-dominant hand.

Then, inject multiple injections of about 2 units each, with the injection points separated by about 2 cm. The needle depth is only sub q or even intradermal; if you go too deep, you miss the platysma.

Dilution Change for Three Places

The dilution for the platysma bands (injection point #10), for necklace lines (injection point #11), and for the mouth (injection point #12) can work better if you use a separate bottle to which you add 2 ml of bacteriostatic saline to 100 units of BoNT (instead of one milliliter).

The reason for the increased dilution (everything else in this course is done with a dilution of 1 ml added to 100 units of BoNT) is that you want the BoNT to spread more. If the BoNT spreads too much when injecting the levator labii (for example), you can create a crooked smile; but if the BoNT spreads more when injecting the platysma or the orbicularis oris, you see a better result.

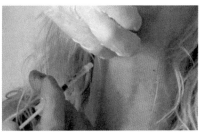

Figure 133. Holding the most prominent part of a platysma band with the non-dominant hand while injecting with the dominant hand (screen shot from video on BoNTClass.com).

With this most conservative method of treating the platysma, you plan the distribution of a total of twenty units (for the entire neck) such that *you treat only the most prominent parts of the four bands and leave the remaining parts of the bands untreated.*

Important: You do not inject more than 20 units in total but inject differently for each patient since *the prominent parts of the bands will vary from person to person and even from treatment to treatment in the same person.* You are truly "tailor making" your BoNT treatment.

The idea with this conservative treatment is that by strategically placing the BoNT, you achieve an excellent result with the least possible amount of BoNT. If you want a more aggressive but still safe method of treatment, then the following "sure strategy" will give a beautiful result.

Where to Put the Needle: "Sure Strategy"

If the patient's platysma bands do not respond to her satisfaction when you use the conservative strategy, then the following strategy by Yi et al. (2022) will give her maximum results.

To inject the bands using this method, inject two units in five points in each of the four bands.

(2 units/point) x (5 points/band) x (4 bands) = 40 units in total

The needle only goes subdermally. There can be some fatty tissue here; still, it is easy to go too deep with your needle and have no effect on the

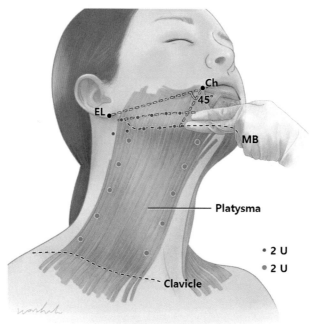

Figure 134. Each green dot represents 2 units of BoNT injected sub q to treat the platysma bands. The red dots represent two units each to lift the jaw line--done less frequently than are platysma bands and described in more detail in Yi et al (2022). Diagram © by and courtesy of Yi et al (2022) under the usual open-source commons.

platysma. If you are at the right depth, you will see a subdermal bleb at each point after you do the injection. If you do not see a bleb after each injection, you are injecting too deep; nothing bad happens, you just do not achieve the intended results.

If you are using the dilution of 2 cc added to 100 units of BoNT, then 2 units would be 0.04 cc in your syringe (4 units in a 30-unit insulin syringe). With the usual dilution of 1 cc added to 100 unites of BoNT (what is used for the other injection points), 2 units is only 0.02 cc on your syringe (2 units on a 30-unit insulin syringe).

You double the volume for the same amount of BoNT when you add 2 cc instead of 1.

Documentation: Why I Prefer Paper & Pen (not iPad)

At the bedside, I have tried many electronic ways of avoiding the use of pen and paper. I have bought tens of thousands of dollars in software and too many devices with their associated pens. Everything I have tried at the bedside (not at my computer) is noticeably slower than a simple pen and paper.

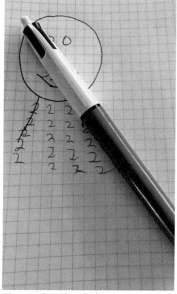

Figure 135. Sketch illustrating 10 units in all 4 platysma bands. Also, note the 4-color Bic pen. I have a few pens that cost an embarrassing amount of money. But this is the pen I prefer to use to make accurate and clear notes. It was invented in 1970, when I was 10 years old. I have used it for the past 50 years. (Available on Amazon.com).

If I want a digital version of my sketch, I snap a photo of it (as in the figure on this page) and save it in the same file as the photos of the patient's face.

When I am at my computer, I may sketch directly onto a photo using iPhoto or Skitch (which integrates with Evernote).

But, when I am at the bedside, I do not like to fiddle with a laptop or iPad; I want to focus on the patient, not stare at a screen. I know that, for insurance purposes, some may need to use an electronic medical record; that need is one of the reasons that I quit accepting insurance of any kind in 2003.

Nothing, for me, is as quick and as accurate as a sketch on paper.

As for using paper in general, I also like the fact that *the smartest computer programmer cannot hack into a paper file in a filing cabinet locked in my office.*

My patients will never get an email from me that says, "I am sorry, someone hacked into your chart."

My office also has a burglar alarm. And I live in Alabama, where (except in Birmingham) crime is very low, so it is very unlikely that anyone will break into my office, partly because a good percentage of us have guns. So, my records are safe, and I do not apologize for the fact that they are on paper; I am relieved and so are my patients.

I also like to use a four-color Bic pen so that I can use a different color for the location of BoNT vs. fillers on the same sketch (or with the units in one color and the face sketch in another), making it easier to document my treatments.

I also use the SketchWow app on my MacBook to make sketches (and used it to make some of the sketches in this course). But I use pen and paper instead of the computer to make sketches when I can.

A Mother is Glad to See Me Write on Paper

Last week, when I was about to BoNT the face of a new patient, I said to her, "I take privacy very seriously. If I meet you in public, I will pretend not to know you. Because many people in my town know that I am a physician, if I even speak to you, then it could prompt questions from onlooking friends and family about why you might be my patient. Also, I keep my records on paper locked in a filing cabinet locked in my office, because no one can use a computer and hack into a paper chart."

She replied, "Thank you very much! I recently received an email notice from my child's dentist that all their records had been hacked and the charts of my children were now compromised and known to other people."

Everyone loves a good secret.

Everyone loves people who can keep secrets. Be outrageously obsessed with your patient's privacy and they will reward you with their respect and gratitude.

If secrets you can keep,
Many patients will for you seek.

When you walk the street,
Do not know the patients you meet.

If they speak first,
To them, you may reply;
But you never mention why
As you look them in the eye.

Or else when they go home,
Their spouse may them stone.

Your Second Husband & Your Computer

Even though I keep patient records on paper, I keep track of photos and write emails and website pages with my computer (to learn more about my marketing strategies, go to BoNTClass.com/marketing).

When I do use a computer (including writing this course), I use a Mac—not a PC. You should do the same.

Have you ever heard anyone say, "I love my PC"?

Absolutely not.

Unfortunately, some of the best financial software still requires a PC. But, for cosmetic physicians, the Mac is the choice.

Note: Have you ever known a woman whose first husband beat her, smashed her cell phone, and kept six girlfriends on the side; then she divorced him, and her second husband cherishes her, does not even know other women exist, and drapes her with diamonds?

That woman loves the second husband with passion and gratitude.

That is what happens when someone divorces their PC and switches to a Mac.

If you are still tolerating your PC's abuse (and you are not doing your own accounting), then let me show you how to swap to a Mac.

Follow these 12 easy steps to divorce your abuser—the PC:

1. **Buy a MacBook Pro.** *Go to* Apple.com *and buy the fastest one with the most memory you can afford, and always buy the fastest possible internet connection for wherever you are working—that saves you loads of time. I am talking about buying the laptop (notebook), not the top-of-the-line desktop; the top Apple desktop runs around $50,000 and is more computing power than you need as a physician.*

2. *When you buy the Mac, choose the option to* **have Word & Excel installed** *before it ships (yes, a Mac will run Windows software). I disdain to concede to putting Microsoft software on my Mac, but you will need your documents to be in* Word *before you can hand them off to most publishing software. And most people still swap numbers using* Excel *(not the Mac version,* Numbers).

3. *Turn on your PC,* **store all your passwords at 1PassWord.com**

4. **Upload all the important files from your PC to DropBox.com.** *Buy the business version of DropBox; it meets the required privacy standards of HIPPA and gives you one more way to not rely on Google.*

5. **When your MacBook Pro arrives, turn it on, log into your WIFI and set up the fingerprint login (follow the instructions on the screen).**

6. **Install 1Password onto your new Mac,** *and you will immediately have access to all the passwords that were on your PC.*

7. *As you go about your work, using the Mac, download any needed files (that were on your old PC) from where you saved them on Dropbox.*

8. **Install the** Chrome **browser on your Mac.** *Safari (which comes on your Mac) works acceptably, but Chrome shows you everything (including your own website) the way most of your patients see them because most of your patients use Chrome.*

9. *Also, **install the** Firefox **browser** for a backup browser and more privacy when you want it.*

10. Stick your old PC on a shelf so that if you need something from it (that you forgot to transfer to DropBox) you will have it. Put it far back on a bottom shelf so you do not experience flashbacks and post traumatic stress disorder from all the hours of abuse it dealt you, requiring you to install updates and antiviral software and sending you searching Google for how to get buggy software to work.

11. Pour your favorite beverage, listen to some great music on iTunes, and celebrate the fact that you will no longer suffer abuse from your PC.

12. Take your MacBook to the office, your home, and when you travel; enjoy the freedom of being able to accomplish your work anywhere in the world.

No software company pays me money, so the preceding tips are nonbiased opinions that will probably change as new software is developed. If you want to see my latest recommendations regarding software that may help you with your cosmetic practice, I update this course at BoNTClass.com within the members-only section.

Much Gratitude to the Authors

I am grateful to the authors of the review paper (Yi, 2022) from which I updated my ideas about treating the platysma bands; Yi et al. provide a source of clear anatomical dissections and explanations and a deep source of references regarding the injection of the platysma. I highly recommend you download their open-source paper and contemplate its content:

Yi KH, Lee JH, Lee K, Hu HW, Lee HJ, Kim HJ. Anatomical Proposal for Botulinum Neurotoxin Injection Targeting the Platysma Muscle for Treating Platysmal Band and Jawline Lifting: A Review. *Toxins (Basel)*. 2022;14(12):868. doi:10.3390/toxins14120868

37. INJECTION POINT #11: NECKLACE LINES

Necklace Lines

The other problem you can help using BoNT in the neck is "necklace lines."

Necklace lines track horizontally around the neck. Any one necklace line usually does not go completely around the neck.

If you inject the platysma muscle directly beneath each necklace line, then the muscle relaxes beneath the line and helps pull it out—softening the appearance of the line.

Of all the injection points covered in this course, this one is the least effective. You must do multiple treatments for this to work, but over time, it will help.

You will see better and faster results in the neck if you combine BoNT treatments with Vampire Facial® techniques—both micro needling the necklace lines and the subcision of individual lines with a 30-gauge needle while injecting small aliquots of platelet-rich plasma (PRP).

Where to Put the Needle

Place sub-q blebs of BoNT, 2 units each, directly into the necklace lines about 2 cm apart. Use only 6 to 10 units per line for no more than twenty units all together in the treatment of all the necklace lines.

Rather than trying to treat the entirety of every line, only inject at the deepest parts of the most prominent lines.

Important: Always alert your patient to the idea that it will take multiple treatments before necklace lines improve. But some people really love the results of treating necklace lines—so do offer it to your patients.

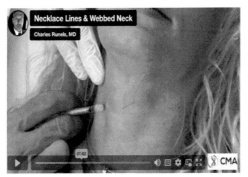

Figure 136. Injection of necklace line with a sub-q bleb of 2 units of BoNT using a 30-unit insulin syringe with a 31-gauge needle. Screen shot from a video demonstration at BoNTClass.com. A green arrow points to one of the lines.

Combine These with BoNT for an Amazing Result

A combination of therapies can greatly improve the neck. Consider offering all the following in combination with your BoNT injections:

- Do our Vampire Facial® (micro-needling combined with PRP).
- Have the patient use our Altar™ cream immediately after the treatment and morning and night for maintenance of a youthful glow (for the rest of their life). You can buy Altar® wholesale if you are one of our Vampire Facial® providers.
- Have the patient use Retin A (more effective than retinol), applied to the face and neck every night.
- You can also inject very small aliquots of hyaluronic acid fillers subdermally to interrupt the necklace lines.

Retin A builds collagen. Altar™ builds collagen, helps heal the micro-needling wounds, and helps prevent the peeling that can be caused by Retin A.

I'm not a big fan of retinol. It works, but it is only Vitamin A. But Retin A (*retinoic acid*) is a vitamin A *derivative* that is much more effective than retinol at building collagen and softening fine lines.

Many people say they cannot tolerate Retin A (because of peeling); but, if they apply Altar™ cream every night immediately after they apply the

Retin A, they will usually tolerate the Retin A and reap the synergy of benefits of using both Retin A and Altar™ cream.

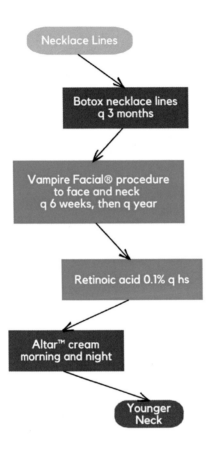

Figure 137. Possible treatment plan to improve the entire neck with targeting the necklace lines includes the following: (1) BoNT, (2) Vampire Facial® techniques every six weeks for three treatments, (3) Retin-A®, & (4) Altar™ (see VampireSkinTherapy.com).

The next lesson will show you one of the most popular BoNT techniques; it improves both the shape of the lips and the texture of the surrounding area.

38. INJECTION POINT #12: LIP GLAMORIZER ("LIP FLIP) & SMOKER'S LINES ERASER

When you BoNT your patient's mouth, they want either (or both) of two things: (1) to create a more glamorous shape or (2) to soften smoker's lines. The first improves the shape; the second improves the texture.

In actual practice, when you treat smoker's lines, you both smooth texture and improve shape. And when you treat shape, you will also smooth texture.

If the person does not yet have smoker's lines, you will delay the creation of smoker's lines when you treat their mouth for shape.

So, when you treat the mouth, you talk with each patient about their concerns (shape or texture), but using the same technique, you will always help them with both.

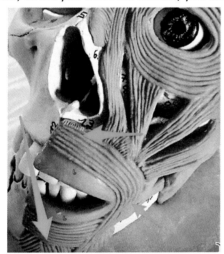

Figure 138. The "lip," as it is commonly defined, is marked by "L". The orbicularis oris extends beyond the lip in every direction (the edges of orbicularis oris distant to the lip are marked by arrows).

The Orbicularis Oris & the Definition of a Kiss

Not Limited to the Lip
The orbicularis oris extends superiorly to the nose; it is not confined to the lips (if you consider the lips as commonly defined). The orbicularis oris also extends beyond the lips both laterally and inferiorly.

Though orbicularis oris functions as one muscle, it actually contains two separate layers. The upper, superficial layer connects to skin; the lower layer connects to the mucosa. The deep fibers of the orbicularis oris run in different directions, but they work together to perform a constricting and releasing action like a sphincter. So, it looks like a sphincter when you see someone drinking from a straw, but the anatomist would say that it is not a true sphincter because it consists of more than one muscle.

The orbicularis oris also keeps food in the mouth and helps with speech and other miscellaneous tasks like whistling, playing the flute, and kissing.

Definition of a Kiss

Memorize the following: *Kiss—The anti-juxtaposition of two orbicularis oris muscles in a state of contraction.*

When at a BoNT party or with a new patient, if you weave that definition of a kiss into your explanation of how BoNT works and say it very quickly, it usually gets a chuckle.

The Only Muscle that Does Not Connect to Bone

Every muscle in the face, other than the orbicularis oris, connects skin to bone or bone to bone (temporalis). The other skeletal muscles of the body (other than the facial muscles) connect bone to bone.

The two functional layers of the orbicularis oris muscle contain fibers originating only from other muscles; so, the *orbicularis oris muscle is the only facial muscle that does not connect to bone at all.*

Lip Strategies: Understanding the Why of the Where

There are two methods for injecting the mouth: (1) the Lip Flip and (2) the Deep Line Eraser.

The Lip Flip

If you keep the part of the orbicularis oris muscle that lies near the nose at its normal resting state, but you relax the orbicularis oris where it lies directly beneath the vermillion border, then the vermillion border both *spreads out* (pulling out the pleats of the smoker's lines) *and rolls up* (creating a more glamorous shape and adding a few millimeters of height to the lip).

If the patient has minimal or no smoker's lines, and you are injecting only to create a more glamorous shape, then do the Lip Flip: thread the needle into the vermilion border and inject as if you were doing an IV push.

The vermillion border is a potential space, and you can feel the needle pop into that space exactly like you feel when the needle pops into a vein when you start an iv or draw blood for lab testing.

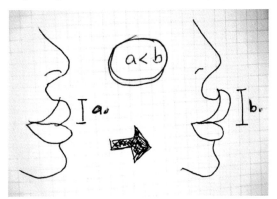

Deep Line Eraser
If your patient shows deep smoker's lines, you can also inject above the lips, putting one unit in multiple places—five or six injections of one unit each, evenly spread across the upper lip, above the vermilion border

Figure 139. Lip Flip: Injecting BoNT along the vermillion border allows the muscle fibers below the border to relax while keeping the fibers near the nose at their usual tension; the result is a pulling out of lines and a flipping up that increases the width of the lip.

(about halfway between the nose and the lip) for a more aggressive relaxation of the orbicularis oris.

Even with deeper lines, most people will eventually see an impressive softening of their lines, even if you inject only the vermillion border (the Lip Flip). The Deep Line Eraser is not usually needed. Either way, softening of the lines is only achieved if the patient consistently undergoes treatment of their mouth every three months for a year or so.

Combination Therapies for Smoker's Lines
A softening of smoker's lines can be hastened by combining BoNT strategies with our Vampire Facial® procedure.

If you do the Vampire Facial and BoNT on the same day, do the BoNT last. In general, when you combine BoNT with any other procedure, you inject BoNT last, so the BoNT does not migrate when you do the other procedure.

As another example, you can routinely inject fillers and BoNT on the same day. But always do the fillers first, followed by the BoNT.

Reconstitution Variation

With most of the face, you want to keep the injected BoNT confined to very near where you insert your needle.

But, with the mouth, you want the BoNT to spread more widely to fill most of the vermillion border (sparing only the corners of the mouth). To facilitate that spreading (for all the orbicularis oris injections), reconstitute the BoNT by adding two ccs of bacteriostatic saline (instead of the usual one cc) to one bottle of one hundred units of cosmetic BoNT.

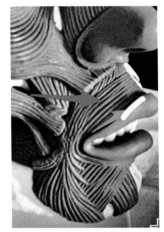

Then take a Sharpie® and mark the BoNT bottle with an "M" for "mouth," and keep this bottle in the refrigerator to use for only mouth injections.

Figure 140. Injection, from a lateral approach, into the vermillion border (green arrow) causes the BoNT to spread along the border (white line). This leaves the surrounding orbicularis oris (blue arrow) untreated— enhancing shape and softening lines.

This dilution, of course, changes the volume you draw into the syringe when measuring units of BoNT. With the more concentrated dilution (used in the other parts of the face), 1 unit of BoNT is 0.01 cc (1 unit on an insulin syringe); with this more dilute mixture for the mouth (where you put 2 ccs in a 100-unit vial), 1 unit of BoNT is now 0.02 cc (or 2 units on an insulin syringe).[7]

---

[7] With Dysport, the volume added is the same and the injections are done in the same, but the number of units will be three times the other products.

Deciding If to Inject for Shape

First, understand desired mouth ratios.

To make the decision about if to treat and how to treat the orbicularis oris, measure the top lip from the vermillion border (at the center of Cupid's bow) to the lower edge of the upper lip, where the lips touch; and measure the bottom lip, from the vermilion border (at the center) to where the lips touch.

Measured in this way, with those of African or Asian descent, the upper lip is usually near the same width as the bottom lip.

With those of Caucasian descent, the upper lip is usually near one-half the width of the lower lip.

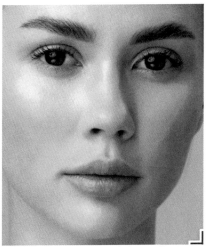

Figure 141. The mouth of those of Asian or of African descent usually shows the upper lip at the same width as the lower lip (when measured in the center from the vermillion border to where the lips touch).

My Mouth Goes from Caucasian to African (& My First Experience of Medicine's Malice)

It was 1975 in a dermatologist's office in Birmingham, Alabama. I was 15 years old. At six-feet two inches tall and only 145 pounds, I had grown into the textbook demonstration of an ectomorph teenager—including glasses and cystic acne.

As I stretched supine on the table, I asked the nurse, "Is this safe?"

She was putting cloth-covered, lead shields over my neck and at the top of my head (where my baseball cap usually sat).

I clearly remember the cold of the table on my forearms, which extended down to my sides, and the weight of the lead over my throat and head.

295

My face remained uncovered.

The nurse answered, "Very safe."

Then, she went behind a lead screen and watched through a tiny window.

I lay very still.

Then, I heard a loud clunk, followed by a quiet buzz that lasted a few minutes.

She was treating me for cystic acne in a way that was common then—x-rays.

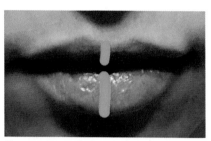

As the x-ray machine buzzed, I remember thinking, "If this is safe, why is she behind that lead screen?"

Figure 142. With the Caucasian mouth, the upper lip is usually near 1/2 the width of the lower lip when measured from the vermillion border (in the center of the mouth) to where the lips touch.

The treatments did very little for my acne, and it felt wrong. So, after going every week for several months, I quit. Years later, I learned that the multiple treatments in that office gifted me with a 25% chance of developing thyroid cancer and guaranteed a future with facial basal cell carcinomas.

Other things physicians taught in the 1970s that we now know did harm included arguments in cardiac journals (and advice to patients) that aerobic exercise is bad for you because it causes ventricular hypertrophy. Dr. Cooper and Dr. Sheehan were (early on) considered quacks in physician's circles, at that time, for teaching that aerobic exercise might be beneficial (even though the research was becoming strong indicating benefit).

Physicians doubted the existence of the "runner's high."

I was running 5 to 15 miles a day and knew there was a runner's high. Years later, the idea of endorphins being released with running became known, and multiple studies have now shown that aerobic exercise does more to prevent heart disease than any diabetes or hypertension drug on the market.

Also, at that time, bodybuilders who took anabolic steroids were not thought by physicians to be made stronger, the drugs just caused "water weight." Not until the late 1980's did the research concede what everyone in the gym knew (I lifted weights at the YMCA), people who take anabolic steroids and lift weights do get extremely strong.

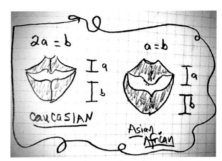

Figure 143. Understanding the usual ratios helps the injector know who to treat (and who to not treat) for a natural result.

Continuing the list of 1970s errors, the diets physicians taught then to those who suffered with diabetes, encouraged foods like pasta and discouraged protein; we now know these diet plans to have been detrimental. And protein-sparing fasts (popularized by Atkins®) were then thought to be detrimental; research now shows that protein-sparing fasts are an effective tool to normalize hemoglobin A1C for those suffering from diabetes. Vince Gironda, a stunt man turned Hollywood gym owner, as early as the 1960s, was teaching protein-sparing fasting to athletes and movie stars (Clint Eastwood in his youth was one of them) as a way to better health—years before Atkins® and years before the medical research supported the idea.

As late as the 1980s, physicians still told men that 85% of those suffering from erectile dysfunction (ED) suffered from a psychogenic etiology; if they would correct their thoughts, they could have good sex. Urologists were encouraged to become sex therapists. Then Viagra came along, and we realized that 85% of men suffer ED from a vascular etiology (not psychological).

So, starting in my teens, I saw a string of errors in medicine, that caused unintended harm, taught by physicians as "proven."

I wonder what we teach now that will be embarrassing twenty years from now.

Still, my encounter with X-rays for acne was good for me (and my patients) because later, as a physician, I knew the current guidelines might be inaccurate; accepted dogma is not to be ignored, but we should always look for new data that blows up the current dogma.

Planck Principle

The Planck Principle says that *"Science advances one funeral at a time."* It is derived from his statements as follows:

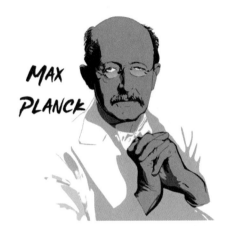

Figure 144. Max Planck, "A new scientific truth does not triumph by convincing its opponents...but rather because its opponents eventually die..."

A new scientific truth does not triumph by convincing its opponents and making them see the light, but rather because its opponents eventually die and a new generation grows up that is familiar with it ...

An important scientific innovation rarely makes its way by gradually winning over and converting its opponents: it rarely happens that Saul becomes Paul. What does happen is that its opponents gradually die out, and that the growing generation is familiarized with the ideas from the beginning: another instance of the fact that the future lies with the youth."

— Max Planck, Scientific autobiography, 1950, p. 33, 97

Further Steps Toward a Mouth Transformation

I worked as a lifeguard for seven summers (during high school and college).

Taken together (lifeguarding plus X-rays for acne), my risks of recurrent basal cell carcinoma go up so much that it is a wonder I still have a nose.

I definitely see my share of basal cell lesions appear on my face (starting at around age 40).

I recently had a basal cell removed with Mohs surgery and had my upper lip rebuilt. The surgeon took part of the wet mucosa on one side and moved it over and outside the mouth to remake an upper lip where the basal cell was removed. He did a beautiful job; but it changed the ratio of the width of my upper lip to my lower lip. Now my upper lip is equal to my lower lip. If you look at older photographs, before surgery, my upper lip was half the width of my lower lip. So, the Mohs surgery changed me from having a Caucasian mouth to having an Asian/African mouth. Which I think is beautiful, but it changed my look.

Now, the wet mucosa is transitioning to dry mucosa. After everything is completely healed and transitioned, I may need to add a few millimeters to my lower lip (using BoNT or fillers), which is now slightly smaller than the upper lip; so I will eventually correct the mouth to what looks best using the Asian/African mouth ratios.

So what? Why did I tell you that story?

The Moral of the Story

I told you about my experience with Mohs surgery and the changes in the ratios of my own mouth and about the fallacy of believing everything you are told is proven for three reasons:

1) As an example of the deeper and more useful and *expert way that you can think about the mouth by simply understanding a few basic ideas about the math* of the face and how to make predictable changes by knowing a few simple injection techniques.
2) Also, *I am not at all unique in that my face has a story; every person can tell you "The Story of My Face"* if you ask enough questions. *You should know the story of the face of every one of your patients.*

   Most people also have a story about when they think a physician, trying to do good, instead did harm. You should know that story too. You never ever criticize the previous doctor (unless there is blatant malpractice with harm), but you should know the story and learn from it.

Until the story you know,
A BoNT needle do not show.

As a part of their story, almost every male patient has a scar on his face by the time he finishes high school. Many women also have scars from trauma or from acne or surgery. *Know the story of every scar on your patient's face and document those scars* and *the stories.*

You and your treatments are becoming part of the story of your patient's face. You should know, understand, and respect the parts of the story that preceded you. Only after you understand what proceeded you are you qualified to become part of the future story of a face.

3) We, as physicians, can be wrong. So, question everything in this book and everything you know. Find ways to show it is all wrong. But, until you do, run with it since it has worked. When you find something that discredits something I am teaching, please write to me; I will be grateful.

To further expand the preceding ideas, if someone visited me with an Asian-ratio mouth (upper lip width equal to lower lip), and I used fillers or injected the orbicularis oris and made their upper and lower lip not equal, then that would look weird to the person treated even if the result made the upper lip half the lower lip (which would look natural on a Caucasian face).

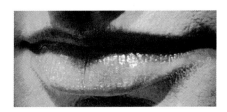

So, if your patient already enjoys an ideal upper to lower lip ratio, and you widen the top lip, you should probably widen the bottom as well.

Figure 145. This upper lip measures less than 1/2 the width of the lower lip (when measured in the center from vermillion border to where the lips touch). This mouth would be an ideal candidate for the Lip Flip (with injection of only the upper lip).

Teaching the Woman (or Man) About Her Face

If the patient is young (without smoker's lines), when I inject the orbicularis oris, it is usually because the upper lip is less than half of the width of the bottom lip. Oftentimes, the patient has not noticed the ratio.

So, with the patient holding a mirror, I use my two thumbs to flip the lip out, and say, "Does that feel better?"

While she watches in the mirror, I roll the upper lip out to the extent of about what the BoNT will do—increasing the top-to-bottom ration so that the upper lip goes *from less than* one-half the width of the lower lip *to equal to* one-half the width of the lower lip. The patient sees the change in the mirror and almost always wants me to do the treatment.

She will feel it more than she sees it; it feels more attractive when the rations are corrected.

The downside to injecting the orbicularis oris is that, for a week or two after you inject, the patient may feel awkward when she drinks from a straw or tries to whistle or do anything that involves puckering the lips.

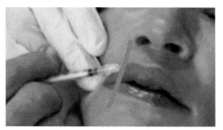

Figure 146. *When injecting the upper lip, the needle approaches from the side and enters the vermillion border in line with the lateral nares. After you feel the needle pop into the space, then you inject the BoNT as if you were doing an iv push.*

Once, I made the mistake of injecting the mouth of a woman who is a newscaster—she could tell I affected her speech (where most people do not notice a difference in speech). *So, if someone speaks or sings for a living, do not inject the mouth with BoNT.*

Where to Put the Needle

For the Lip Flip for the upper lip, put three separate injections into the vermillion border.

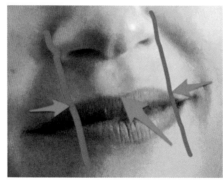

Injection Point #1
In general, you can mark any location by where two lines intersect: "x marks the spot." The lines that mark the spot to inject orbicularis oris are easy to find.

Figure 147. *The three injection points along the upper vermillion border.*

Imagine a line that drops straight down from the lateral edge of the nares; where the line crosses the vermilion border (the second line) is the location of the first injection point.

Injection Point #2
Next, you repeat the injection on the other side.

When you inject the upper lip laterally, the BoNT will spread over the lateral part of the mouth but will not cross into the center of Cupid's bow.

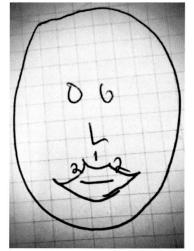

Figure 148. Shorthand notation indicating treatment of the upper vermillion border with 5 units total of BoNT (2 on each side and 1 in the center).

Injection Point #3

After injecting each side of the upper lip into the vermillion border in line with the lateral edge of the nares, then for the last injection, you inject 1 unit (0.02 ccs) into the vermillion border in the center of Cupid's bow.

This center injection is best done by approaching the mouth from directly in front of the patient instead of from the side.

This injection usually bleeds more than the lateral injections, so I ask the patient to hold pressure with one finger pressed onto a gauze held in the center of their upper lip until the bleeding stops.

Because I put two ccs instead of one into the bottle when I mixed the BoNT for the mouth, it changes the volume—two units now will be four units on the syringe and one unit will be two units on the syringe.

So, for the upper Lip Flip, inject two, one, and two units (left, middle, and right), but it will be 0.04, 0.02, and 0.04 ccs on the syringe. (If this seems confusing, read this section with a BoNT needle in hand).

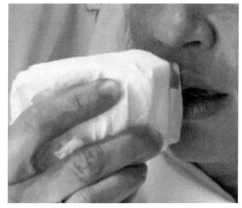

Figure 149. Holding a large ice cube (wrapped with a paper towel) on the upper lip for anesthesia and to decrease bruising. A cloth towel is draped across the chest to help with the dripping water from the ice.

303

Now you have done the "Lip Flip."

Pain Control

Injecting orbicularis oris is the one BoNT injection that I do in the face that hurts without numbing cream (the rest of the face does not need numbing cream if you follow the instructions in Modules I & II).

So, for the mouth injections, I ask the patient to hold ice for about 30 seconds to 1 minute (depending on their pain threshold) at the site where I plan to do the injection.

If they rub the ice back and forth across their entire lip, that does not give adequate anesthesia; instead, ask them to hold the ice in one place—only where you intend to do the next injection. If you have them hold it for a good minute or so, then they will hardly feel your needle at all.

Repeat the ice for every mouth injection point.

The Homunculus Predicts Your Bedroom Behavior

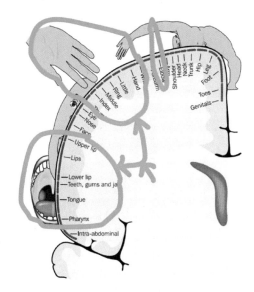

When you map how much of your brain is devoted to sensation in the tongue and mouth (versus the rest of your body), you see that your mouth, your

Figure 150. If you consider the homunculus and the relative amount of brain devoted to the mouth and the hand, compared with the amount of brain devoted to other body parts (like the elbow), a reason for kissing and hand holding becomes apparent.

tongue, and your hand take up most of your sensate brain—hence the reason we kiss instead of rubbing elbows and the reason for ice before injecting the mouth with BoNT.

But anesthesia from ice is only effective for a second or two after you remove the ice; so as soon as the ice comes off the patient's mouth, you must be ready to do the injection.

That is why I have the patient hold the ice—so there is less delay. As soon as the ice comes away, I do the injection.

Your patient will see a change in the mouth immediately after you inject the vermillion border, even though BoNT does not work instantly (the full effect of BoNT is two weeks, and it usually does not start to work until the second day after injection).

But the volumetric effect from the diluent (when injecting the vermillion border) gives your patient a preview of what the mouth will look like in a couple of weeks.

And usually, they love it; the mouth looks sassier and more glamorous when you roll it out a millimeter or two.

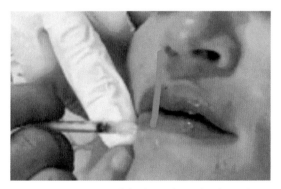

Where to Put the Needle to Inject the Lower Lip

When you do a Lip Flip on the lower lip, you also look for the intersection of two easy-to-find lines: (1) the vermillion border of the lower lip and (2) a line dropped from the lateral edge of the nose.

Figure 151. Injection of the lower lip with a lateral approach in line with the lateral edge of the nares. Only two injections are needed (left and right) since there is no cupid's bow on the lower lip.

But, for the lower lip, you omit the injection in the center since there's no Cupid's bow to inhibit the spread of BoNT to the center of the lip.

So, you only inject the vermillion border of the bottom lip twice—each injection is 2 units (0.04 cc in the mouth mixture previously described), injected as if you are pushing it into a vein, in line with the lateral-most edge of the nares on each side.

For some, I do the Lip Flip on both the upper and lower lips, but most only want their top lip treated because their top lip is less than 1/2 the width of the lower lip.

For some reason, I see fewer women whose bottom lip is too small to match the upper lip, but it happens. When it does, I treat only the lower lip and not the upper lip.

A Beauty Clue

You do not see many celebrities whose top lip is larger than the bottom lip. Usually, creating a ratio where the top lip equals the lower lip, or the top lip is one-half the width of the lower lip, is considered more attractive.

For more about the ratios of the top lip to the bottom and for other ideas about the math of the face, study Dr. Marquardt's website BeautyAnalysis.com. The ideas found there have been extremely helpful to me. You can also find more about these ideas in my Vampire Facelift® book at VampireFacelift.com.

What if you Miss

When you inject the vermillion, if you see a circular configuration of the fluid as it flows subdermally, nothing bad happens; but you really did not do the procedure the way I am recommending. If you see a circular configuration, you went too deep, injecting the muscle rather than threading the vermillion border. In that case, you will still see a pretty effect; but to really see the beautiful flipping effect and the glamorous shape that I am describing, the liquid from your injection should travel in a linear configuration along the vermilion border.

Do not panic if you do not do it perfectly and you see a circular configuration of the fluid you injected; it does not work every time perfectly for me either; it still creates a beautiful effect.

If you get it right, though, they truly love it, and they always come back.

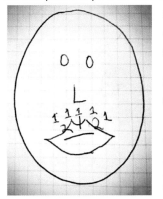

Figure 152. Documenting a more aggressive treatment:

First, inject the vermillion border (2 units on each side and 1 unit in the center).

Then, inject 1 unit 5 times, distributed evenly across the upper lip, between the vermillion border & the nose.

For all lip injections, use a mixture of 2 cc of bacteriostatic saline added to 100 units of cosmetic BoNT.

Where to Put the Needle for a More Aggressive Smoker's Lines Treatment

Usually, the only time I am asked to do a more aggressive treatment of smoker's lines is when the person already has smoker's lines. In this case, I do the usual treatment of the vermillion border (as described in the previous section) and add to that a second row of injections.

For the second row, I inject 5 points with one unit each. Each injection is about halfway between the nose and the lips.

One injection goes directly under the nose, and then two more injections are placed on each side of the nose.

The needle only goes subdermally, and I always use ice to decrease the pain. But, in this case, you could apply ice, then do two or three of the five injections before reapplying the ice.

Another Peek at the BoNT Board

Even in my office, on every patient, I use the board that I described when we talked about BoNT parties. The board keeps me organized and being organized means I do the treatments faster and better.

The inverted BoNT bottle caps (glued to the board) hold the syringes, but, the syringes can even lie on a table and still stay clean because the needle is not touching. I use my board as a clean surface and syringes can lie on the board, even if they are not in one of the holders.

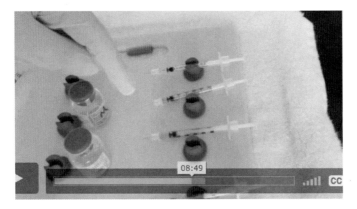

Figure 153. Syringes organized on the board for injecting the lip (screenshot from videos at BoNTClass.com)

Nothing dirty/used ever goes back onto the board. Once I use a needle, it goes into a needle disposal (always within reach of where I stand when I do BoNT treatments).

Mark Bailey and his group in Toronto taught me to use the BoNT Board to organize my BoNT syringes nearly 2 decades ago, and I have not found a better way yet.

If you find a better way, I hope you will write to me and teach me about it at DrRunels@Runels.com.

References

Planck, Max, and Max von Laue. *Scientific Autobiography and Other Papers*. Translated by Frank Gaynor. New York: Philosophical Library, 1949.

Paluch, Amanda E, Shivangi Bajpai, David R Bassett, Mercedes R Carnethon, Ulf Ekelund, Kelly R Evenson, Deborah A Galuska, et al. "Daily Steps and All-Cause Mortality: A Meta-Analysis of 15

International Cohorts." *The Lancet Public Health* 7, no. 3 (March 2022): e219–28. https://doi.org/10.1016/S2468-2667(21)00302-9.

Finkle, Alex L. "Sexual Impotency: Current Knowledge and Treatment I. Urology/Sexuality Clinic." *Urology* 16, no. 5 (November 1980): 449–52. https://doi.org/10.1016/0090-4295(80)90592-0.

Quote from the article:

"Investigative and therapeutic measures for evaluating sexual impotency are rather recent. Psychogenic and organic problems may overlap. Thorough clinical appraisal and objective tests are currently affording better differentiation of etiology and, consequently, appropriate treatment. Causes of and tests for sexual impotency guide the choice of treatment. Surgical intervention can be offered for irreversible organic impotency. However, most instances of acquired impotence are psychogenic. Any nonjudgmental, competent practitioner can aid victims of psychogenic impotence by a "listening and encouragement" method. Urologists, in particular, are commonly confronted with genital/sexual problems and may be best suited as primary therapists by developing interest in urologic counseling. A newly formed Urology/Sexuality Clinic at the University of California in San Francisco provides therapy for patients and offers training for resident physicians."

Module IV.

How to Use BoNT to Help with Four Difficult-to-Treat Medical Problems

Depression, Migraines, Bruxism, & Erectile Dysfunction

39. TREATING MEDICAL PROBLEMS WITH BONT

In this module, you will learn how to use BoNT to treat four medical problems: (1) depression, (2) migraines, (3) bruxism, and (4) erectile dysfunction.

There are other medical problems that may be helped with BoNT. I chose these four because they are strongly supported by the research, and they are commonly seen in every physician's office.

The medical uses of BoNT are not effective for all people (like everything else in medicine). But for those for whom it works, BoNT can be life changing.

She Did not Cry Because of Pain

Recently, a woman sat in my office and sobbed. She had suffered from migraines for many years. In her late sixties, she had visited multiple headache clinics.

She had received from me a combination of BoNT and testosterone pellets. I first learned in 1999 (from a gynecologist who had published in *Neurology)* about testosterone pellets helping women with migraines.

This woman had been weeks without a migraine and was sobbing with joy and gratitude and with remorse—with remorse because her daughter had committed suicide out of desperation from migraines; her daughter had never been offered the same treatment.

The Insurance-Tail Wagging the Doctor-Dog

Sadly, most of our colleagues determine that if insurance does not pay for a medical treatment, then that treatment is likely quackery; that attitude is the tail wagging the dog.

For example, strong research supports BoNT as an effective treatment for both bruxism and depression, but these two treatment strategies are not yet covered by insurance, so BoNT is usually not offered or even considered by many primary care physicians for the treatment of bruxism and depression.

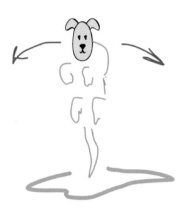

Can You Do a Double-Blind, Placebo-Controlled Study of Parachutes, Birth Control Pills, or BoNT?

Figure 154. Doctor allowing insurance to define the standard of care.

Many physicians will use the lack of a double-blind, placebo-controlled studies as a reason for not recommending treatments not covered by insurance. Often, that is a legitimate criticism; but you cannot do a double-blinded, placebo-controlled study of everything.

For example, walking 10,000 steps a day in multiple studies has been shown to cut all-cause mortality in the coming year in half. But there is no way to confirm that with a double-blind, placebo-controlled study.

Similarly, if you inject saline as a placebo in a study of BoNT for depression, the patient will know if they received BoNT or a placebo because (if in the placebo group) he will still see movement of the procerus. People feign double-blind, placebo-controlled studies of BoNT, but such studies are usually impossible.

If you are waiting for a legitimate double-blind, prospective, placebo-controlled study of parachutes, birth control pills, or BoNT for depression—you have a long time to wait, and your patients will never benefit from what could be a life-changing therapy.

What to Do for a BoNT Treatment Covered by Insurance if You Do Not Accept Insurance

If your practice is all cash (not insurance-based) and someone wants their migraines treated with BoNT, you face a dilemma: you want to treat them, but you know that they could have it done much cheaper by their neurologist—but you think you can, perhaps, achieve a better result.

The following is what I do in that situation (where insurance will pay for the treatment, but I do not accept insurance); when someone asks, "Can you help my migraines with BoNT?"

I answer, "If you have it done by your neurologist, your insurance will likely pay for it. But I will make it look pretty and help your migraines."

And most of them choose to go to their neurologist and have it paid for completely by insurance. That is how it should be. I am happy that I helped them find an effective migraine therapy even if another doctor provides it.

But often they will come back to me and say, "I want you to do it, so it looks pretty because my neurologist drooped my brow," or "My eye was crooked after my neurologist treated me," or something similar.

The cash price to treat migraines with BoNT is within the budget of most; usually, all it takes to make migraines disappear is to treat the glabella (procerus and the corrugators). Many of my patients are even reminded that it is time for their BoNT treatment by the recurrence of their migraines.

Never Keep the Money If the Patient Does Not Love the Result

To date, BoNT is not registered for any psychiatric indication. Thus, it is currently used on a "compassionate" basis: for free to the patient, at the doctor's expense, or for cash to the patient. I do both.

You could say to yourself, "I want to help the patient, but I am afraid to take their money for fear the treatment will not help? "

313

Should you think that and chose not to treat the patient, the patient loses the possible benefit of the treatment. So, I prefer, in that situation, to own the risk: *If the patient does not love the result of any cash procedure, I give all their money back*—every dime, every time, every day since I started taking cash payments in 2003 (twenty years ago).

But, to keep from going broke, when possible, I price the procedure high enough that I receive at least two to three times the cost of goods so that if the patient is not helped, I can refund all her money. Then, because of adequate markup, if I have over a 60 to 70% success rate, I still make enough profit that I'm not paying to go to work, and no one feels duped out of their money.

If you do not decide that you will always give money back to anybody who does not see the desired benefits from your procedure, I think you become afraid to help your patient.

So, *if you are accepting cash, make sure you have a procedure that is at least 70% successful, and at worst, if it does not help, it still carries very little risk of causing harm. Then, always give all the money back every time your patient does not love the results.*

In effect, *your successes finance your ability to refund money to those whom you cannot help.*

The research regarding the use of BoNT to treat medical problems changes quickly. But, for the following four problems covered in this course, the success rate is high enough that you can afford to refund all the money of those who are not helped.

Now, let us think about four conditions for which you can use low-risk BoNT treatments to dramatically improve the lives of many of your patients: (1) depression, (2) migraines, (3) bruxism, and (4) erectile dysfunction.

40. TREATING DEPRESSION WITH BONT

Three hundred million people worldwide suffer the mental and physical pain and comorbidities of depression. According to the World Health Organization (WHO), *depression is the leading cause of disability worldwide.* (Whitcup,2019) And since many do not respond completely to our current therapies, millions suffer from chronic depression. (Whitcup,2019)

With our best therapies, depression is becoming more prevalent, not less. Depression is even growing more prevalent among teens. (CDC,2019) According to the Centers for Disease Control and Prevention (CDC), the suicide rate for teenagers (ages 15-19) in the United States was 9.9 per 100,000 individuals in 2020. This represents a significant increase from previous years, with the rate for this age group increasing by 2.2% from 2019.

That means around 1 in 10,000 teens in the U.S. self-destructed in 2020. Said another way, during that same time, according to the National Center for Education Statistics (NCES), the average size of a public high school in the United States was approximately 839 students; so, on average, about 1 in every 12 high schools in the U.S. lost a student to suicide during *that year alone. Therefore, over the course of the four-year high school tenure of an individual student (assuming the same suicide rate), an average of one in three high school students would lose a classmate to suicide. And suicide rates worsened after the pandemic.* (NCES,2023)

Holy Serotonin—And the Hindrance to a Better Way

A recent review article, which covered *the past two decades of research* regarding the treatment of depression, showed that even though selective serotonin reuptake inhibitors (SSRIs) improve the symptoms of depression, *SSRIs also increase the risk of suicide.* The article also showed that *the accepted dogma of a "chemical imbalance" of serotonin in the brain causing depression is wrong*; low levels of serotonin do not cause depression. (Moncrieff,2022) (Wise,2022) (Zhang,2021)

That does not mean that SSRIs do not help; it means that SSRIs do not help in the way we thought.

What happens when we prescribe SSRIs?
There is no clear answer in the literature to how SSRIs help those who suffer from depression, but *anorgasmia, continued dysphoria, anhedonia, and an increased risk of suicide and maybe homicide—those are known effects of SSRIs.*

Possibly SSRIs dull the senses (more about how they do so later). People feel their depression; they just do not worry about it as much. Perhaps depression is not felt as much, but also fear is not felt as much, which could explain why people are more prone to suicide.

I am not proposing that we throw away antidepressants, but *we should acknowledge that we do not completely understand depression and that we need something better. Acknowledgment that we do not know an ideal way to treat depression could be the first step to finding a better way. The hindrance to learning is not ignorance; it is the illusion of already knowing.*

Not a "Magic Bullet"

BoNT is not a magic bullet that cures all depression. The many etiologies for depression include all the following and more: life events, hypothyroidism, low growth hormone, malnutrition, postpartum hormonal changes, hyperprolactinemia from pituitary microadenomas, head trauma, stroke, and as a side effect of medications. BoNT would not be the best *sole* treatment in such cases. But BoNT might help in all of them. (Khademi,2021)

Darwin & Depression

How BoNT might help with depression can be found in ideas proposed by Charles Darwin, who described specific muscles that express depression.

"Omega Melancholicum"

Darwin described the *omega melancholicum:* when one is worried, anxious, or sad, those emotions create the "number 11" sign (from contraction of the corrugators), and a "furrowed brow" (contraction of the medial frontalis), which completes the *omega melancholicum* configuration.

Veraguth's Folds

A depressed person also demonstrates *Veraguth's Folds,* lines that go from *the lateral corner of the eye to the medial ipsilateral eyebrow.* When you draw Omega Melancholicum and Veraguth's Folds, you demonstrate a face that looks worried, sad, tearful, and depressed.

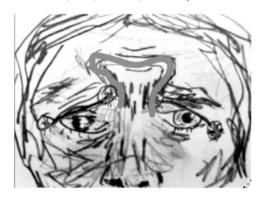

"Veraguth's Folds" (*) and "Omega Melancholicum".

Demonstrating the muscles used to express sadness is the first step to knowing how BoNT helps depression. The next step involves the examination of cold and warm emotions.

Cold Emotions & Warm Emotions

Consider the difference between cold and warm emotions.

Cold Emotion

First, a thought enters consciousness; you hear it, see it, and think about it. *Psychological or cognitive information enters your consciousness*; this is a *cold emotion.*

With a *cold emotion*, you know the depressing idea and are aware of emotion regarding the idea, but the emotion is only cerebral. Somatic physiology is not engaged, only mind.

Warm Emotion

When cold emotion escalates into warm emotion—the emotion

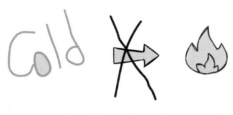

becomes visceral; you feel "heartache," you feel "gut-punched," you sob, and experience tachycardia and fatigue. You may become so full of emotion that you "explode" by seeking a physical outlet—

Figure 155. Blocking the transformation from cold emotion into warm emotion is what antidepressants do.

possibly a destructive one. You pace or punch a wall (or a person); you curse, or you hurt yourself or another.

Block to Rock

*When transformation
of cold depression
into warm,
you block;
patients, to you,
will flock.*

In short: *Warm emotions manifest extracerebral signs and symptoms.*

As an example of the power of warm emotion, consider that in couples who have been married for over 50 years, when one of the two dies, the surviving partner is cursed with a 50% increased chance of dying from cardiac arrest within a year (Ytterstad,2015). In another study, the mortality rate from both *circulatory disease* and *cancer* increased 25% in men in the first six months after losing a spouse to death. (Martikainen,1996)

Warm emotion not only hurts—it kills.

"Selective Blocking" ...A Hypothesis for Why SSRIs Increase Suicide & BoNT Does Not

One Hypothesis, *non-selective blocking*, says that SSRIs stop depression in the cold emotion stage but increase the risk of suicide because they also stop other emotions in the cold emotion phase; the person is also blocked from warm emotions associated with sex (causing anorgasmia) and from the warm emotion of fear associated with self-destruction. As part of their depression, they may feel sad enough for suicide (cold emotion) but not feel fear as a warm emotion associated with the act. Feeling only the cold emotion commanding suicide (or homicide) but blocked from the warm emotion of fear—the cold-emotion, robot-like person becomes dangerous to self and others.

Selective blocking of only depression in the cold emotion phase while allowing other warm emotions, like sex and fear, to remain intact offers an improvement over the effects of SSRIs.

Can BoNT accomplish selective blocking of depression while preserving warm emotions of happiness? Studies suggest so. (Alum,2008)

To understand how BoNT might accomplish selective blocking, consider the *Facial Feedback Hypothesis*.

The Warming of an Emotion & the "Facial Feedback Hypothesis"

According to the Facial Feedback Hypothesis, when an idea enters consciousness (A in the following diagram), then that idea triggers (through *efferent nerves*) facial musculature activation that matches the cold emotion—creating a facial expression of sadness (B).

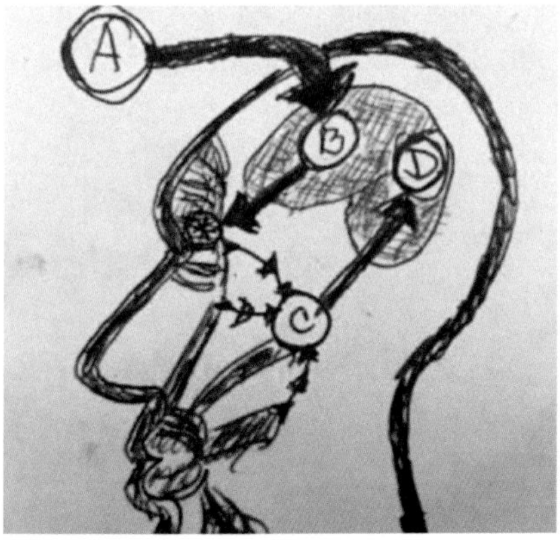

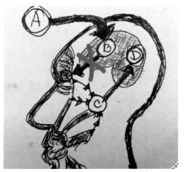

Figure 156. *an idea enters consciousness (A); efferent nerves signal facial muscles to express emotion related to the idea (B); afferent nerves tell the brain the configuration of the facial muscles, emotional proprioception (C); the brain discerns the muscle configuration & cold emotion goes to warm emotion (D).*

The muscles that are triggered to move with depression cause the configurations of Veraguth's Folds and Omega Melancholicum.

Afferent nerves then sense that the muscles have moved into an expression of sadness and relay that message back to the brain (C); the awareness of the facial muscles expressing emotion is called *emotional proprioception*.

The emotional proprioception signals of depression are acknowledged by the brain (D); the cold emotion (A) becomes a warm emotion (D).

Cold emotion, somatically enhanced, becomes warm emotion.

BoNT Blocks the Facial Feedback Loop

The diagram of the Facial Feedback Loop explains how BoNT helps with depression. By blocking the signals of the efferent nerves going to the glabella region, idea (A) is perceived, then it stops. There is no effective efferent signal (B). (Alam,2008)

Figure 157. *With BoNT, the efferent nerves cannot activate facial muscles to express the cold emotion (A). So, emotional proprioception keeps telling the brain "Happy" and the warm emotion of "depressed" is attenuated. (Alam,2008)*

The cold emotion, not somatically enhanced, stays cold.

Multiple studies support this idea of BoNT helping depression by blocking the facial feedback loop. (Alam,2008)

For example, studies show that if someone is exposed to a stimulant that should cause sadness, after BoNT, there is a delayed response in the perception—it takes longer to even acknowledge sadness after receiving BoNT in the glabellar region. (Bulnes,2019) (Davis,2010)

Facial Feedback Can Cause a Death Spiral

What is not illustrated in the Facial Feedback loop diagram is that (without BoNT) D causes B to tell your muscles to make again the sad face (Omega Melancholicum and Veraguth's folds)—which goes back to C, which cycles back to D, over and over and over.

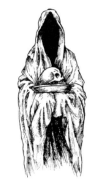

So, when *one is stuck in the Facial Feedback Loop as applied to the emotion of depression, that continuous loop can spiral down, way down—with the sufferer prone on the floor, in tears, vomiting, and putting a pistol to their head. Their*

Figure 158. When the cold emotion of depression becomes warm, the risk of suicide goes up.

loved ones find them. Children grow up without parents. Parents bury their children.

Summary of How BoNT Helps the Depressed

When BoNT is used in the corrugators and procerus, not only do the facial muscles not react to enhance the cold emotions (sadness, anger, and fear) into warm emotions, but because the feedback loop is broken, now *there continue to be signals (by afferent nerves from the facial muscles) of calm and happiness—not only blocking the negative*

321

feedback loop but also providing continuing emotional proprioception of peace to help neutralize the cold emotion of depression!

So, the brain perceives "sad" (A).

But after BoNT, the facial muscles ignore the brain's cold emotion of sad and repeat to the brain, "No, you are not sad; you are happy."

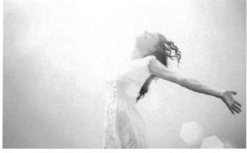

Figure 159. With BoNT, even though the brain perceives "sad," the muscles keep saying, "happy"--breaking the Facial Feedback loop.

But *there could be more.* BoNT might work for depression in ways even more powerful than what is implied by the facial feedback hypothesis.

BoNT, Depression, & the CNS

We also know from pain studies (including the treatment of bruxism and migraines) and from animal studies that *BoNT is taken into the peripheral nerves by endocytosis and travels (at about one-half centimeter per day) along the axon to the more central ganglion.* (Ramachandran,2014)

For example, the relief of migraines by BoNT (one of the FDA indications for Botox) is thought **not** to be the result of relieving muscle tension in the face. Instead, it is thought that BoNT relieves migraines by migrating along afferent neurons from the glabellar region to the *trigeminal ganglion* and then to the *trigeminal nucleus caudalis*, both of which are *shared by afferents from the meninges.* The glabella acts as a port through which BoNT can be injected to affect neurotransmitters within the ganglion to attenuate the sensation of pain from the meninges—relieving migraine. (Ramachandran,2014)

So, BoNT not only blocks acetylcholine at the muscle-nerve synapse but also blocks neurotransmitters of pain at the ganglion level. (Mazzochio,2015) (Caleo,2018)

The effect of BoNT on the ganglion can also *increase parasympathetic tone and decreases sympathetic tone.* (Giuliano,2022)

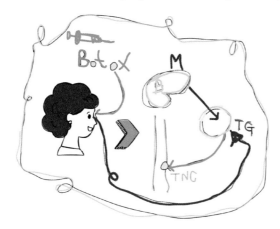

As with migraines, also with the treatment of depression, after injecting the glabella, the BoNT migrates along the cranial nerves, moving centrally to block neurotransmitters of pain and to increase parasympathetic tone.

Figure 160. BoNT injected into the glabellar region migrates along the afferent nerves to the trigeminal ganglion (TG) and then to the trigeminal nucleus caudalis (TNC). Both the TG and the TNC are shared by the afferent pain fibers coming from the meninges (M) surrounding the brain (B). The signals from these pain fibers are blocked at the TG and the TNC by the effects of the BoNT that migrates there. This is thought to be the mechanism by which BoNT relieves migraines. (Ramachandran,2014) Could it also have an effect in the treatment of depression?

Knowing this demands the question, "Does the migration along the afferent nerves, centrally, to the trigeminal ganglion give additional help with depression beyond what is provided by the facial feedback loop?"

Strong research says, "Yes, it does." (Marchand-Pauvert,2013)

More research is needed. But even though we do not yet know exactly how BoNT helps depression, we do know that those who suffer from mild depressive state and those with depression so severe they do not respond to antidepressant medications are helped by injecting the corrugators and procerus with BoNT.

And we now know from good studies that BoNT can even help some who suffer from personality disorders associated with depression. [Kruger2016]

Should Insurance Define Standard of Care?

Considering the previously discussed ideas, in my opinion, we should offer BoNT as a first-line pharmaceutical option to a significant portion of those who are clinically sad and not responding to non-pharmacological measures.

So, what keeps us from routinely offering BoNT for depression?

Some might say, "I do not offer BoNT for depression because insurance does not pay for it."

I would answer, "And?"

This is a treatment that costs less than a new set of tires or two nights in a hotel room (every three months) or filling up a car with gas a few times. The patient should, at least, be offered the option.

And if the patient cannot afford it, I would say, "Give it to them and let those who have finance those who have not."

That was the idea behind insurance (not to define what is good medicine and what is quackery, as it has become). If insurance does not pay, then each physician should treat a reasonable number of people for free.

What seems tragic is when physicians are hesitant to admit that the *best medicine is often denied by allowing insurance to define what is best.*

Profit Governs Altruism

You, as a physician, can only afford to give away treatments to the less fortunate if you make enough money to pay your bills *with leftovers*.

You cannot stay in practice if you get pushed into a no-profit zone. And you cannot self-finance your treatment of the financially poor if you have no surplus money—that is, if you are not making enough profit.

If you are helping others solely with resources paid for by government safety nets, then *those nets were also constructed with someone's surplus—taxes on the profit of others*. You can use the same strategy in your office to help the unfortunate (in addition to what your government finances), but only if you make enough profit.

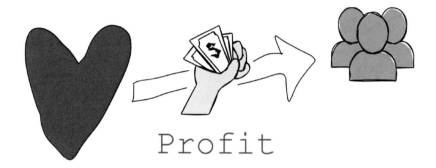

Figure 161. Love, knowledge, and skill are concretized by profit. Someone's surplus (yours or another's) must buy the resources used to help others. Profit is the conduit through which your altruism passes.

Profit is ethical if made with the right intention (giving value worth more than the money received); not making a profit can be both wasteful and unethical (not creating value).

One strategy for the primary care physician is to offer cosmetic BoNT for profit and use some of those profits to help finance the free care of those who suffer migraines or depression but who cannot afford BoNT.

Where to Put the Needle

As a reminder, in the treatment of depression, all you know about good medical diagnosis and treatment still applies to the treatment of depression, even if using BoNT as a treatment option.

All I am suggesting is that (especially with the recent debunking of one of the sacred beliefs about serotonin) we do need more combination therapies for depression, and BoNT is a research-supported option.

For the actual injection of BoNT to treat depression, *the same techniques that help people look better also help them feel better*

(Alum,2008). The mechanics of mixing and injecting in a way that avoids pain is described in detail in Module II of this course. Study that module first.

Then, to treat depression, simply inject *the glabella (corrugators and procerus) in the locations and with the amounts as explained in Chapter*

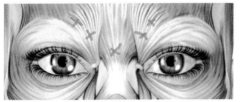

27. That is all it takes for most people.

The whole treatment takes less than 5 minutes.

Easy.

Figure 162. Injection points for BoNT for depression (covered in more detail in Chapter 27).

Assuming you do not inappropriately treat pregnant women or people with myasthenia gravis, *the worst you can do with BoNT (if you follow my instructions) is to cause a bruise, droop an eyelid for a few weeks, or cause a mild headache for a day or two.* I know few therapies for depression that have the potential for as much good with such a strong safety profile.

A Request & an Offer for You

I want to know where you think I might be wrong and where you think more research is needed (especially if you are qualified to do that research). We (members of the Cellular Medicine Association) use two nonprofits and one for-profit organization to help finance research—so telling me where I am wrong could prompt ideas for future studies.

Not counting family, nothing gives me more pleasure than to hear that some little something I said was of help to one of your patients.

Please let me know how it goes when you implement the ideas in this chapter.

References

Al Abdulmohsen T, Kruger THC. The contribution of muscular and auditory pathologies to the symptomatology of autism. *Medical Hypotheses*. 2011;77(6):1038-1047. doi:10.1016/j.mehy.2011.08.044

Alam M, Barrett KC, Hodapp RM, Arndt KA. Botulinum toxin and the facial feedback hypothesis: Can looking better make you feel happier?

Bulnes LC, Mariën P, Vandekerckhove M, Cleeremans A. The effects of Botulinum toxin on the detection of gradual changes in facial emotion. *Sci Rep*. 2019;9(1):11734. doi:10.1038/s41598-019-48275-1

Centers for Disease Control & Prevention (CDC), Youth Risk Behavior Survey https://runels.com/yrbs

Davis JI, Senghas A, Brandt F, Ochsner KN. The effects of BOTOX injections on emotional experience. *Emotion*. 2010;10(3):433-440. doi:10.1037/a0018690

Giuliano F, Denys P, Joussain C. Effectiveness and Safety of Intracavernosal IncobotulinumtoxinA (Xeomin®) 100 U as an Add-on Therapy to Standard Pharmacological Treatment for Difficult-to-Treat Erectile Dysfunction: A Case Series. *Toxins*. 2022;14(4):286. doi:10.3390/toxins14040286

Journal of the American Academy of Dermatology. 2008;58(6):1061-1072. doi:10.1016/j.jaad.2007.10.649

Khademi M, Roohaninasab M, Goodarzi A, Seirafianpour F, Dodangeh M, Khademi A. The healing effects of facial BOTOX injection on symptoms of depression alongside its effects on beauty preservation. *Journal of Cosmetic Dermatology*. 2021;20(5):1411-1415. doi:10.1111/jocd.13990

Kruger THC, Magid M, Wollmer MA. Can Botulinum Toxin Help Patients With Borderline Personality Disorder? *AJP*. 2016;173(9):940-941. doi:10.1176/appi.ajp.2016.16020174

Marchand-Pauvert V, Aymard C, Giboin LS, Dominici F, Rossi A, Mazzocchio R. Beyond muscular effects: depression of spinal recurrent inhibition after botulinum neurotoxin A: Recurrent inhibition after BoNT-A. *The Journal of Physiology.* 2013;591(4):1017-1029. doi:10.1113/jphysiol.2012.239178

Martikainen P, Valkonen T. Mortality after the death of a spouse: rates and causes of death in a large Finnish cohort. *Am J Public Health.* 1996;86(8_Pt_1):1087-1093. doi:10.2105/AJPH.86.8_Pt_1.1087

Moncrieff J, Cooper RE, Stockmann T, Amendola S, Hengartner MP, Horowitz MA. The serotonin theory of depression: a systematic umbrella review of the evidence. *Mol Psychiatry.* Published online July 20, 2022. doi:10.1038/s41380-022-01661-0

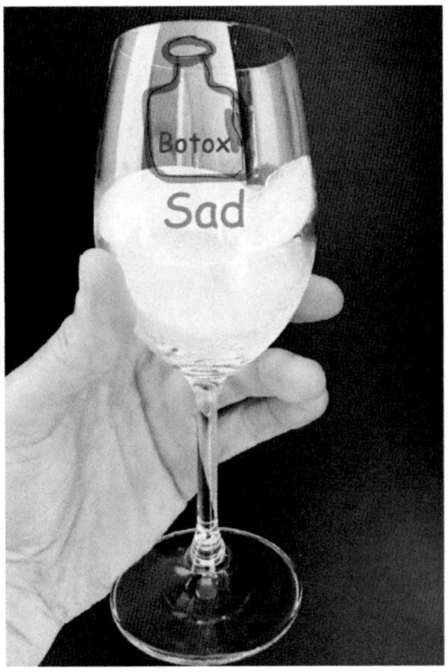

Figure 163. Blocking the facial feedback loop by BoNT can make the brain blind to the emotional proprioception of depression while keeping it aware of happiness proprioception. Therefore, by keeping depression from changing from a cold to warm emotion, BoNT keeps depression cold.

National Center for Health Statistics. U.S. Census Bureau, Household Pulse Survey, 2020–2023. Anxiety and Depression. Generated interactively: from https://www.cdc.gov/nchs/covid19/pulse/mental-health.htm

Ramachandran R, Yaksh TL. Therapeutic use of botulinum toxin in migraine: mechanisms of action. *Br J Pharmacol.* 2014;171(18):4177-4192. doi:10.1111/bph.12763

Wise J. "No convincing evidence" that depression is caused by low serotonin levels, say study authors. *BMJ.* Published online July 19, 2022:o1808. doi:10.1136/bmj.o1808

Wollmer MA, Magid M, Kruger THC, Finzi E. The Use of Botulinum Toxin for Treatment of Depression. In: Whitcup SM, Hallett M, eds. *Botulinum*

328

Toxin Therapy. Vol 263. Handbook of Experimental Pharmacology. Springer International Publishing; 2019:265-278. doi:10.1007/164_2019_272

Ytterstad E, Brenn T. Mortality after the death of a spouse in Norway. *Epidemiology*. 2015;26(3):289-294.doi:10.1097/EDE.0000000000000266

Zamanian A, Jolfaei AG, Mehran G. Efficacy of Botox versus Placebo for Treatment of Patients with Major Depression. :3.

Zhang Q, Wu W, Fan Y, et al. The safety and efficacy of botulinum toxin A on the treatment of depression. *Brain and Behavior*. 2021;11(9):e2333. doi:10.1002/brb3.2333

You know,
you feel,
the feeling is cold.

Then,
Emotional proprioception,
Makes you reel.

Cold emotion warns,
Hot emotion burns.

Cold emotion feels,
Hot emotion kills.

But
a little BoNT,
and no scowl.

Brain says, "Sad."
Face says,
"Glad!"

And Brain
Replies, "OK."
And smiles too.

41. TREATING MIGRAINES WITH BONT

The Theory of Migraines

Though migraines are not completely understood, the condition is thought to be triggered by environmental and hormonal factors; genetics also plays a role (90% of those who suffer from migraines have a relative who suffers from the same). Neurotransmitter imbalances may also play a role in the etiology. (Escher, 2017)

With every postulated etiology, it is the trigeminal nerve that carries the afferent pain signal. (Escher, 2017)

Even though BoNT has been shown to improve the lives of migraine sufferers, migraines are thought *not* to originate from muscle tension; instead, with all causes, there is thought to be a loss of the accurate regulation of vasodilatation of the meninges with resultant activation of the afferent nerves that project from the meninges to the trigeminal nucleus caudalis (TNC). (Ramachandran, 2014)

How Does BoNT Help Migraines?

Since the afferent nerves from the meninges converge on the same trigeminal ganglion (TG) and TNC as do the afferent nerves from the extracranial face and scalp, the pain feels as if it originates from those extracranial areas (referred pain).

This convergence of afferent pain fibers from the face and scalp and the meninges offers a clue to the mechanism of action of BoNT for migraines.

When BoNT is injected into the face and scalp, it is absorbed by local afferent nerve terminals; there BoNT cleaves soluble N-ethylmaleimide-sensitive factor attachment protein receptor (SNARE) proteins and prevents local terminal release. But this local effect does not fully explain how it works to help migraines; BoNT is also *taken up by endocytosis into sensory afferents nerves and transported to cleave*

SNARE proteins at the TG and the TNC, attenuating the transmission of converging pain signals from the meninges.

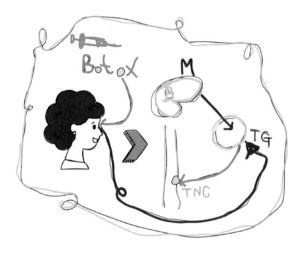

A Wonderful Side Effect of Treating Migraines with BoNT

Figure 164. BoNT may improve migraine by blocking the transmission of pain signals of afferent nerves from the meninges--which share the trigeminal ganglion and trigeminal nucleus caudalis with the afferent nerves from the extracranial face and scalp.

In the last chapter (Chapter 40), we discussed the way BoNT can help those suffering from depression. Since those who suffer from migraines have a two to three times increased incidence of depression (Wang, 2010), it is handy to have one treatment that helps with both problems.

Also, the relationship between depression and migraine seems to be bidirectional, with each causing the other in a negative feedback loop. (Minen, 2016). So, treating someone with BoNT can break the downward spiral of depression causing migraine, causing depression, causing migraine, etc. to save a life from chronic pain.

A Simple Secret about Treating Migraines with BoNT

The rest of this chapter describes the standard, FDA-approved method for mixing BoNT and injecting it for the treatment of migraines; this protocol requires a significant amount of BoNT (155 to 200 units, depending on the author) and a different method of mixing and injecting than what was taught in Modules 2 and 3 in the cosmetic portion of this course.

The secret is *that for many who suffer from migraines, you do not need to use the standard migraine protocol; every experienced BoNT injector enjoys the accolades of patients who receive complete relief of their migraines after only treating the glabella (procerus and corrugators), as in Chapter 27 of this course.*

For many, that is all it takes.

In other words, you could throw this whole chapter away (Chapter 41), and many of your patients would experience complete relief from their migraines if you simply injected their glabella.

Moreover, of those who experience complete relief from their migraines after BoNT is injected by their neurologist for free (since it is often covered by insurance), many will leave their neurologist and *go back to their cosmetic doctor and pay cash—pay for something they could receive for free, for the following three reasons:*

1. The outcome of the cosmetic method looks better than that of the neurologist-provided migraine protocol (which can cause a *droopy look*).
2. When treated with the full migraine protocol, the change in muscle function of the neck can create odd and uncomfortable *"floppy" feelings* (because supportive muscles of the neck become noticeably more relaxed).
3. For many, *cosmetic methods provide complete relief* from migraines. The less aggressive, cosmetic protocol works.

Still, there are many who will not find relief from the cosmetic injection methods. For those, you should learn the specific, FDA-approved methods of treating migraines with BoNT as described in this chapter.

Setting Expectations

Though for some people, BoNT will make their migraines go completely away, research shows that, on average, the result of treating chronic, severe migraines with BoNT is two fewer headaches per month—only two.

So, for those with severe, life-limiting, frequent migraines, set the patient's expectations by saying to the patient something like the following:

"Though I am hopeful that your headaches will
forever go,
the more likely outcome
is
a decrease in severity
& two fewer headaches
per month."

Then, if they express understanding and sign your consent form, proceed as described in this chapter.

People suffering from chronic pain have many reasons to feel angry at the stars; so, more than ever (even though you will likely do no harm with a BoNT injection), before you treat them, you need strong informed consent to help assure that, at worst, they remain angry at the stars and not at you.

Mixing BoNT to Treat Migraines

When I inject cosmetic BoNT (see Module 2 in this course), I put only one cc. of bacteriostatic saline into a 100-unit vial of cosmetic BoNT. When treating only migraines, without regard to cosmetic purposes, I want a broader spread, so I add two ccs of bacteriostatic saline to 100 units of cosmetic BoNT.

First, pull up one cc of bacteriostatic saline using a one cc syringe (more accurate than measuring a small amount with a five or ten-cc syringe). Then add that one cc to a 100-unit vial of cosmetic BoNT. Then repeat the process with another one cc for a total of 2 cc added to the vial.

BoNT comes vacuum-packed. If the vacuum doesn't pull the plunger down when you insert the first syringe, then the seal has been broken, and you should discard the vial. I have never had that happen, but that is the safety check on the vial.

The package insert tells you to use non-bacteriostatic saline, but non-bacteriostatic saline hurts more. So, use the bacteriostatic saline, it works, and it hurts less.

After I add the saline, I use a beer bottle opener to remove the metal band securing the stopper. There is a knack for taking the top off using a beer bottle opener, but it is not difficult and more convenient than the expensive tools made for that purpose. If you inject BoNT regularly, keep a beer bottle opener on your key chain; it will save you the time and the inconvenience of searching for the opener.

You remove the top because you want the needle to touch nothing until it touches the person's skin—that keeps the needle sharp and greatly decreases the pain of the injection. (You will *find more about mixing and injecting BoNT in a way that provides a comfortable experience in Module 2 of this course and at* BoNTClass.com.)

Also, as when injecting cosmetic BoNT, when you inject BoNT for migraines, there is no need to wipe off makeup or cleanse the areas. You can even go right through makeup. When you inject fillers, this is not the case because you are injecting an implant that can become infected. But, with BoNT, you can inject without cleansing the face.

How to Inject Seven Muscle Groups to Treat Chronic Migraines

The seven muscle groups to inject when you treat chronic migraines are as follows (listed in the order that I usually inject them):

1. Procerus
2. Corrugators
3. Frontalis
4. Occipitofrontais (Occipitais)
5. Temporalis

6. Trapezius
7. Splenius Capitis

With all seven of the muscle groups, each injection point is five units.

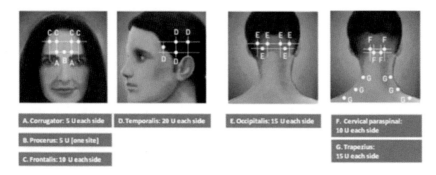

Figure 165. A summary of where to inject all seven muscle groups as approved by the FDA for the treatment of migraines with BoNT.

Normally when we mix cosmetic BoNT, we put 1 ml of bacteriostatic saline into a 100-unit bottle of BoNT, so five units on an insulin syringe (0.05 ml) contain five units of BoNT.

But, as described above, when treating migraines (for a better spread of the BoNT throughout the muscles), you add two ccs of bacteriostatic saline to a 100-unit vial; therefore, five units of BoNT will be contained in 10 units (0.1 ml) on an insulin syringe.

Use a 30-unit, BD brand, 31-gauge insulin syringe (as with cosmetic injections); they hurt less than any other syringe, and there is no residual in the hub of the needle (which wastes money). For comfort, in addition to not touching the needle to anything before it touches the face, do not use one needle more than three times, four at most, because, after that, the needle hurts.

It is muscle anatomy, not wrinkles or tenderness.

As you inject for migraines, you might be tempted to inject based on where the muscles are tender. Research shows that injecting where the muscle is tender is not as effective as what I am about to show you; the main thing is to inject the muscles that will affect the trigeminal ganglion so that the afferent nerves from the meninges are blocked.

Remember, migraines are now thought *not* to be associated with somatic muscle tenderness. Also, even when I inject BoNT for cosmetic reasons, I am not injecting wrinkles. I *use the movement of the face and the associated wrinkles to find the individual muscles that I want to relax, but I do not inject wrinkles. The same applies to both wrinkles and tenderness with migraines*; you use both tenderness and wrinkles to help you find the muscles (the 7 groups you intend to inject), but you do not try to inject trigger points.

1. Injecting Procerus

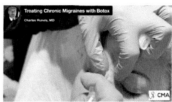

The glabella region includes the corrugators and procerus. Start by putting five units in the center of the procerus. Start with the procerus because it is the least painful.

Figure 166. Injecting procerus with 5 units at the intersection of the "x" imagined by imagining two lines that go from the medial corner of each eye to the contralateral brow.

To find the procerus, imagine a line that goes from the medial canthus of one eye to the medial end of the opposite brow.

Imagine that same line with both eyes. Then, inject five units in the center of the X formed by those two lines.

Always inject facial muscles in the same order so that you develop a routine that assures you do not forget an area; a routine also makes you more time efficient. After injecting procerus, it seems logical to finish the face before moving to the other muscles, so next inject the corrugators.

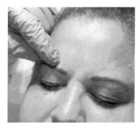

Figure 167. A fingertip lightly placed at the insertion site (marked by a dimple) helps with visualization of the corrugator.

2. Injecting the Corrugators

First, ask the patient to knit their brows together. When she does, you will see a dimple on each side just above the brow with "pleats" medial to the dimple. That dimple (one on each side) represents the insertion site of the corrugator.

From the insertion site, each corrugator pulls the skin toward the midline of the face. I like to put the index finger of my nondominant hand into the insertion site. Then, I can both "see" and feel the muscle belly traveling medially from my finger. I imagine the medial end of each corrugator attaching to the same place where I injected the procerus. I realize this medial insertion may not be the exact anatomy, but it helps me see where to inject.

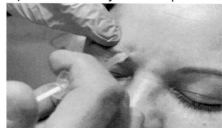

After you ask the patient to knit her brows together and you find the corrugators, then ask her to relax her face before you do the injection. When doing BoNT for cosmetic purposes, I often

Figure 168. Unlike with cosmetic BoNT injections (see Module 3), with the treatment of migraines, you simply inject 5 units in the center of the muscle belly (10 units on your syringe).

use 7 to 15 in each corrugator—divided into two injections into each corrugator. But for migraines, just put five units in the center of the muscle belly (which will be ten units or 0.10 ml on your insulin syringe).

Do that whole process (knit the brow, touch the dimple, find the corrugator, relax the brow, inject the corrugator) with each side.

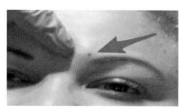

Figure 169. If you see an active "dot" of blood, if it looks like you need a BAND-AID, you are making a bruise; so, hold pressure.

That is a total of 15 units for the whole glabella region (5 in procerus, 5 in each corrugator). After the three injections, lightly massage the area for a few seconds to spread the material.

Note about bruising and Band-Aids. With every injection point, if you see bleeding, hold light pressure until the bleeding stops. If the bleeding is brisk, it can take up to a minute, but usually, you only must hold each area for a few seconds. If the skin looks like you need a BAND-AID, you are making a bruise. So, stop and hold pressure.

3. Injecting Frontalis

If you look at the distribution of the BoNT injections for migraines as diagrammed in the research, the center of the frontalis is spared. The reason is that many people have a split frontalis, but not everybody. Put an extra five in the center if they do not have a split.

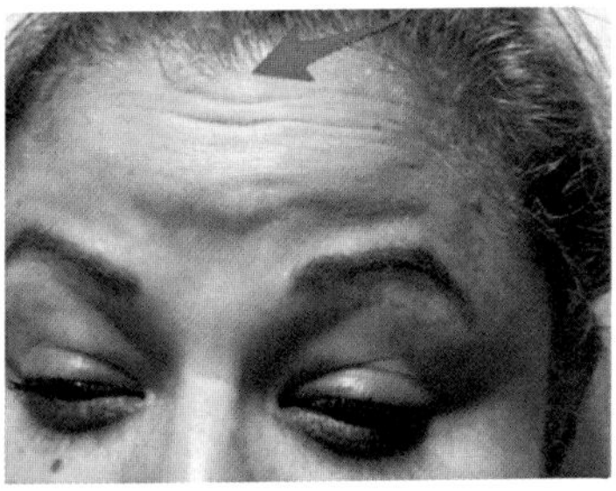

Figure 170. The "U" shaped dip in the superior edge of the frontalis indicates a split frontalis.

To see the frontalis, say to your patient, "Lift your brow as high as you can."

Then, you can see the distribution of her frontalis (and if she has a split); you can see the muscle belly. You are looking for the muscle; the wrinkles are a guide, but *so is the protrusion of the muscle and the depression where there is no muscle.*

Your patient does not die if you put BoNT in the depressed area where there is no muscle, but it wastes her money.

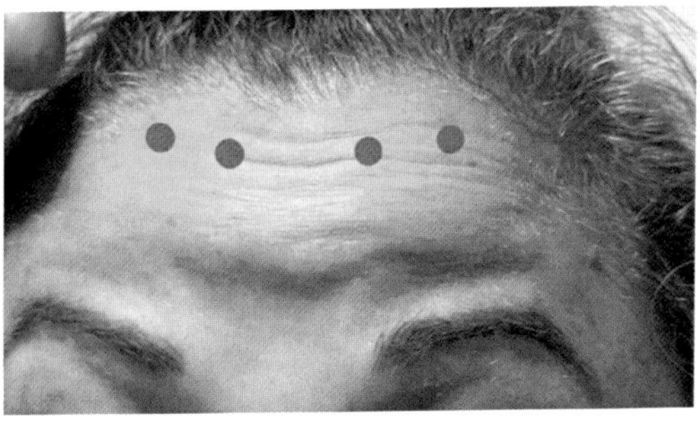

Figure 171. For migraines, inject 4 locations, each injection site receives 5 units, for a total of 20 units.

Each injection point is five units—four injection points for a total of 20 units in the frontalis.

Put the most lateral injection slightly lateral to *an imaginary line going up from the lateral edge of the iris to the top of the frontalis.*

Put the next injection of 5 units in line with the medial canthus at the top of the frontalis. Repeat on the other side.

Massage each muscle area for a few seconds after every injection when treating migraines (which I do not do when I inject the face for cosmetic purposes except with the frontalis and the glabella region). You massage the muscles when treating migraines because it is comforting, and in all seven locations, it helps to spread the BoNT, and (unlike as happens with cosmetic injections) you do not risk ill effects of inadvertently affecting unintended muscles.

Then, after the two or three-second massage, look for active bleeding; only when you see no bleeding do you move to the next muscle group.

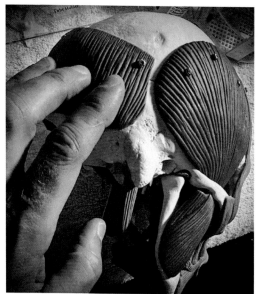

Figure 172. Occipitalis (Occipitofrontalis, Fronto occipitalis) receives 15 units divided into three locations, where my fingertips rest. Notice my very short fingernails--clipped short to (1) look cleaner, and (2) to avoid scratching patients.

4. Injecting Occipitofrontalis (Occipitalis, Frontalis, Fronto Occipitalis)

Nomenclature reflects function.

It took a while for me to decipher that *reference books and research papers use four different names to mean the same muscle—occipitalis.* Unless you know all four names and why there are four of them, you may find further reading on the injection of BoNT for migraines to be confusing. So, a review of each of the four synonyms and the rationale for each name is worth the five minutes it takes to review them: (1) Frontalis, (2) Occipitofrontalis, (3) Fronto Occipitalis, and (4) Occipitalis.

Synonym 1: Frontalis

In some books, you will see this muscle (which overlies the occiput) labeled as simply the *"frontalis,"* which makes no sense if you only look at an anatomy diagram, because this part of it is not in the front—it is in the back. And we are already calling the front part the frontalis.

But, because the occiput section is connected by aponeurosis to the section over the forehead, and since they both function in synchrony to lift the brow, some call both parts of it the frontalis.

So, it is the occipital part of the frontalis—which to me means the "back of the front" but you can just call them both the frontalis.

If that seems confusing to you, then we are in the same club.

Synonym 2: Occipitofrontalis

This name, I suppose, makes more sense because it is the back part of a muscle in the front (frontalis), so why not give it a name that implies the same: Occipitofrontalis—the *back of the front?*

Still seems confusing to me, but I am not a part of the supreme court of nomenclature judges. I think this name is most preferred by those who take pleasure in feeling smarter than others by speaking in code.

Name 3: Fronto Occipitalis

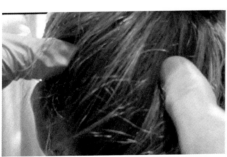

Why not call it fronto occipitalis instead of occipitofrontalis (the front of the back, instead of the back of the front)?

Some people do—still the same muscle.

Figure 173. The occipitofrontalis will extend from a centimeter or so medial to the center of the occiput to just posterior to the ear (at about 2 centimeters above the ear).

This name is most preferred by those who are vigilant about equity. I like this one better than the first two.

We have listed three names so far for the same muscle; one more to go.

In some books, the muscle is simply called *"occipitalis."*

I like this name best. No confusion.

In fairness to those who prefer one of the first three names (and you must vote for one of the four names every time you speak or write about the muscle), the confusion arose in the past because the occipitalis and the occipitofrontalis were considered two separate muscles: both overlying the occiput, but the occipitalis was the more inferior part of the posterior part. Now all the muscle overlying the occiput is considered one muscle. (Whitmore, 2011)

The reason that occipitalis was previously considered to be two muscles is because it has two muscle bellies joined by the galea aponeurotica, with each of the two parts doing something slightly different (the inferior part even contracting involuntarily). (Kushima, 2005).

But now, occipitofrontalis and occipitalis are considered synonymous. (Whitmore, 2011)

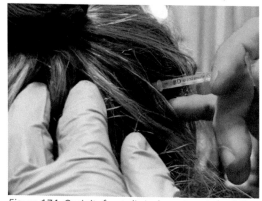

Figure 174. Occipitofrontalis is deep; insert the full length of your needle. No need to give them a shampoo or cleanse with alcohol--just go through the hair down to the scalp.

Maybe that exercise in semantics was unwarranted, but it seems to me that if you are going to inject a muscle, you do not need to buy it dinner, but you should respect it enough to know its name.

Where to Put the Needle

Find the occipitofrontalis by palpating just superior to the top of the ear and just lateral to the midline of the occiput.

Inject 5 units, then, moving horizontally and laterally, inject twice more with 5 units each (a total of 3 injections); repeat on the other side for a total of 30 units and 6 injections. The three injections on each side should cover most of the occiput of that side and spare the center of the occiput.

5. Injecting Temporalis

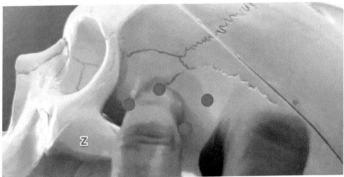

To find the temporalis, start by finding the cheekbone and then feel just above the posterior aspect.

Figure 175. My index finger rests on where temporalis resides. The dots mark the rhomboid-shaped injection points. The "z" marks the zygoma.

Remember you grind your teeth with your masseters but move your teeth up and down with your temporalis. So, if you ask her to clench her teeth, you can feel the temporalis contract.

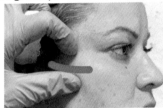

Figure 177. If you grasp the "cheekbone" with your index finger and thumb, your index finger will touch the temporalis.

Go just above the cheekbone and inject 5 units into the temporalis, then move posteriorly 2 cm and inject another 5 units.

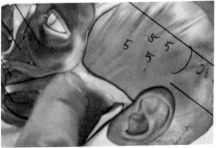

Figure 176. Find the temporalis by finding the zygoma and then inject 4 injection points in a rhomboid configuration. Each injection point is 5 units (10 units on your syringe).

343

Imagine a rhombus (think of a rectangle with the upper edge moved posteriorly by 1/2 to a full centimeter); then inject the top two corners of the rhombus.

Repeat on the contralateral side—20 units per side, for a total of 40 units.

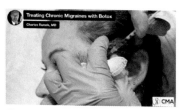

Figure 178. Injecting temporalis from screen shot of video on BoNTClass.com

6. Injecting Trapezius

We have two more (of the seven muscle groups treated when treating migraine) to complete the treatment: (1) the trapezius, and (2) the splenius capitis.

For the trapezius, find where the vertical part of the neck sweeps horizontally and becomes the shoulder—find that inflection point.

Inject the inflection point (slightly posteriorly). Then inject about an inch or two above the first injection, and again about an inch or two below—

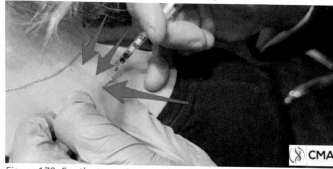

Figure 179. For the trapezius, use three injection points of 5 units per injection on each side; 15 units per side; a total of 30 units.

5 units in each of the three injection points. That is 15 units total which will be all the contents of a full 30-unit insulin syringe (since you did the dilution for migraines with 2 ccs of saline).

Then repeat on the other trapezius, with another 15 units distributed into 3 injection points.

7. Injecting Splenius Cap

For the treatment of migraines, the splenius capitis muscle is the label used on some instructional diagrams; other diagrams label this area as the "paraspinal muscles."

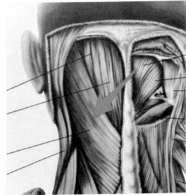

I think your injections work better if you imagine a specific and strategic target. So, aim for the splenius capitis (not a vague group of paraspinal muscles).

The splenius capitis attaches inferiorly to the nuchal ligament and to the spinous processes of the lowest cervical vertebrae (C7), and to the most superior three thoracic vertebrae (T1-T3).

T1, T2, & T3. Injecting BoNT into the mastoid notch and then medial and inferior to the notch will relax it.

It attaches superiorly to the mastoid process. So, when it contracts, it turns the head and flexes the neck.

Injecting on Rounds

As a resident in internal medicine, I worked with a mentor who suffered from severe migraines. And because he suffered from migraines, he was especially motivated to understand migraines. Some thought he was the best migraine doctor in town. Best ideas often come from the worst pain.

Sometimes, while making rounds, he would sit, bow his head, put his forehead against the desk at the nurse's station, and say, "Charles, inject me right here." (In the 1980s, we were injecting lidocaine or steroids; it was less effective than BoNT, but it helped.)

Then he would take my index finger and (pressing the tip of my finger against the back of his head) he would show me the following (after which we would go back to making internal medicine rounds):

First, find the ear. (Did I not warn you in the introduction to this course that injecting BoNT is easy?)

345

Found the ear?

Great! Now, *gently* with your index finger, palpate the skull behind the ear, near the upper part of the lobule—gently. If you imagine you are treating a fearful six-year-old, the pressure will be appropriate.

You can palpate
You can feel,
But if you poke,
patients will squeal.

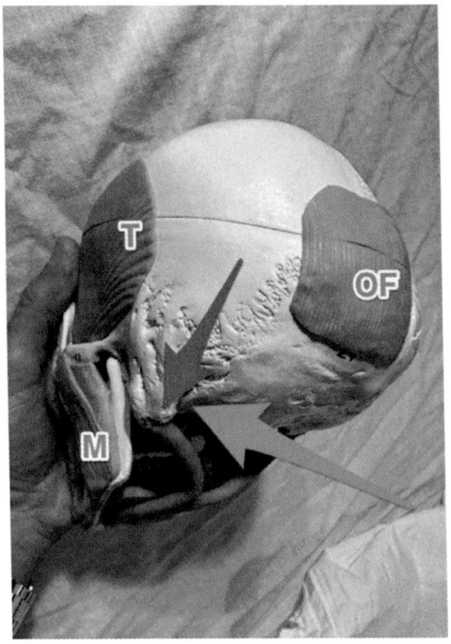

Figure 181. Red points to the mastoid process; blue to the mastoid notch; T labels the temporalis; M-masseter; OF-occipitofrontalis

Next, with your finger, follow the skull posteriorly, and you will find the posterior edge of the mastoid process.

Move your finger slightly more posteriorly; your finger will fall into a soft space—that is the mastoid notch.

Inject five units of BoNT, deep, just posteriorly to the mastoid process, into the mastoid notch; you nailed the splenius capitis near its superior insertion site.

Now, stop, take a breath, and say a silent prayer of gratitude for a way to help your patients find a better life without risking serious harm (using a procedure this easy for you to do).

Then move your finger another two centimeters medially and another four centimeters inferiorly and inject another five units.

Done!

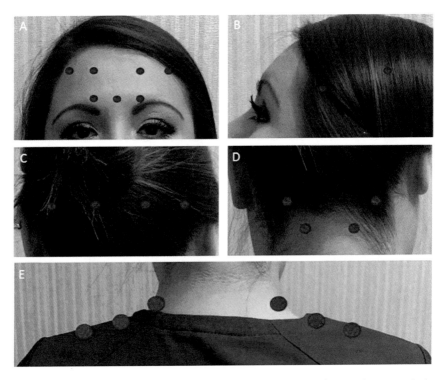

Figure 182. An alternate injection pattern for BoNT for migraines (uses only 2 instead of 4 injection points for the temporalis): A, procerus, corrugators, and frontalis; B, temporalis; C, occipitalis; D, splenius capitis; E, trapezius.

That was the Last of the Seven

Now you know how to inject all seven muscle groups with BoNT to treat migraines.

Treat yourself to your favorite beverage and look forward to many grateful patients.

An Extra Injection to Keep It Pretty

When you do the strict migraine protocol and treat the frontalis and stop without lifting the brow, you could droop the brows. So, with all women and with those men who want it, I always add in an extra three units to lift the brow, even if I am treating just for migraines. (See Chapter 28 of this course for detailed techniques for lifting the brow.)

The brow lift likely does not help with migraines; it is only because I do not want to droop her. Most neurologists will not do the brow lift because that is not part of the migraine treatment.

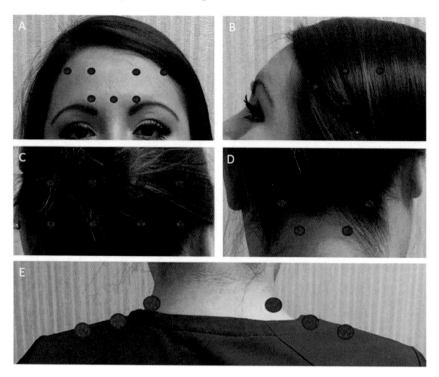

Figure 183. An alternate map of the injection sites for the treatment of migraines. D shows injection sites for the splenius muscle (paraspinal muscles); A shows sites for the procerus, corrugators, and frontalis; B, temporalis; C, occipitofrontalis (occipitalis), shows an extra row of injections; D, splenius capitis, & E, trapezius (Zandieh, 2022)

For the brow lift, I use a separate vial with my usual dilution of one cc to one hundred units, which gives me one unit of BoNT per one unit on my syringe. If I use the more voluminous dilution that I use to treat migraines, I am more likely to cause ptosis when the BoNT spreads down onto the lid.

First, I find the anterior protrusion of the zygoma or what I call the "corner of the head." And then I put my finger medial to that, grab the brow, and inject five units between my fingers.

This is the part that would make her eyelids droop if she rubbed it. So, tell her to wait 4 hours before she touches her brows.

Now, we are finally done. We treated migraines, and we threw in extra, so eyebrows do not droop.

Another Word about Cash vs. Insurance as It Specifically Applies to Migraine Treatment

When people see me for other problems and ask if I can treat their migraines with BoNT, I tell them I can, but that their neurologist can charge their insurance, and they can get it for free.

But, if they want me to treat their migraines, then I will make the results pretty and treat their migraines.

I think it is unethical to charge cash for the treatment of migraines with BoNT without informing your patient that they may be able to receive the treatment for free using their insurance.

If you accept insurance (I do not), then, of course, treat them and charge their insurance.

Surprisingly, many people, without treating anything other than the procerus, the corrugators, and the frontalis, will enjoy complete relief from their migraines.

If they choose to pay (cash, credit card, or check) instead using their insurance, the cosmetic-only strategy (not treating temporalis, occipitalis, trapezius, or splenius capitis) is worth trying since that is much less expensive for them than paying for the complete migraine protocol; and if you add in crow's feet and a brow lift, they will see a great cosmetic effect as well.

Further Help to Make it Even Easier than Easy

For detailed videos that demonstrate the injections for migraine treatment—which you can watch over and over (even, if you are smart, right before you treat a patient), see my online version of this course at

BoNTClass.com—it costs less than you will make from two BoNT patients and will bring to you patients wet (with tears of gratitude); and those grateful people will gladly give you many thousands of dollars.

References

1. Chan TLH. OnabotulinumtoxinA Improves Quality of Life in Chronic Migraine: The PREDICT Study. *Can J Neurol Sci.* 2022;49(4):477-478. doi:10.1017/cjn.2021.159

2. Escher CM, Paracka L, Dressler D, Kollewe K. Botulinum toxin in the management of chronic migraine: clinical evidence and experience. *Ther Adv Neurol Disord.* 2017;10(2):127-135. doi:10.1177/1756285616677005

3. FDA official recommendations regarding Botox. https://www.accessdata.fda.gov/ drugsatfda_docs/label/2011/103000s5236lbl.pdf

4. Kushima, Hideo, Kiyoshi Matsuo, Shunshuke Yuzuriha, Takeshi Kitazawa, and Tetsuji Moriizumi. "The Occipitofrontalis Muscle Is Composed of Two Physiologically and Anatomically Different Muscles Separately Affecting the Positions of the Eyebrow and Hairline." *British Journal of Plastic Surgery* 58, no. 5 (July 2005): 681–87. https://doi.org/10.1016/j.bjps.2005.01.006.

5. Minen MT, Begasse De Dhaem O, Kroon Van Diest A, et al. Migraine and its psychiatric comorbidities. *J Neurol Neurosurg Psychiatry.* 2016;87(7):741-749. doi:10.1136/jnnp-2015-312233

6. Ramachandran R, Yaksh TL. Therapeutic use of botulinum toxin in migraine: mechanisms of action. *Br J Pharmacol.* 2014;171(18):4177-4192. doi:10.1111/bph.12763

7. Wang SJ. Comorbidities of migraine. *Front Neur.* 2010;4. doi:10.3389/fneur.2010.00016

8. Whitmore, Ian, Federative Committee on Anatomical Terminology, and Federative International Programme on Anatomical Terminologies, eds. *Terminologia anatomica: = International anatomical terminology ;*

FIPAT, federative international programme on anatomical terminologies. 2nd ed. Stuttgart: Thieme, 2011.

9. Zandieh A, Cutrer FM. OnabotulinumtoxinA in chronic migraine: is the response dose-dependent? *BMC Neurol*. 2022;22(1):218. doi:10.1186/s12883-022-02742-x

42. TREATING BRUXISM (& ASSOCIATED HEADACHES) WITH BONT

A Quick & Easy Miracle

People suffer tremendously from bruxism, but you can quickly and safely make life better for them. (Ågren, 2020) They are happy; you feel good about what you did; and you are rewarded handsomely for helping (and never lose sleep worrying that you hurt someone). You are going to love treating bruxism.

Bruxism is another condition (in addition to a gummy smile, Chapter 33) for which the dentist would be the most appropriate person to treat the problem—if the dentists knew how. Unfortunately, many states in the U.S. do not allow dentists to inject BoNT. So, I cannot blame dentists for being unaware of the possibilities. Therefore, their patients are often treated for bruxism and associated headaches (sometimes severe and life-limiting) with uncomfortable devices when you can usually relieve bruxism with only 30 units of BoNT.

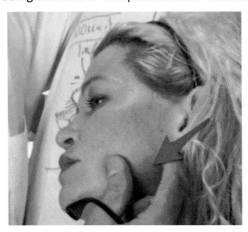

Figure 184. Index finger placed lightly on the mandible and the thumb on the anterior edge of the masseter (easily palpated when the patient clenches her teeth).

The relief is so dramatic that people will return when they realize their headaches are back, and say, "Oh, it's time for more BoNT."

Some will come to you just for bruxism but then want other services. They will remember to come to see you when their headache returns. Then you also do the other things you know how to do. So, you make their headaches better and keep their face youthful. Most, however, will visit you for cosmetic treatments and then will be delighted and grateful when they discover you can also treat their bruxism.

And it is easy to do. I have never seen anybody made to look stupid by this treatment. Of all the techniques in this course, injecting the masseters for bruxism may be the safest regarding your risk of making a weird-looking face.

How to Spot the Person Who Needs You

If you see a Caucasian woman who demonstrates the following, she almost always suffers from bruxism: when you look at her from the

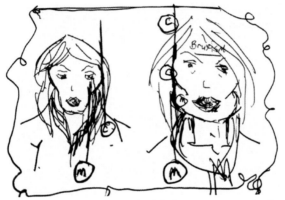

front, her jaw (at the masseter) is wider than her cheek (at the widest point).

This sign (the jaw wider than the cheek in a Caucasian female) is called the *Runels Sign*.

Figure 185. The woman on the left demonstrates a cheek (c) that is wider than her jaw at the masseter (m). The woman on the right demonstrates a jaw that is wider than the cheek; therefore, if she is Caucasian, she demonstrates Runels Sign and likely suffers from bruxism. I do not know a similar sign that applies to other ethnicities. This sign is sensitive but not specific.

I do not know of a similar sign that applies to other ethnicities. For women of Asian descent, the jaw is often wider than the cheek without the condition of bruxism. In the case of an Asian woman, one might affect a narrowing of the jaw, if she wants, by injecting each masseter with 50 units of BoNT, per side, divided into three different locations (for a total of 100 units to treat both sides.)

Men also usually have a jaw that is wider than the cheek; so, in men, this rule does not apply.

Those of other ethnicities (African, Indian, Native American, etc.) who suffer from bruxism also seem less reliably identified by this rule.

But, for women of European descent, the Runels Sign almost always applies.

So, from across the room, if you see a woman of Caucasian descent who demonstrates a jaw wider than the cheek, she likely suffers from Bruxism.

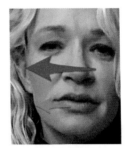

Figure 186. Cheek wider than jaw and Caucasian—she does not demonstrate the Runels Sign; thus, she is less likely to suffer from bruxism.

Therefore, if you want to be a hero, do the following: When you are treating a Caucasian woman with cosmetic BoNT, and you see that she demonstrates the Runels Sign, and you want to help her and easily encourage her devotion to you and your practice for life, simply say the following, "I notice that your face seems to demonstrate signs of bruxism. Do you grind your teeth at night or suffer from headaches?"

The woman answers, "Yes! My husband says it sometimes sounds like I am going to crack my teeth when I am sleeping. The dentist made a device for me to wear at night, and that helps, but I do not really like wearing it. How did you know?"

You then hand her a mirror and say (while she looks at her face), "Often, when someone grinds their teeth at night, their masseter muscle becomes hypertrophied. The shape can be glamourous, but it can also be a sign that the woman suffers from bruxism. If you want, I can usually make that better with only 30 units of BoNT. If you do not think it helps, I will give you 30 units for free at your next BoNT treatment. But I think you will love it."

She smiles and says, "Yes! Let's try it!"

I have had that conversation, as if scripted, almost word for word, so many times over the past decade that I have lost count. And many women have found relief.

Simply by asking that question every time you see the Runels Sign, you will pay for this course many times over and help many to a better life.

Where to Put the Needle

Find the Masseter Muscle

First, ask them to clench their teeth, then you can easily palpate the masseter muscle's anterior edge; it is close to halfway along the jaw.

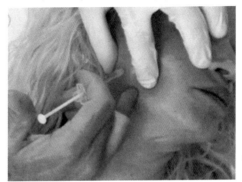

The posterior part is also the posterior edge of the jaw. So, when you follow their mandible posteriorly, you go around the curve, and you are at the posterior edge of the masseter.

Figure 187. Injecting 15 units into the masseter muscle to help with bruxism. Use a simple bolus of cosmetic BoNT (mixed with 1 cc to a 100-unit vial).

I am holding her masseter muscle by the anterior and posterior edges while doing the injection (in the photo).

Injecting

Draw up 30 units of BoNT, with the recommended dilution (1cc/100 units), which will be one completely full syringe using our 30-unit, 31-gauge insulin syringes.

Now, put your needle in the center of the rectangle-shaped masseter, and if you are a little off-center, it won't matter.

After the needle is all the way in (the skin is flush with the base of the needle), inject 15 units.

You inject half of the 30 units on one side and half on the other.

As a rule, I ask people to contract their muscles (whether it is the corrugator, the frontalis, or whatever) to find where I want to inject, but then I ask them to relax the muscle when doing the injection.

Hollywood Tip

To really understand the masseter, watch the best-looking masseter muscle ever filmed; watch Brad Pitt in *Legend of the Fall* when he is angry, drinking his coffee on the front porch after he just had sex with his late brother's wife, and he is arguing with the older brother—and he clenches his teeth.

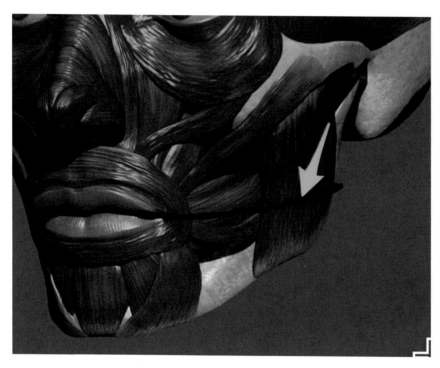

Figure 188. To find the injection point for bruxism, imagine a line from the corner of the mouth, horizontally to the back of the jaw; a needle inserted into this line in the center of the masseter muscle will deliver the BoNT in the correct place.

Part of what makes Pitt (and other leading men) a sex symbol is his huge masseter muscle. A prominent masseter is a very masculine shape.

Study the structure and shape of faces when at the movies and let Hollywood teach you about beauty. What makes a face look strong, angry, old, sad, exhausted, smart, drunk? The plot teaches you the topography of the faces—and knowing the topography of faces makes you a better injector.

Further Help

- You can watch a video of me injecting the masseter for bruxism at BoNTClass.com
- You can see a more detailed topographic map that demonstrates that the female has a cheek is wider than the masseter and that men show a masseter that is wider than the cheek at the following website (which I recommend that you study): BeautyAnalysis.com

References

Ågren M, Sahin C, Pettersson M. The effect of botulinum toxin injections on bruxism: A systematic review. *Journal of Oral Rehabilitation*. 2020;47(3):395-402. doi:10.1111/joor.12914

Caleo M, Restani L. Direct central nervous system effects of botulinum neurotoxin. *Toxicon*. 2018;147:68-72. doi:10.1016/j.toxicon.2017.10.027

Fernández-Núñez T, Amghar-Maach S, Gay-Escoda C. Efficacy of botulinum toxin in the treatment of bruxism: Systematic review. *Med Oral Patol Oral Cir Bucal*. 2019;24(4):e416-e424. doi:10.4317/medoral.22923

43. TREATING ERECTILE DYSFUNCTION WITH BONT

In my view, you could teach a reasonably attentive fourteen-year-old how to treat frown lines with BoNT. Without knowing anything else, she could treat frown lines, see excellent results, and not hurt anyone.

Such is *not* the case with erectile dysfunction (ED).

Though it is true that (as with facial BoNT injections) the chance of doing harm by injecting the penis is near zero, seeing excellent results treating ED with BoNT (unlike with cosmetic injections) requires understanding all the following: the pathology and anatomy of ED, patient selection and follow-up, other options for the treatment of ED, and how to integrate BoNT injections with the other therapies.

This chapter will demonstrate why BoNT might help some men with ED, but the practitioner should either understand all of the other aspects of the treatment of ED, or work closely with another practitioner who does.

BoNT for ED—Why & Why Not?

Also, before considering the specifics of how to treat erectile dysfunction with BoNT, it is useful to consider the strongest arguments for *not* using BoNT to treat ED.[8]

For that purpose, consider the argument for not using BoNT to treat ED, presented by the authors of an editorial in the *Journal of Sexual Medicine*: "*Given the multitude of treatment options currently available for the management of ED (PDE5i, VED, IU alprostadil, ICI, prostheses) and the many treatment options currently under investigation (LiSWT,*

---

[8] In general, before doing or recommending the doing of anything, it is useful to consider the reasons for not doing. Not only does such an exercise strengthen understanding, bit it also helps assure the practice of "first do no harm."

SCT, PRP), a substantial advantage of BoNT-A use would need to be demonstrated to warrant its inclusion in the treatment algorithms." (Habashy, 2022)

In other words, "We already have good ways to treat ED, so we do not need a better way."

The preceding statement echoes Dr. Barry Marshall's observation when accepting the Nobel Prize:

"The greatest obstacle to discovery is not ignorance—it is the illusion of knowledge."

When Dr. Marshall did his research, doctors already "knew" that ulcers were caused by acid and stress, and the best treatments were H2

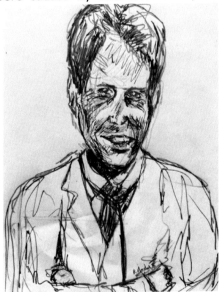

Figure 189. *"The greatest obstacle to discovery is not ignorance—it is the illusion of knowledge."—Dr. Barry Marshall*

blockers and surgery, so they thought there was no need for something new and better (and completely rejected the idea that ulcers may be caused by helicobacter pylori and helped with antibiotics).

Similarly, Habashy et al do not mention in their editorial that the long-standing therapies for ED do nothing to reverse the pathology causing the ED. Neither do they mention that we should not only consider the advantages of BoNT for ED but also *consider the disadvantages of the "multitude" of currently*

available treatment options for ED (the actual number of options that comprise the "multitude" is eight).

In other words, the need for new may be because the new accomplishes more *while also avoiding the unwanted side effects of the old.*

Five Long-Standing Therapies

Consider the following list of unwanted effects for each of the five long-standing treatments for ED (in the order presented by Habashy et. al):

1. **PDE5Is** can increase the risk of blindness, melanoma, and cause decreased hearing, they can be costly, and must be taken long-term. (Etminan , 2022) (Gul, 2019)

   All but one formulation must be taken an hour or so before sexual intercourse—hindering spontaneity.

   Also, PDE5Is show decreased effectiveness over time, they do not work for some and cannot be tolerated by others.

   Reasons for intolerance include all the following: Headache (9–16%); Dyspepsia (4–12%); Flushing (3–10%); Nasal congestion (1–10%); Abnormal vision (1–2%); Myalgia (< 5%); and Backpain (< 6.5%). (Gul, 2019)

   Most importantly, *PDE5is do little to improve the health of the penile tissue.*

2. **Vacuum erection devices (VED)** must be used before each encounter, which can take time and be awkward in the bedroom.

   They also require the use of a constrictor band, which can be uncomfortable (for both the man and his lover) and may not maintain adequate erection hardness. (Cayetano-Alcaraz, 2023)

   There is, however, evidence that VEDs may help improve the health of the penis. (Welliver, 2014)

3. **IU alprostadil** requires use before each encounter, can be painful, and becomes less effective with time. It also does

nothing to improve the health of the penile tissue.

4. **Intracavernosal injections** (ICI) require an injection before each sexual encounter, risk priapism, and fibrosis, and present an ongoing cost. (Gul, 2019) They also become less effective with time and do not work for all men, with some men becoming resistant to their effects in less than a year.

5. **Penile implant** satisfaction rates vary from 79 to 98% depending on the cohort, with most studies showing satisfaction with the procedure at around 80%. But one study showed that only 69% would "definitely do the procedure again." (Wong, 2022)

    Complaints by the 20% who said they would definitely *not* do the procedure again and the 11% who were *unsure* if they would do the procedure again include all the following: Loss of length 4.39/5 (1.05); loss of use of penis 4.67/5 (0.84); appearance 3.78/5 (1.07); unnatural feel of implant 4.05/5 (1.04); hard glans 3.62/5 (0.87); surgical complications 3.63/5 (1.40); concealment of implant 3.50/5 (1.10); indiscrete erection 4.0/5 (1.14). (Wong, 2022)

    Unlike with drugs or other therapies, the 20% or so who are unhappy with penile implants cannot simply "discontinue" their use (as with an ineffective or intolerable drug); instead, discontinuation requires an additional surgery to remove the device (along with associated risks and discomfort).

    For all the foregoing reasons, most agree that *implants should be reserved for those who do not respond to less invasive modalities.*

6. **Every penile implant surgery represents a man for whom conservative therapy did not work. Said another way, if the current standard non-surgical options were adequate, there would be no penile implant surgery.**

Since the current less aggressive options are often inadequate, why would we not incorporate additional conservative therapies (assuming the additions are helpful for at least some who are treated)?

7. *None of the current long-standing therapies do anything to slow the progression or reverse the pathology of ED other than perhaps the penis vacuum device.*

Three Relatively New *Adjunctive* [9] Therapies

Shock wave therapy, stem cells, and platelet-rich plasma (PRP), are three relatively new strategies (within the past ten years) for improving erectile function that *work by improving the health of penile tissue.* (Habashy, 2022)

1. **Low-intensity shock wave therapy (LiSWT)** has the potential to improve the health of the tissue. It usually requires a series of six treatments spread out over three weeks, each session requiring 20 minutes or so of the time of a provider and the patient. Sessions need to be repeated periodically.

2. Since the FDA has classified **stem cells** as a drug, stem-cell therapy (SCT) for ED is not currently available in the United States without the umbrella of an IRB-approved research protocol. Therefore, SCT is not available to most men in the United States.

3. The use of **platelet-rich plasma (PRP)** for ED was first introduced by the author in 2010 with his **P-Shot® (Priapus Shot®) procedure**

---

[9] Alternative implies "instead of." Adjunctive implies "in addition to," or "integrated into an overall treatment strategy;" therefore, "adjunctive" is the term preferred over "alternative" when considering new therapies backed by strong science. But even the term "adjunctive" implies bias against the use of a new idea just because it is new. Therapy supported by science is simply medicine; that which is supported by science is simply another therapy. Labeling the new as "alternative" or "adjunctive" implies second best only because it is a recently considered treatment option.

(registered with the US Patent & Trademark Office)[10]—a specific method of preparing and injecting PRP for the improvement of erectile function. (https://uspto.gov)

PRP has been shown to help both ED and Peyronie's disease. It is a shot that must be repeated every year or so. It helps improve the health of the tissue of the penis as demonstrated by doppler flow studies and ultrasound. But it is not sufficient alone to completely cure ED in all men (it improves erection by about seven, on average, on a 5-25 point ED scale). PriapusShot.com/research lists a collection of research regarding the P-Shot® procedure.

The Fourth & Much Needed Regenerative Option—BoNT

Considering the previously discussed eight options and their limitations, and considering that even with these options, still, some men are not helped sufficiently and proceed to penile implant (of which around 20% regret the implant), one reaches the obvious conclusion that we could use additional non-surgical strategies.

The very fact that some men progress to the need for a penile implant shows that our current non-surgical options are not sufficient; we need something new and helpful in our toolbox for treating ED.

Moreover, *BoNT has been shown to improve erection even in some who no longer respond to PDE5is* (including those with spinal cord injury and long-standing diabetes). (El-Shaer, 2021) (Abdelrahman, 2022)

---

[10] The P-Shot® (also known as the Priapus Shot®) is a particular type of trademark known as a "service mark." The use of a service mark indicates that physicians licensed by the Cellular Medicine Association to use the name P-Shot® have agreed to follow a specific protocol that includes patient selection, how platelet-rich plasma is prepared, how it is activated, how it is injected, and how the patient is cared for after the procedure.

Synergy Improves Results

Of the currently available options, four potentially improve the health of the penis: VED, the P-Shot® procedure, shock wave, and BoNT. (Mykoniatis, 2021) (El-Shaer, 2021) (Abdelrahman, 2022)

Moreover, even though studies most strongly support an individual treatment when only one treatment is compared with a placebo or control arm, in the clinic, with individual patients, for best results, multiple therapies can be combined for a synergistic effect. (Mykoniatis, 2021)

Research to prove the relative effectiveness of a variety of combination treatments involving 4 or more variables is mathematically difficult. As with other diseases, however, *clinicians are free to combine multiple therapies for ED when each component of the combinatio has been shown to be effective and science supports the synergy of the combination.* (Mykoniatis, 2021)

For example, for a decade, the P-Shot® procedure has been used in combination with VED and PDE5is; multiple studies show that each works well alone. More recently, LiSWT, VED, and BoNT are combined with the P-Shot® for effects beyond what the research demonstrates for any one of those therapies alone.

Why would one only treat symptoms
(PDEIs, alprostadil, ICI)
when the possibility of reversing or slowing the
progression of pathology exists
(P-Shot®, VED, BoNT, LiSWT)?

For the individual patient (not for research), when regenerative therapies exist, even when non-regenerative therapies are effective, to use only non-regenerative therapies for treatment and give up the possibility of slowing or reversing pathology seems to the author to be less than optimal care.

For example, since both PRP and BoNT have decades of research showing the possibility of neovascularization and neurogenesis, why would one not offer the P-Shot® procedure or BoNT (for their regenerative effects) as part of an overall treatment plan even when PDE5Is might work alone to sufficiently treat the symptoms of ED?

A Suggested Algorithm for Combined Therapies (How BoNT Fits in the Treatment Plan)

Considering that eight options exist for the treatment of ED, a need arises for a way to structure the various options as a treatment plan.

The following is a suggested treatment algorithm that is supported by multiple studies:

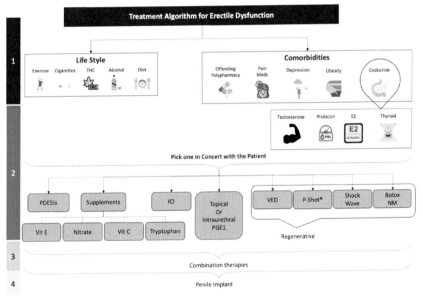

Figure 190. Erectile dysfunction treatment algorithm: Exercise helps; cigarettes, marijuana, & alcohol hinder. Diet can help or hinder. PDE5i (phosphodiesterase type 5 inhibitor); ICI (Intracavernosal injections); VED (vacuum erection device); P-Shot® (specific method for the preparation and injection of PRP); BoNT & other Neuromodulators (NM). (Cayetano-Alcaraz, 2023), (PriapusShot.com/research) ©2023, Charles Runels, MD

Three Ways BoNT Improves Erection (Mechanism of Action)

The last subject to consider before examining the methods for the Intracavernosal injection of BoNT is the possible mechanism of action. BoNT is thought to improve erectile function in three ways:

1. The relaxation of smooth muscle, with resultant increased arterial *blood flow*.
2. An increased ratio of *parasympathetic* to sympathetic tone, resulting in increased blood flow.
3. The *regenerative* effects of BoNT (neovascularization, neurogenesis, and the remodeling of fibrotic tissue)—also improving blood flow as well as possibly helping with Peyronie's disease.

1. The *Relaxation of Smooth Muscle* by BoNT

BoNT relaxes smooth muscle; it has been used for over a decade to treat overactive bladder (with detrusor spasms and urge incontinence) by the relaxation of smooth muscle. (Ibrahim, 2022)

In the same way, BoNT can relax the smooth muscle governing the arterial blood flow of the penis, resulting in a harder erection. (Abdelrahman, 2022)

By comparison, relaxing smooth muscle to increase penile arterial blood flow is thought to also be the primary mechanism of action of PDE5Is to improve ED.

2. The Increase in *Parasympathetic Tone* and Decrease in Sympathetic Tone Afforded by BoNT

BoNT is thought to block the release of norepinephrine from the presynaptic terminal—causing a "chemical sympathectomy" of the treated area (in this case, the penis). (Morris, 2002) (Aru, 2017)

BoNT is taken up by endocytosis into afferent neurons. It then migrates centrally to the ganglion where it can both (1) affect the signal of other afferent neurons converging on the same ganglion and (2) change the balance of parasympathetic and sympathetic tone—essentially affecting a sympathectomy. (Ramachandran, 2014)

366

This same central migration (not relief of muscle tension) is thought to be crucial to the mechanism by which BoNT relieves migraine. (Ramachandran, 2014)

Since erection is improved by increased parasympathetic tone, when BoNT decreases sympathetic tone, erection is enhanced by the relative increased parasympathetic tone (this in addition to the direct increased arterial blood flow secondary to smooth muscle relaxation). (Giuliano, 2019)

The effect of BoNT to improve erection (mostly studied thus far in combination with PDE5Is) can be seen even in those who have suffered spinal cord injury and those effects can last six months or longer. (Giuliano, 2019) This impressive effect could be largely from the synergy of smooth muscle relaxation and a chemical sympathectomy.

3. BoNT is thought to demonstrate *regenerative* effects through neurogenesis, neovascularization, and fibrotic tissue remodeling.

Neurogenesis
The physiology literature has discussed the neurogenesis effects of botulinum toxin for over fifty years.

For example, since (like BoNT) myasthenia gravis blocks communication between nerve and muscle; and since motor end plates have long been known to enlarge in adaptation to myasthenia gravis (Woolf, 1964), investigators wondered if BoNT would precipitate similar changes.

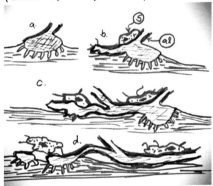

Figure 191. Diagram of possible sequence of events after the injection of botulinum toxin. (a) The toxin becomes fixed to the motor nerve terminal (blue cross hatching); (b) axonal sprouting from the terminal, supported by Swann cells (S) which form the axolemma (al); (c) the bound toxin is diluted, and the axon forms new contacts with the muscle fiber at some distance from the site of the original end plate; (d) the contacts develop subneural folds of the sarcolemma—the result is an expansion of the innervation network. (Duchen, 1972)

As expected, researchers demonstrated that when BoNT blocks the motor end plate, new axons sprout, which Schwann cells support—resulting in significant new innervation. (Duchen, 1968)

Also, the initial muscle atrophy seen after botulinum toxin is temporary, but the new axons (which rapidly proliferate and quickly establish function by new neuromuscular junctions) can be permanent. (Duchen, 1968)

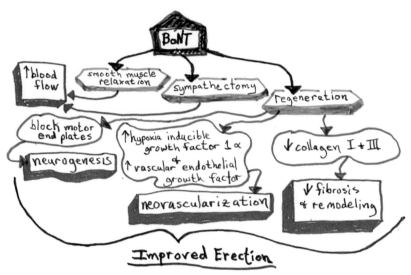

Figure 192. Research supports the improvement in erection by BoNT in a variety of ways: smooth muscle relaxation and decreased sympathetic tone increase blood flow; blocking end plates triggers neurogenesis; increased hypoxia inducible factor-1α (HIF-1α) and increased vascular endothelial growth factor (VEGF) triggers neovascularization; decreased collagen I and III production triggers decreased fibrosis and remodeling of scar tissue.

Other studies demonstrating the neurogenesis effect of BoNT abound. For example, more recently, Xeomin® was shown to help with regeneration in spinal cord injury. (Mastrorilli, 2023)

Neovascularization

Most of the research regarding the angiogenesis effects of BoNT have been studied towards the goal of improved flap survival in plastic surgery. (Fasano, 2022) In that arena, BoNT has been shown to improve blood flow in both skin and muscle. (Fasano, 2022)

The mechanism of action has been postulated to be at least partly from BoNT-promoted increased levels of both hypoxia-inducible factor (HIF) 1α and vascular endothelial growth factor (VEGF). (Aru, 2017) (Park, 2016)[11]

With one of many possible expanded applications, BoNT injected into the endometrium of the uterus of rats caused angiogenesis and a resultant improvement in fertility. (Koo, 2021)

Though angiogenesis is not a proven mechanism of action for the demonstrable improvement in erection seen with the injection of BoNT into the corpus cavernosum, such a mechanism would be consistent with effects demonstrated in all other tissues thus far studied.

With PDE5Is, there is vasodilatation of existing blood vessels; and (as mentioned previously) this is also thought to be one of the effects of BoNT. But neovascularization is much more than vasodilatation: here, the idea is that BoNT not only dilates existing arterial blood flow but also adds new blood vessels and dilates those new blood vessels as well.[12]

Decreased Fibrosis

One review article looked at 1,000 papers regarding the use of BoNT both to treat and prevent scar formation (Carrero, 2018); so, the research regarding the ability of BoNT to treat fibrosis has been extensive.

The way that BoNT helps prevent or treat scar formation is not well understood. One possible mechanism is the ability of BoNT to decrease the activity of hypertrophic-scar-forming fibroblasts, with the resultant

---

[11] Platelet-rich plasma (used in the P-Shot® procedure) also contains VEGF as well as over 20 other cytokines and growth factors, (Pavlovic, 2016) so one might expect a synergy between Intracavernosal BoNT and the P-Shot® procedure.

[12] Obvious, but worth highlighting simply because it is beautiful and profound.

decrease in the production of Type I and Type III collagen (the primary components of scars). (Zhibo, 2008)

BoNT may also decrease scar formation by decreasing wound tension. (Carrero, 2018)

If BoNT promotes new axons & new blood vessels,
& decreased fibrosis
not simply the dilatation of existing blood vessels,
then,
along with shock waves, stem cells, and
the P-Shot® procedure,
BoNT takes its place as a regenerative treatment
for erectile dysfunction
to reverse or slow the disease process.

Specific applications of using BoNT to improve scars range from decreasing scars after breast surgery to remodeling fully mature keloid scars. (Wang, 2023) (Carrero, 2018) (Disphanurat, 2021)

Therapies to decrease scaring combining BoNT with a variety of modalities, including lasers and stem cells, show promising synergy. (Wang, 2023) (Rahman, 2021)

Using BoNT for the prevention and remodeling of fibrosis and scar tissue in the penis has not been directly studied. *But should BoNT demonstrate the same effects on fibrosis in the penis as has been demonstrated in every other tissue studied, the result would be an improvement in blood flow and increased pliability (a balloon that is easier to expand), resulting in improved erection.*

Multiple studies have demonstrated the usefulness of PRP to help with Peyronie's disease. (Virag, 2017) (Culha, 2019) *If the same synergy of combination therapies seen in other tissues were seen in the penis, combining BoNT with the P-Shot® would be both effective and synergistic for the treatment of Peyronie's disease.*

Two Questions You Answer Every Time You Treat Erectile Dysfunction (Even if You Do Not Know the Questions)

The first recurring question follows: *"Why would one forego the possibility of safely reversing or slowing the progression of disease (ED or Peyronie's) simply because treating only the symptoms of ED with PDE5Is (in an individual patient) happens to be effective?"*

Another relevant question now in the mind of well-read men follows: *"If safe regenerative therapies exist, why wait until PDE5Is quit working before deploying them?"*

The answer to those two questions is answered, by your choices, every time a treatment plan is offered to a man suffering from ED. The answers seem obvious and explain why many men are demanding, and many physicians are providing combination therapies using both symptom-treating therapies and regenerative therapies from the onset of ED symptoms.

A more profound question would be this: *"Why wait until symptoms appear before offering regenerative therapies that might prevent ED?"*[13]

How to Prepare for the Treatment of ED with BoNT

To prepare to inject BoNT, first, discuss the patient's history with consideration of all the factors in the erectile dysfunction treatment algorithm.

If the decision is made to inject BoNT into the penis, then possible benefits and side effects are discussed, and a consent form should be signed. *Only use a consent form that your attorney has approved*, but you can use as a guide the consent form at BoNTPenis.com/consent .

---

[13] Avenues for future research multiply (not shrink) when knowledge grows. Another question becomes: "Is it desirable or is it unethical to treat normal functiontioning men in order to prevent disease in the arena of sexual dysfunction?"

Anesthetic

For anesthetic, I use either numbing cream or a penile block.

Numbing Cream

I use a cream that is 20% benzocaine, 8% lidocaine, & 8% tetracaine that a local pharmacy compounds. I put around five ccs of this cream on a 4x4-inch gauze pad. Then I give the patient the gauze (with the numbing cream), and a clean (but non-sterile) glove.

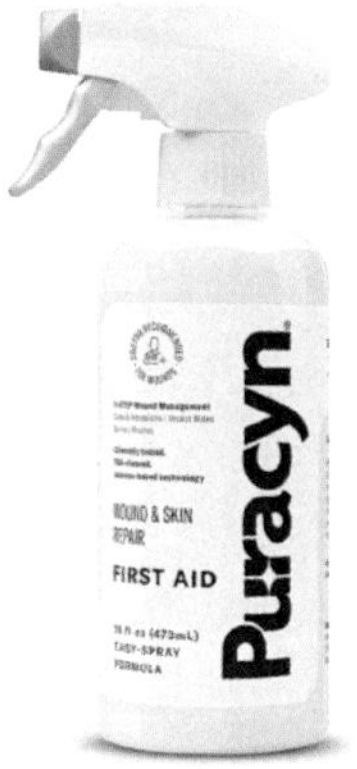

Then I tell the patient to go to the restroom and apply the cream to the penis, then put their clothes back on.

Then the numbing cream absorbs while I talk with the patient and prepare the BoNT for injection. For best effect, the cream should be in place for twenty minutes before injecting the BoNT.

Lidocaine Block

For the penis block, fill a 5-cc syringe with two ccs of 2% lidocaine without epinephrine. Use a 27-gauge or 30-gauge ½ inch needle.

Figure 193. I use the Purasyn® brand of hypochlorous solution (sold on Amazon) to cleanse the penis before injecting.

Then inject one cc on each side of the penis, at the base of the penis, at 10 O'clock and 2 O'clock: insert the needle through the skin quickly, but then advance the needle slowly until you feel it bump into Buck's fascia; inject one cc; repeat on the other side.

Give the block 10 minutes to take effect before injecting the BoNT into the corpus cavernosum.

Mix the BoNT

Using a one cc syringe and an 18-gauge needle, add one cc of bacteriostatic saline to 1 vial of 100-unit cosmetic BoNT.

Gently swirl the liquid in the bottle.

Withdraw the 1cc of fluid back into the one cc syringe.

Change the needle on the syringe from an 18 gauge to a 1/2-inch 27-gauge needle.[14]

How to Inject BoNT into the Penis for ED

Cleansing the Penis Before Injection

To cleanse the penis for injection, soak a 4x4-gauze by spraying it with hypochlorous solution (I use Purasyn®). Then use the soaked gauze to wipe away the numbing cream at the injection site before each injection.

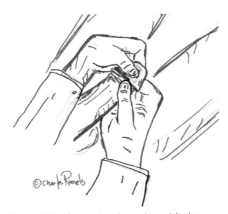

Figure 194. The patient is supine with the injector standing on the patient's right. The right (dominant hand) retracts the foreskin. Then, the left (non-dominant hand) grasps the glans. A gauze pad is used to help secure grip and provide more comfort.

Positioning the Penis for Injection

Both your accuracy and the patient's comfort will improve if you take time to carefully position the penis before injection.

This step, positioning, is extremely important—do not be in the least haphazard; if the penis is twisted or not stable, then the needle is more likely to miss the corpus cavernosum causing more pain and less effectiveness.

The BoNT will cause little effect if it is deposited subdermally rather than in the corpus cavernosum. And, with poor positioning and an unstable grip, you will justifiably lose the confidence of your patient as you frantically chase a floppy snake with your needle.

Instead, you should *establish complete stability of the penis and be able to point exactly to the dorsal nerve and to each corpus cavernosum*

---

[14]A tip for cosmetic injectors: the Juvéderm syringe comes with two 27-gauge needles. I usually only use one of these. I save the remainder for injecting the penis.

throughout the length of the penis (with your eyes closed) before you even think about injecting.

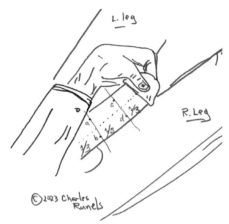

Figure 195. Imagine the penis divided into thirds. Inject into the dividing lines at 2 O'clock and 10 O'clock. If the penis is less than 3 inches erect, inject only at points (a) and (b)--the other two injections are not needed. A total of 100 units is injected: if four injection points, then each injection site receives 25 units (0.25 ccs); if two injection points, then each injection site receives 50 units (0.5 ccs).

Here are the steps to that aim:

1.   Study penile anatomy until you can (with your mind's eye) see each corpus cavernosum and the dorsal neurovascular bundle (it is not complicated).

2.   If the man is uncircumcised, first retract the foreskin with your dominant hand. If you try to grasp the penis using the foreskin as your handle, you will not provide a secure and accurate injection.

3.   (For the uncircumcised man, this would be the first step.) With the foreskin retracted, use your non-dominant hand to grasp the glans with your thumb and forefinger. Using a 4x4 gauze to help with the grip (less slippery than your gloved fingers) and to comfort of the patient (softer than the material of your glove) will make your life easier.[15]

The dorsal nerve and blood supply are at 12 O'clock; so, *place your thumb at 12 O'clock when you grasp the glans so that you keep track* of where those structures reside.

4.   Then, pulling the glans with your non-dominant hand, gently stretch the penis: straight, down, and between the legs— *without twisting it.*

---

[15] Thomas Jefferson said, "Always take hold of things by the smooth handle."

Only stretch the penis one or two inches longer than its unstretched flaccid length. If you stretch the penis too much, you overly thin the diameter of the corpus cavernous, making it more difficult to accurately inject the BoNT therein.

Moses threw down his rod
and it became a snake.
Before injecting,
stretch the snake
so it becomes a rod.

Injecting the BoNT

1. Identify the spot at 1/3 the length of the penis (measuring from the base to the tip of the glans), and at 2 O'clock. This is at point "b" on the diagram.

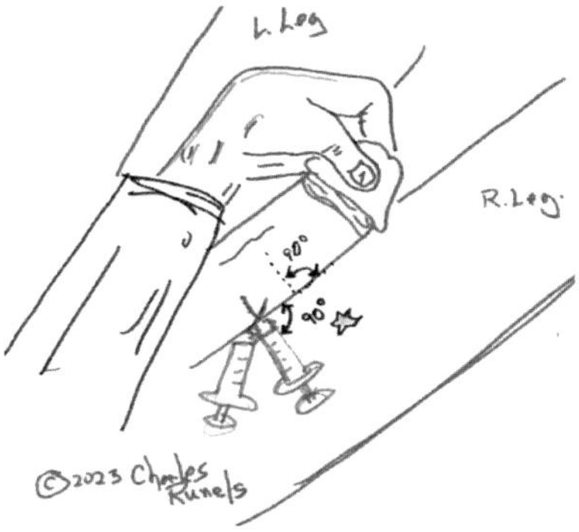

With the penis secured with your non-dominant hand and with the dorsal neurovascular bundle marked by the thumb of your non-dominant hand, *position the syringe at ninety degrees to the penis and forty-five degrees to the bed.*

Figure 196. The needle & barrel of the syringe should be at 90 degrees to the axis of the penis. Changing the angle changes the depth of the injection.

Then, touch the penis lightly with the needle, and pause a second or two; this touch offers a non-verbal notification to your patient that you are about to inject and so avoids surprise.

If instead of the light touch, you say something like, "One, two, three…", you only increase the anxiety.

If, before injection, you offer the man a rubber ball to squeeze while you inject him, you are putting him into a trance that says, "This is going to hurt."[16]

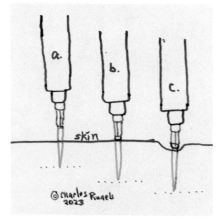

Figure 197. For depth of insertion, for most men, when using a 1/2 inch needle, (a) if the hub is hovering above the skin, the needle will likely not be fully inserted into the corpus cavernosum; (b) when the hub of the needle lightly touches the skin, and the angle of the needle is correct, the lumen of the needle will be in the corpus cavernosum in the best position for injecting; (c) when the needle is advanced until the hub depresses the skin, the lumen will often be too deep—decreasing accuracy and increasing pain.

So, without speaking, lightly touch the needle to the skin, then quickly insert the needle.

Stop the progression of the needle's penetration as soon as the hub of the needle touches the skin.

A ½ inch needle, when advanced exactly to where the hub *touches but does not depress the skin, will be at exactly the proper depth for men.*

If you hold the syringe like a dart when you insert the needle, you will hurt the patient with the movement that must occur when you reposition your hand to inject. So, instead, hold the syringe between your index and middle fingers (of your dominant hand) and position your thumb over the plunger when you insert the needle; then there will be no unneeded movement to reposition your hand (to put your thumb on the plunger) after inserting the needle.

The goal is to insert the needle as quickly and as accurately as possible and then hold it as still as possible while you next push the plunger to inject the BoNT.

Important
When you push the plunger, the tendency may be to advance the

---

[16] For more on how words can make your patient hurt more or hurt less, study the writings of Milton Erickson (Erickson, 1992)

needle, pushing the needle deeper as you push the syringe plunger—causing unwarranted pain. So, don't. Instead, keep the needle perfectly still while you inject 0.25 cc (25 units).

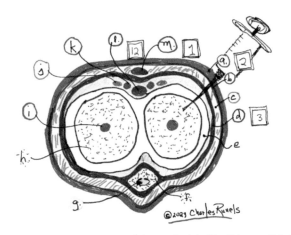

Figure 198. Cross section of the penis: (a) skin; (b) superficial (Dartos or Colle's) fascia; (c) areolar tissue; (d) deep (Buck's) fascia; (e) tunica albuginea; (f) corpus spongiosum; (g) urethra; (h) corpus cavernosum; (i) deep artery; (j) dorsal nerve; (k) dorsal artery; (l) deep dorsal vein; (m) superficial dorsal vein. A ½-inch needle advanced at 2 O'clock until hub lightly touches skin, at a 90-degree angle to the long axis of the peins, will position the lumen of the needle in an ideal position to inject the corpus cavernosum.

Then, *quickly* remove the needle. There is no benefit, only prolonged and amplified pain, if you slowly (rather than quickly) remove the needle.

2. Repeat the injection in the same way at points "a," "c," and "d" (see the diagram).

When injecting, stand on the ipsilateral side of the corpus cavernosum that you intend to inject; inject one side, then walk to the other side, reposition the penis, and inject again.[17]

---

[17] Details like where to stand, in my view, play an important part in both accuracy and grace while doing the procedure. Grace may seem irrelevant, but grace contributes significantly both to your patient's confidence and to your accuracy. An ungraceful procedure is metaphorically like having your office furniture in disarray, only worse. So, details about positioning of both the patient, your torso, and your hands are important.

I realize that an experienced physician may think it unnecessary to walk to the other side of the bed in order to inject both sides of the penis. Without exaggeration, I am sure that an experienced physician could also do this

Note

At this time, there is no research comparing the possible locations of injection or the number of injection points to determine the method that affords superior distribution or results (which may not be the same). When doing the P-Shot® procedure, our group (the <u>Cellular Medicine Association</u>) has found that dividing the penis into thirds and injecting a total of four times (at both dividing lines on both sides), instead of two times or at other locations, provides the most complete distribution of the material injected.

If you do four injections of BoNT, then each injection site would receive 0.25 ccs containing 25 units—for a total of 100 units.

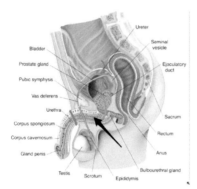

Figure 199. Securing a tourniquet at the base of the penis (blue line) before injecting the corpus cavernosum would prevent diffusion of the material injected into the more proximal penis (black arrow).

For more details, ***videos of the injection techniques can be seen at <u>BoNTClass.com</u>.***

Frequently Asked Questions

Do you need a tourniquet?

If the purpose of the tourniquet is to prevent systemic effects, it seems unnecessary considering the LD50 of BoNT and the history of much greater dosages being used elsewhere in the body.

For example, cosmetic physicians and neurologists routinely and effectively inject BoNT (much more than recommended for the penis) into other body areas, and no tourniquet is used. For example, 150 to

---

procedure while hanging blindfolded from a trapeze suspended from the ceiling of the exam room. But why would she? If you find a better method of positioning than described, then use it; but *the simplest and least awkward technique that gets the job done will usually be the most elegant and the most effective.*

200 units of BoNT is routinely injected into the head (face, scalp & neck) when treating migraines, and no tourniquet is placed around the neck.

If the purpose of the tourniquet is to keep the BoNT in the penis, why would one not want to allow the BoNT to diffuse proximally a small distance in order to treat that more proximal root of the penis that lies deep to where the tourniquet would constrict?

Do you need to massage the penis afterward?
In one study of BoNT for ED, the investigators did a "fine massage" to each injection point for 5 minutes after each injection. Reading the study, I wonder if (with four injection points) there was a total of 5 minutes or of 20 minutes massage. (Abdelrahman, 2022).

Though the study by Abdelrahman et al (Abdelrahman, 2022) is brilliant and adds tremendously to the support for BoNT for ED, I am not convinced of the necessity of the massage; here is why: when I inject the glabella region (procerus and corrugators) with BoNT, I massage the area (to facilitate even distribution) for about 5 *seconds*, but *not* for 5 to 20 *minutes*. I do not know of anyone who does facial aesthetics who does a 5-minute facial massage after the entire treatment and certainly not after each injection point—yet cosmetic BoNT works wonderfully well without the massage.

I concede that a 5-minute to 20-minute penis massage may increase patient demand for the procedure. Still, because of the experience of two decades of thousands of physicians successfully doing millions of cosmetic injections without massage, I do not see a medical need for massaging the penis after injection of BoNT for ED. If such a massage is thought to be needed, in my view, patients can massage their own penis while I treat the next patient.

In short, massaging the penis can be a very good thing; but that is not my job.

Priapus Sh⚲t®

Can you combine BoNT with the P-Shot® procedure?

To combine BoNT with the P-Shot® (Priapus Shot®) procedure, simply follow the instructions for preparation of the BoNT as described in this chapter.

Then, after preparing the PRP as per the protocols for the P-Shot® procedure, add ½ of the BoNT to one of the 5cc syringes of PRP and ½ of the BoNT to the other.

Then, follow the usual procedure for the P-Shot® (PriapusShot.com/members). Members can login there to see a step-by-step video on that website for both the P-Shot® alone and the P-Shot® combined with BoNT.

Can you further explain the choice of the needle size?

Most people can push an aqueous solution from a one cc syringe through a 30-gauge needle, but it becomes difficult if pushing from a 5cc syringe through a 30-gauge; this would be the case when injecting only BoNT. Therefore, you could use a 30-gauge needle if only injecting BoNT into the corpus cavernous but would need a one cc syringe.

But when combining BoNT with the P-Shot® procedure, the situation changes since PRP comprises most of the material in the syringe. PRP is more viscous than saline, so some people have trouble pushing PRP through a 30-gauge needle.

You can always try a 30-gauge needle, but if the injection is too difficult, return to a 27-gauge. Always use the smallest gauge through which you can comfortably push the material.[18]

---

[18] When combining the P-Shot with BoNT, keep 25-gauge needles within reach while doing the procedure because occasionally PRP quickly becomes too viscous to push through even a 27-gauge needle. If you inject in less than 3 minutes after activating the PRP, then this extreme viscosity happens rarely; but if you delay the injection more than 3 minutes after activating the PRP, the platelet-rich fibrin matrix can sometimes make it near impossible to inject. So, never rush, but move quickly.

Further Help with Both *Injection Technique* and *Marketing* BoNT for ED

For detailed videos demonstrating the injection of both platelet-rich plasma and BoNT for erectile dysfunction, see free materials and consider further training at BoNTPenis.com/physicians ,and at PriapusShot.com/members.

For free materials regarding the use of PRP for ED, see PriapusShot.com/physicians

For further understanding and training regarding treating sexual dysfunction in men, see free materials at PriapusShot.com/research.

References Regarding BoNT for ED

Abdelrahman IFS, Raheem AA, Elkhiat Y, Aburahma AA, Abdel-Raheem T, Ghanem H. Safety and efficacy of botulinum neurotoxin in the treatment of erectile dysfunction refractory to phosphodiesterase inhibitors: Results of a randomized controlled trial. *Andrology*. 2022;10(2):254-261. doi:10.1111/andr.13104

Aru RG, Songcharoen SJ, Seals SR, Arnold PB, Hester RL. Microcirculatory Effects of Botulinum Toxin A in the Rat: Acute and Chronic Vasodilation. *Annals of Plastic Surgery*. 2017;79(1):82-85. doi:10.1097/SAP.0000000000001054

Cayetano-Alcaraz AA, Tharakan T, Chen R, Sofikitis N, Minhas S. The management of erectile dysfunction in men with diabetes mellitus unresponsive to phosphodiesterase type 5 inhibitors. *Andrology*. 2023;11(2):257-269. doi:10.1111/andr.13257

El-Shaer W, Ghanem H, Diab T, Abo-Taleb A, Kandeel W. Intra-cavernous injection of BOTOX® (50 and 100 Units) for treatment of vasculogenic erectile dysfunction: Randomized controlled trial. *Andrology*. 2021;9(4):1166-1175. doi:10.1111/andr.13010

Emura F, Peura D. Interview with Barry J. Marshall. Winner of the Nobel Prize in Medicine for the Discovery of Helicobacter pylori. :8.

Etminan M, Sodhi M, Mikelberg FS, Maberley D. Risk of Ocular Adverse Events Associated With Use of Phosphodiesterase 5 Inhibitors in Men in the US. *JAMA Ophthalmol*. 2022;140(5):480. doi:10.1001/jamaophthalmol.2022.0663

Giuliano F, Denys P, Joussain C. Effectiveness and Safety of Intracavernosal IncobotulinumtoxinA (Xeomin®) 100 U as an Add-on Therapy to Standard Pharmacological Treatment for Difficult-to-Treat Erectile Dysfunction: A Case Series. *Toxins*. 2022;14(4):286. doi:10.3390/toxins14040286

Giuliano F, Joussain C, Denys P. Safety and Efficacy of Intracavernosal Injections of AbobotulinumtoxinA (Dysport®) as Add on Therapy to Phosphosdiesterase Type 5 Inhibitors or Prostaglandin E1 for Erectile

Dysfunction—Case Studies. *Toxins*. 2019;11(5):283. doi:10.3390/toxins11050283

Gul M, Serefoglu EC. An update on the drug safety of treating erectile dysfunction. *Expert Opinion on Drug Safety*. 2019;18(10):965-975. doi:10.1080/14740338.2019.1659244

Habashy E, Köhler TS. Botox for Erectile Dysfunction. *The Journal of Sexual Medicine*. 2022;19(7):1061-1063. doi:10.1016/j.jsxm.2022.03.216

Ibrahim H, Maignel J, Hornby F, Daly D, Beard M. BoNT/A in the Urinary Bladder—More to the Story than Silencing of Cholinergic Nerves. *Toxins*. 2022;14(1):53. doi:10.3390/toxins14010053

Lin H, Wang R. The science of vacuum erectile device in penile rehabilitation after radical prostatectomy. Transl Androl Urol 2013;2(1):61-66. doi: 10.3978/j.issn.2223-4683.2013.01.04

Morris JL, Jobling P, Gibbins IL. Botulinum neurotoxin A attenuates release of norepinephrine but not NPY from vasoconstrictor neurons. *American Journal of Physiology-Heart and Circulatory Physiology*. 2002;283(6):H2627-H2635. doi:10.1152/ajpheart.00477.2002

Mykoniatis I, Pyrgidis N, Sokolakis I, et al. Assessment of Combination Therapies vs Monotherapy for Erectile Dysfunction: A Systematic Review and Meta-analysis. *JAMA Netw Open*. 2021;4(2):e2036337. doi:10.1001/jamanetworkopen.2020.36337

Porter DM. Botox: the new Viagra? It's one way to treat erectile dysfunction.https://www.thetimes.co.uk/article/botox-could-help-men-beat-erectile-dysfunction-here-s-what-to-know-8x2vvt9c7. Accessed November 8, 2022.

Ramachandran R, Yaksh TL. Therapeutic use of botulinum toxin in migraine: mechanisms of action. *Br J Pharmacol*. 2014;171(18):4177-4192. doi:10.1111/bph.12763

Stolerman IP, ed. *Encyclopedia of Psychopharmacology*. Springer Berlin Heidelberg; 2010. doi:10.1007/978-3-540-68706-1

Welliver RC, Mechlin C, Goodwin B, Alukal JP, McCullough AR. A Pilot Study to Determine Penile Oxygen Saturation Before and After Vacuum Therapy in Patients with Erectile Dysfunction After Radical Prostatectomy. *The Journal of Sexual Medicine*. 2014;11(4):1071-1077. doi:10.1111/jsm.12445

Wong J, Witherspoon L, Flannigan R. Under-recognized factors affecting penile implant satisfaction in patients. *CUAJ*. 2022;16(8). doi:10.5489/cuaj.7720

Research Regarding the Regenerative Effects of BoNT

Aru RG, Songcharoen SJ, Seals SR, Arnold PB, Hester RL. Microcirculatory Effects of Botulinum Toxin A in the Rat: Acute and Chronic Vasodilation. *Annals of Plastic Surgery*. 2017;79(1):82-85. doi:10.1097/SAP.0000000000001054

Bushnell JY, Cates LN, Hyde JE, Hofstetter CP, Yang CC, Khaing ZZ. Early Detrusor Application of Botulinum Toxin A Results in Reduced Bladder Hypertrophy and Fibrosis after Spinal Cord Injury in a Rodent Model. *Toxins*. 2022;14(11):777. doi:10.3390/toxins14110777

Chernoff G. Combining topical dermal infused exosomes with injected calcium hydroxylapatite for enhanced tissue biostimulation. *J of Cosmetic Dermatology*. 2023;22(S1):15-27. doi:10.1111/jocd.15695

Disphanurat W, Viarasilpa W, Thienpaitoon P. Efficacy of Botulinum Toxin A for Scar Prevention After Breast Augmentation: A Randomized Double-Blind Intraindividual Controlled Trial. *Dermatol Surg*. 2021;47(12):1573-1578. doi:10.1097/DSS.0000000000003198

Duchen, LW. Motor Nerve Growth Induced by Botulinum Toxin as a Regenerative Phenomenon. Proc. Roy. Soc. Med. 1972;10;196-7.

Duchen LW, Strich SJ. THE EFFECTS OF BOTULINUM TOXIN ON THE PATTERN OF INNERVATION OF SKELETAL MUSCLE IN THE MOUSE. *Exp Physiol*. 1968;53(1):84-89. doi:10.1113/expphysiol.1968.sp001948

Erickson MH, Rossi EL, Ryan MO, Sharp FA. *Healing in Hypnosis*. Irvington Publishers; 1992.

Fasano G, Grimaldi L, Nisi G, Calomino N, Cuomo R. The Regenerative Effects of Botulinum Toxin A: New Perspectives. *Journal of Investigative Surgery*. 2022;35(5):1074-1075. doi:10.1080/08941939.2021.2008553

Franz CK, Puritz A, Jordan LA, et al. Botulinum Toxin Conditioning Enhances Motor Axon Regeneration in Mouse and Human Preclinical Models. *Neurorehabil Neural Repair*. 2018;32(8):735-745. doi:10.1177/1545968318790020

Mastrorilli V, De Angelis F, Vacca V, Pavone F, Luvisetto S, Marinelli S. Xeomin®, a Commercial Formulation of Botulinum Neurotoxin Type A, Promotes Regeneration in a Preclinical Model of Spinal Cord Injury. *Toxins*. 2023;15(4):248. doi:10.3390/toxins15040248

Matak, Bölcskei, Bach-Rojecky, Helyes. Mechanisms of Botulinum Toxin Type A Action on Pain. *Toxins*. 2019;11(8):459. doi:10.3390/toxins11080459

Park TH, Lee SH, Park YJ, Lee YS, Rah DK, Kim SY. Presurgical Botulinum Toxin A Treatment Increases Angiogenesis by Hypoxia-Inducible Factor-1α/Vascular Endothelial Growth Factor and Subsequent Superiorly Based Transverse Rectus Abdominis Myocutaneous Flap Survival in a Rat Model. *Annals of Plastic Surgery*. 2016;76(6):723-728. doi:10.1097/SAP.0000000000000435

Wang YX, Wang Y, Zhang Q, Zhang RD. Current Research of Botulinum Toxin Type A in Prevention and Treatment on Pathological Scars. *Dermatol Surg*. 2023;49(5S):S34-S40. doi:10.1097/DSS.0000000000003770

Woolf, A. L. (1964). 'Pathological anatomy of the intramuscular nerve endings', in *Disorders of Voluntary Muscle*, pp. 163-193. Ed. J. N. Walton. London: Churchill.

References Regarding BoNT for Fibrosis and Scaring

Bushnell JY, Cates LN, Hyde JE, Hofstetter CP, Yang CC, Khaing ZZ. Early Detrusor Application of Botulinum Toxin A Results in Reduced Bladder

Hypertrophy and Fibrosis after Spinal Cord Injury in a Rodent Model. *Toxins*. 2022;14(11):777. doi:10.3390/toxins14110777

Disphanurat W, Viarasilpa W, Thienpaitoon P. Efficacy of Botulinum Toxin A for Scar Prevention After Breast Augmentation: A Randomized Double-Blind Intraindividual Controlled Trial. *Dermatol Surg*. 2021;47(12):1573-1578. doi:10.1097/DSS.0000000000003198

Kasyanju Carrero LM, Ma W, Liu H, Yin X, Zhou B. Botulinum toxin type A for the treatment and prevention of hypertrophic scars and keloids: Updated review. *J Cosmet Dermatol*. 2019;18(1):10-15. doi:10.1111/jocd.12828

Rahman SHA, Mohamed MS, Hamed AM. Efficacy and safety of Nd:YAG laser alone compared with combined Nd:YAG laser with intralesional steroid or botulinum toxin A in the treatment of hypertrophic scars. *Lasers Med Sci*. 2021;36(4):837-842. doi:10.1007/s10103-020-03120-0

Wang YX, Wang Y, Zhang Q, Zhang RD. Current Research of Botulinum Toxin Type A in Prevention and Treatment on Pathological Scars. *Dermatol Surg*. 2023;49(5S):S34-S40. doi:10.1097/DSS.0000000000003770

Zhibo X, Miaobo Z. Botulinum toxin type A affects cell cycle distribution of fibroblasts derived from hypertrophic scar. *Journal of Plastic, Reconstructive & Aesthetic Surgery*. 2008;61(9):1128-1129. doi:10.1016/j.bjps.2008.05.003

Representative References Regarding the P-Shot® Procedure

Kumar CS. 265 Combined Treatment of Injecting Platelet Rich Plasma With Vacuum Pump for Penile Enlargement. *The Journal of Sexual Medicine*. 2017;14(1):S78. doi:10.1016/j.jsxm.2016.11.174

Lee PJ, Jiang YH, Kuo HC. A novel management for postprostatectomy urinary incontinence: platelet-rich plasma urethral sphincter injection. *Scientific Reports |*. 123AD;11:5371. doi:10.1038/s41598-021-84923-1

Chung. A Review of Current and Emerging Therapeutic Options for Erectile Dysfunction. *Medical Sciences*. 2019;7(9):91. doi:10.3390/medsci7090091

Casabona F, Gambelli I, Casabona F, Santi P, Santori G, Baldelli I. Autologous platelet-rich plasma (PRP) in chronic penile lichen sclerosus: the impact on tissue repair and patient quality of life. *Int Urol Nephrol*. 2017;49(4):573-580. doi:10.1007/s11255-017-1523-0

Pavlovic V, Ciric M, Jovanovic V, Stojanovic P. Platelet Rich Plasma: a short overview of certain bioactive components. *Open Medicine*. 2016;11(1):242-247. doi:10.1515/med-2016-0048

Ruffo A, Franco M, Illiano E, Stanojevic N. Effectiveness and safety of Platelet rich Plasma (PrP) cavernosal injections plus external shock wave treatment for penile erectile dysfunction: First results from a prospective, randomized, controlled, interventional study. *European Urology Supplements*. 2019;18(1):e1622-e1623. doi:10.1016/S1569-9056(19)31175-3

Shaher H, Fathi A, Elbashir S, Abdelbaki SA, Soliman T. Is Platelet Rich Plasma Safe And Effective In Treatment Of Erectile Dysfunction? Randomized Controlled Study. *Urology*. Published online February 2023:S0090429523000742. doi:10.1016/j.urology.2023.01.028

Chung E. medical sciences A Review of Current and Emerging Therapeutic Options for Erectile Dysfunction. Published online 2019:1-11.

Schirmann A, Boutin E, Faix A, Yiou R. Pilot study of intra-cavernous injections of platelet-rich plasma (P-shot®) in the treatment of vascular erectile dysfunction. *Progrès en Urologie*. Published online June 2022:S1166708722001300. doi:10.1016/j.purol.2022.05.002

Poulios E, Mykoniatis I, Pyrgidis N, et al. Platelet-Rich Plasma (PRP) Improves Erectile Function: A Double-Blind, Randomized, Placebo-Controlled Clinical Trial. *Journal of Sexual Medicine*. 2021;18(5):926-935. doi:10.1016/j.jsxm.2021.03.008

Masterson TA, Molina M, Ledesma B, et al. Platelet-rich Plasma for the Treatment of Erectile Dysfunction: A Prospective, Randomized, Double-blind, Placebo-controlled Clinical Trial. *Journal of Urology*. Published online April 30, 2023:10.1097/JU.0000000000003481. doi:10.1097/JU.0000000000003481

Everts P, Onishi K, Jayaram P, Lana JF, Mautner K. Platelet-Rich Plasma: New Performance Understandings and Therapeutic Considerations in 2020. *Int J Mol Sci*. 2020;21(20):7794. doi:10.3390/ijms21207794

Liu MC, Chang ML, Wang YC, Chen WH, Wu CC, Yeh SD. Revisiting the Regenerative Therapeutic Advances Towards Erectile Dysfunction. *Cells*. 2020;9(5):1250. doi:10.3390/cells9051250

Matz EL, Pearlman AM, Terlecki RP. Safety and feasibility of platelet rich fibrin matrix injections for treatment of common urologic conditions. *Investig Clin Urol*. 2018;59(1):61-65. doi:10.4111/icu.2018.59.1.61

Israeli JM, Lokeshwar SD, Efimenko IV, Masterson TA, Ramasamy R. The potential of platelet-rich plasma injections and stem cell therapy for penile rejuvenation. *Int J Impot Res*. Published online November 6, 2021:1-8. doi:10.1038/s41443-021-00482-z

Raheem AA, Garaffa G, Raheem TA, et al. The role of vacuum pump therapy to mechanically straighten the penis in Peyronie's disease. *BJU International*. 2010;106(8):1178-1180. doi:10.1111/j.1464-410X.2010.09365.x

Towe M, Peta A, Saltzman RG, Balaji N, Chu K, Ramasamy R. The use of combination regenerative therapies for erectile dysfunction: rationale and current status. *Int J Impot Res*. Published online July 12, 2021:1-4. doi:10.1038/s41443-021-00456-1

Garcia M, Fandel T, Lin G, et al. Treatment of erectile dysfunction in the obese type 2 diabetic ZDF rat with adipose tissue-derived stem cells. *J Sex Med*. 2010;7(1 Pt 1):89-98. Accessed June 14, 2022. https://www.ncbi.nlm.nih.gov/pmc/articles/PMC2904063/

Siroky MB, Azadzoi KM. Vasculogenic Erectile Dysfunction: Newer Therapeutic Strategies. *Journal of Urology*. 2003;170(2S). doi:10.1097/01.ju.0000075361.35942.17

References Regarding PRP for Peyronie's Disease

Virag R, Sussman H, Lambion S, de Fourmestraux V. Evaluation of the benefit of using a combination of autologous platelet rich-plasma and hyaluronic acid for the treatment of Peyronie's disease. *Sex Health Issues*. 2017;1(1). doi:10.15761/SHI.1000102

Levine LA. Peyronie's disease: contemporary review of non-surgical treatment. *Translational andrology and urology*. 2013;2(1):39-44. doi:10.3978/j.issn.2223-4683.2013.01.01

Culha MG, Erkan E, Cay T, Yücetaş U. The Effect of Platelet-Rich Plasma on Peyronie's Disease in Rat Model. *Urologia Internationalis*. 2019;102(2):218-223. doi:10.1159/000492755

References Regarding PRP for Neovascularization

Bindal P, Gnanasegaran N, Bindal U, et al. Angiogenic effect of platelet-rich concentrates on dental pulp stem cells in inflamed microenvironment. *Clin Oral Investig*. 2019;23(10):3821-3831. doi:10.1007/s00784-019-02811-5

Norooznezhad AH. Decreased Pain in Patients Undergoing Pilonidal Sinus Surgery Treated with Platelet-Rich Plasma Therapy: The Role of Angiogenesis. *Advances in Skin & Wound Care*. 2020;33(1):8. doi:10.1097/01.ASW.0000615376.97232.0a

Li Y, Mou S, Xiao P, et al. Delayed two steps PRP injection strategy for the improvement of fat graft survival with superior angiogenesis. *Sci Rep*. 2020;10:5231. doi:10.1038/s41598-020-61891-6

Zhang XL, Shi KQ, Jia PT, et al. Effects of platelet-rich plasma on angiogenesis and osteogenesis-associated factors in rabbits with avascular necrosis of the femoral head. *Eur Rev Med Pharmacol Sci*. 2018;22(7):2143-2152. doi:10.26355/eurrev_201804_14748

Nolan GS, Smith OJ, Heavey S, Jell G, Mosahebi A. Histological analysis of fat grafting with platelet-rich plasma for diabetic foot ulcers—A randomised controlled trial. *Int Wound J.* 2021;19(2):389-398. doi:10.1111/iwj.13640

Sclafani AP, McCormick SA. Induction of dermal collagenesis, angiogenesis, and adipogenesis in human skin by injection of platelet-rich fibrin matrix. *Arch Facial Plast Surg.* 2012;14(2):132-136. doi:10.1001/archfacial.2011.784

Araujo-Gutierrez R, Van Eps JL, Scherba JC, et al. Platelet rich plasma concentration improves biologic mesh incorporation and decreases multinucleated giant cells in a dose dependent fashion. *Journal of Tissue Engineering and Regenerative Medicine.* 2021;15(11):1037-1046. doi:10.1002/term.3247

Saputro ID, Rizaliyana S, Noverta DA. The effect of allogenic freeze-dried platelet-rich plasma in increasing the number of fibroblasts and neovascularization in wound healing. *Ann Med Surg (Lond).* 2022;73:103217. doi:10.1016/j.amsu.2021.103217

References Regarding PRP for Neurogenesis

Pandunugrahadi M, Irianto KA, Sindrawati O. The Optimal Timing of Platelet-Rich Plasma (PRP) Injection for Nerve Lesion Recovery: A Preliminary Study. *Int J Biomater.* 2022;2022:9601547. doi:10.1155/2022/9601547

Chung E. Regenerative technology to restore and preserve erectile function in men following prostate cancer treatment: evidence for penile rehabilitation in the context of prostate cancer survivorship. *Therapeutic Advances in Urology.* 2021;13:17562872211026420. doi:10.1177/17562872211026421

Sánchez M, Anitua E, Delgado D, et al. Platelet-rich plasma, a source of autologous growth factors and biomimetic scaffold for peripheral nerve regeneration. *Expert Opinion on Biological Therapy.* 2017;17(2):197-212. doi:10.1080/14712598.2017.1259409

Kuffler DP. Platelet-Rich Plasma and the Elimination of Neuropathic Pain. *Mol Neurobiol*. 2013;48(2):315-332. doi:10.1007/s12035-013-8494-7

Foy CA, Micheo WF, Kuffler DP. Functional Recovery following Repair of Long Nerve Gaps in Senior Patient 2.6 Years Posttrauma. *Plast Reconstr Surg Glob Open*. 2021;9(9):e3831. doi:10.1097/GOX.0000000000003831

Yasak T, Özkaya Ö, Ergan Şahin A, Çolak Ö. Electromyographic and Clinical Investigation of the Effect of Platelet-Rich Plasma on Peripheral Nerve Regeneration in Patients with Diabetes after Surgery for Carpal Tunnel Syndrome. *Arch Plast Surg*. 2022;49(02):200-206. doi:10.1055/s-0042-1744410

Wu YN, Liao CH, Chen KC, Chiang HS. Dual effect of chitosan activated platelet rich plasma (cPRP) improved erectile function after cavernous nerve injury. *Journal of the Formosan Medical Association*. Published online March 27, 2021. doi:10.1016/j.jfma.2021.01.019

References Regarding the Use of PRP for Muscle Repair

Bernuzzi G, Petraglia F, Pedrini MF, et al. Use of platelet-rich plasma in the care of sports injuries: our experience with ultrasound-guided injection. *Blood Transfus*. 2014;12(Suppl 1):s229-s234. doi:10.2450/2013.0293-12

Bubnov R, Yevseenko V, Semeniv I. Ultrasound guided injections of Platelets Rich Plasma for muscle injury in professional athletes. Comparative study. :5.

Moraes VY, Lenza M, Tamaoki MJ, Faloppa F, Belloti JC. Platelet-rich therapies for musculoskeletal soft tissue injuries. *The Cochrane database of systematic reviews*. 2013;12:CD010071. doi:10.1002/14651858.CD010071.pub2

Le ADK, Enweze L, DeBaun MR, Dragoo JL. Platelet-Rich Plasma. *Clinics in Sports Medicine*. 2019;38(1):17-44. doi:10.1016/j.csm.2018.08.001

Graca FA, Stephan A, Minden-Birkenmaier BA, et al. Platelet-derived chemokines promote skeletal muscle regeneration by guiding neutrophil recruitment to injured muscles. *Nat Commun*. 2023;14(1):2900. doi:10.1038/s41467-023-38624-0

Aguilar-García D, Fernández-Sarmiento JA, del Mar Granados Machuca M, et al. Histological and biochemical evaluation of plasma rich in growth factors treatment for grade II muscle injuries in sheep. *BMC Veterinary Research*. 2022;18(1):400. doi:10.1186/s12917-022-03491-2

Middleton KK, Barro V, Muller B, Terada S, Fu FH. Evaluation of the effects of platelet-rich plasma (PRP) therapy involved in the healing of sports-related soft tissue injuries. *The Iowa orthopaedic journal*. 2012;32:150-163. Accessed June 10, 2017. http://www.ncbi.nlm.nih.gov/pubmed/23576936

Agarwal V, Gupta A, Singh H, Kamboj M, Popli H, Saroha S. Comparative Efficacy of Platelet-Rich Plasma and Dry Needling for Management of Trigger Points in Masseter Muscle in Myofascial Pain Syndrome Patients: A Randomized Controlled Trial. *J Oral Facial Pain Headache*. Published online November 28, 2022. doi:10.11607/ofph.3188

TABLE OF FIGURES

Figure 1. The (1) connector invites (2) you and the (3) members of her group to a party. You come to the party (enter their group) and meet people you could have never reached with paid advertising. The people receive your services. The connector receives a higher standing with her group. 33

Figure 2. Most patients want to stay in their friend-bubble and most physicians want to stay in their office bubble. The smart doctor finds ways to enter the patient's bubble and does not spend a fortune trying to "get" people to leave theirs to enter hers. 44

Figure 3. Is it ethical to keep your knowledge of the healing arts a secret? Is it your **patient's** responsibility to know what you are able to do? Or is **it your** responsibility to teach people what you can do for them? 53

Figure 4. Is it ethical to use bait to lure people to something of great benefit? 55

Figure 5. My favorite syringe to use with BoNT treatments: 31-gauge, 30-unit, 8mm, BD-brand, insulin syringe. 62

Figure 6. A stranger should be able to walk into the room and know by your attire and demeanor that you are the speaker. It is a show of respect to be dressed up (slightly more formal than your attendees) for the occasion. 66

Figure 7. It is not my job to become the sobriety police. 67

Figure 8. George Winston's December Album is full of magic that will calm your patients. 68

Figure 9. Parties grow your practice like multi-level marketing on steroids. 69

Figure 10. The BoNT-Board 72

Figure 11. Bottle opener to remove the caps from BoNT vials. 72

Figure 12. Removing the cap from the BoNT vial. 73

Figure 13. Insulated picnic bag is the BoNT toolbox. Frozen blocks go into the bag. 73

Figure 14. Large-cube, ice cube tray..74

Figure 15. Plastic bag with ice cubes goes into the tool bag. 74

Figure 16. BoNT board loaded with prefilled syringes. 75

Figure 17. A simple drawing to document injections. 77

Figure 18. The red numbers indicate the number of units usually given for repeat visit for a female. Black numbers show order of injection.... 78

Figure 19. BoNT parties bring you new patients who give you stacks of money. 86

Figure 20. After the party, go home and put each name, birthday, and email into your computer. Their face photos go into a file with the photos of (1) the consent form and (2) the diagram of their treatment plan. 88

Figure 21. Give away door prizes at the party and bring extras to sell to those who do not win the prize. 98

Figure 22. The hostess should have simple refreshments or else she will spend more on refreshments than her BoNT would have cost. 100

Figure 23. The part of medicine that makes doctors squirm with guilt. 111

Figure 24. Be very careful of the other crabs; they will try to pull you back into the bucket when you start to crawl out. 114

Figure 25. A club requires automatic billing and (if possible) automatic delivery.. 116

Figure 26. The steps to building your own club are known and easy. Just follow the steps instead of trying to invent a new staircase................ 118

Figure 27. If you really care about your patients, you will listen carefully with every visit with the intent to know them better when they leave than you did when they arrived. 137

Figure 28. When you provide BoNT, you become a part of the most important ceremonies in the lives of your patients............................. 139

Figure 29. If you only do what people pay you to do, even if you do it in an excellent way, you lose. 140

Figure 30. Giving your patients a way to give discount coupons to their friends for your services implements multilevel marketing into your practice... 141

Figure 31. Even if no one is looking at the phone, a phone on the table changes the conversation by introducing the possibility of interruption (even if no interruption occurs). 144

Figure 32. You may be distracted more than you think. Read Deep Work to rediscover your best work. 145

Figure 33. How Schultz made a coffee shop into a healing place (and made huge profits). Every doctor should read this book..................... 148

Figure 34. My office should be a place of peace and contemplation; it then becomes a more powerful place of healing. 151

Figure 35. Wind chimes by the door bring peace and prosperity. 157

Figure 36. The most relaxing album ever made: George Winston's December Album...159

Figure 37. I need a red second hand to prevent bruising.....................160

Figure 38. I use cotton sheets, not paper, for covering the treatment bed and the patient...160

Figure 39. Adding 1 cc of bacteriostatic saline to 100 units of BoNT using a one cc syringe. 166

Figure 40. Beer-bottle opener removes the metal cap so that you can remove the rubber stopper to avoid dulling the needle when you extract the BoNT...167

Figure 41. The last drops of BoNT in the vial are impossible to extract without dulling your needle. 169

Figure 42. Adding the remnant from the almost-empty bottle to the newly mixed 100-unit bottle. 170

Figure 43. For best control, hold the syringe between the pointer and middle fingers, with the thumb near the plunger and the fifth finger lightly touching the skin of the patient. 171

Figure 44. If you do not offer same-day appointments for your BoNT patients, you will lose many patients. 174

Figure 45. Caring for the body temple involves not only medicine but also magic...177

Figure 46. The way I hold the syringe & the vial for a quick & accurate extraction of the BoNT from the vial. (A screenshot from a video on BoNTClass.com) 180

Figure 47. Close view of the approximately 0.01 ml bubble (in a 30-unit insulin syringe) that happens every time you draw up BoNT. You remove the bubble by pushing the fluid back out of the syringe with the needle submerged; then drawing the fluid back in..181

Figure 48. Demonstration of the tiny volume of 2 units of BoNT using the dilution of 1 cc per 100 units of BoNT. This dilution allows for increased accuracy (needed when injecting the lower face). 182

Figure 49. Slightly more than 7 units of BoNT in a 30-unit insulin syringe (using a 1-cc-to-100-units dilution) 183

Figure 50. BoNT holding board loaded with one syringe. 185

Figure 51. The "12 Apostles" in Australia represent the 12 injection points (even though there may not be exactly 12 of either). 188

Figure 52. Belts go horizontally and pleats go vertically. 189

Figure 53. The pleats (wrinkles) run perpendicular to the belt (muscles). 190

Figure 54. The skin appears "corrugated" medial to the insertion site (at the tip of the arrow) and smooth lateral to the insertion site. 193

Figure 55. It helps to stop and swap brains when you think about faces. 194

Figure 56. All parts of the brain are used when you think about faces (left, right, and lizard). 195

Figure 57. Always use your "lizard brain" when you study the faces you inject. 197

Figure 58. By thinking about the faces when you watch movies, you become a better injector by understanding the traits of old, young, angry, kind, evil, and 10,000 other things. 201

Figure 59. I can only do a facial aesthetic consult if I have a mirror, a small hand-held mirror that stays within reach of my treatment bed. I also keep a mirror on the wall for the patient to look into after the treatment (as they leave the room). The treatment bed has an overhead light, so I can see shapes. The mirror on the wall is in a place with a soft diffuse light. If they like my treatment when looking into the mirror with the harsh overhead light, they will love what they see in the mirror with the soft light. 203

Figure 60. Bright lights from multiple directions take away shadows; without shadows, it becomes more difficult to see the shapes and lines that you want to erase (which is exactly why the glamour photographer uses multiple lights). 204

Figure 61. Canned speeches make life better for my patients and me. 206

Figure 62. Every person deserves that you find their perfect recipe. ... 207

Figure 63. All my patients have my cell phone. But I encourage text instead of calling when possible. They can text selfies as an option for follow-up. 209

Figure 64. No body dies from cosmetic BoNT. But still do the consent and do not treat those with myasthenia gravis or who may be pregnant or if they feel too demanding. 210

Figure 65. Comfort the patient with the idea that they are doing you a favor when they ask you to make it better. 212

Figure 66. Those with enough hair to block the forehead put on a disposable head band before I begin taking photos or injecting. 214

Figure 67. Example of a split frontalis showing a lack of muscle superomedial. Also, there is less muscle on the patient's left superolateral. 215

Figure 68. Absence of frontalis in the superomedial forehead. 216

Figure 69. Screenshot (from BoNTClass.com) showing how I document injections with a simple diagram. I usually only write the red numbers (the number of units). The black numbers show the usual sequential order that I follow when injecting. 216

Figure 70. The vertical creases caused by the corrugators: the 11s. 218

Figure 71. Gloved non-dominant hand (holding gauze); non-gloved dominant hand holding syringe. 221

Figure 72. Procerus connects to the bone (inferior) to the skin (superior). It weaves into the occipitofrontalis, making it challenging to distinguish the two muscles in the inferomedial forehead. 222

Figure 73. The "dash" or "-" caused by the procerus muscle is usually more prominent in men. 223

Figure 74. The intersection of the lines drawn from the medial end of each brow to the medial corner of each eye...223

Figure 75. Procerus injection at the intersection of imaginary lines connecting the medial corner of each eye and the medial end of the opposing brow...224

Figure 76. If you see brisk bleeding, holding pressure for a full minute decreases the chances of a bruise. A second hand on the wall and George Winston's December album help you wait the full minute. 225

Figure 77. The music should be whatever relaxes the injector. 226

Figure 78. Arrows mark the insertion sites of both left and right corrugators. The site varies from face to face and sometimes from side to side. 228

Figure 79. Fingertip palpating the insertion-site dimple. 228

Figure 80. The arrows mark the insertion sites for both the left and right corrugators. After seeing and palpating each corrugator insertion site, I ask the patient to relax her face. Then, after the face relaxes, I inject the corrugator at the dots. 229

Figure 81. Injecting the more medial of the two injection sites for the left corrugator. 229

Figure 82. Blue dots mark the injection points for the corrugators. 230

Figure 83. A simple diagram documents the injection amounts without slowing me down with unneeded software. 231

Figure 84. (A) Frontalis lifts the brow. The (B) Procerus, (C) Corrugator, & (D) Orbicularis oculi lower the brow. 232

Figure 85. Before treatment, in the relaxed state, the brow will rest where the force from the pull up (frontalis) equals the pull downs. If the pull up happens to be much stronger than the pull downs, then if you fully relax all of them, the brow will drop. It is nearly impossible to predict what will happen if you fully relax them all; hence, the best results will be seen if you fully relax the pull downs (achieve maximal lift), and then tailor make the treatment of the pull up on a second visit two to four weeks after the first visit. 233

Figure 86. If you relax the frontalis (treat the forehead) without relaxing the pull-down muscles, then all the vectors pull down and you almost always create a neanderthal look. 234

Figure 87. The shape of a seagull's wings in flight reflects the shape of a woman's brows. 235

Figure 88. Finding the "corner of the head" or the lateral process of the zygoma. 235

Figure 89. The injection point (marked by the arrow) is between my fingers which are holding the brow while simultaneously abutting the lateral process of the zygoma (indicated by the blue line). 236

Figure 90. The tetrahydrozoline in Visine® is a sympathomimetic amine that will open the lid and counteract at least some of the droop from a BoNT-associated ptosis. 237

Figure 91. Documenting three units on each side to lift the brow. 238

Figure 92. When the orbicularis oculi shorten, they make pleats that are the crow's feet. 239

Figure 93. The orbicularis oculi cause crow's feet. 239

Figure 94. "Smile muscles" make lines that overlap with crow's feet. .. 240

Figure 95. The lines from the "smile muscles" overlap with the crow's feet and do not go away when you treat orbicularis oculi. 240

Figure 96. Palpating the orbital rim very gently. Then the injections are placed about 1/2 to 1 cm lateral to the orbital rim. 241

Figure 97. Injecting crow's feet: shallow and tangential orientation of the needle about ½ cm from the orbital rim. 241

Figure 98. Documentation of the injection of six units on each side to treat crow's feet. to decrease pain, use two separate syringes (one for each side), each with six units. 242

Figure 99. Changing the injection location by only a few millimeters can be the difference between a gorgeous result and a crazy face. But do not worry: the landmarks are easy..244

Figure 100. The frontalis acts as the only suspenders holding up the brows...245

Figure 101. To preserve movement and to avoid dropping the brow, with a split frontalis in the person over forty, I often inject only two units at each of the blue dots (and do not inject the split in the center). 246

Figure 102. Documentation of treatment of the frontalis with a total of eight units with a split frontalis. 246

Figure 103. For a person over forty with a non-split frontalis, I usually inject five points with two units each (at the blue dots) to preserve some movement. 247

Figure 104. Documentation of a more aggressive, three-row, treatment of a non-split frontalis. 247

Figure 105. Both the person with an over-treated frontalis and the Neanderthal man will demonstrate a heavy and drooped brow. 248

Figure 106. An even shorter, short-hand notation for a three-row treatment of the frontalis. 249

Figure 107. When an attempted gull's wing goes too high, the person looks "Spocked Out."..251

Figure 108. If someone "Spocks Out," simply add 2 units of BoNT at the peak of the "A" formed by the frontalis wrinkles. The brow and the wrinkles will relax to a gorgeous shape...251

Figure 109. The orbicularis oculi are injected in line with the lateral edge of the iris about 1-2mm below the lash line using a lateral-tangential approach. 257

Figure 110. To widen the eye in the resting or smiling position, inject in line with the lateral edge of the iris; use a tangential approach while the patient looks up; only the lumen of the needle is inserted to create a small bleb (done properly, there will be no pain or bruising). 258

Figure 111. Documenting injecting one unit of BoNT into the patient's right orbicularis oculi...259

Figure 112. Bunny lines, appear even with the face at rest in someone who has gotten BoNT for several years. 260

Figure 113. Showing disgust with contraction of the corrugators, procerus, and nasalis...261

Figure 114. Injection point for nasalis is 1/2 cm from the center of the nose at the location of the bridge made with nasalis contracted. Find the injection point with the muscle contracted. Then ask the patient to relax the muscle before doing the injection. 261

Figure 115. The orientation & location of the needle when treating the nasalis. Use two separate syringes, each with two units. 262

Figure 116. The gummy smile can be endearing, and some would rather not treat it. If the person is bothered by their gummy smile, they are usually most displeased about their smile in photos. 263

Figure 117. Where to insert the needle when treating levator labii.....264

Figure 118. To relax the gummy smile, follow the nasolabial fold until it reaches the nose. Then, with the syringe touching the nose, insert the needle. Aim the needle neither left, right, up, or down; aim straight at the back of the patient's head. Inject 2 units on each side for a total of 4 units. 265

Figure 119. A simple sketch in chart to document two units on each side to treat gummy smile...266

Figure 120. Depressor anguli oris (triangularis) muscle......................268

Figure 121. Injection point of the depressor anguli oris. 269

Figure 122. The starting point for measuring to inject the DAO's........270

Figure 123. Wrapping the syringe around to find the place where you will insert the needle...270

Figure 124. Injecting the broad base of the DAO................................271

Figure 125. A simple diagram for chart documenting five units in each triangularis. 272

Figure 126. Orange-peel chin caused by the mentalis muscle..............275

Figure 127. One of the two injection points for the mentalis (inject both sides of the center of the chin). 276

Figure 128. The large yellow arrow points to where the mentalis attaches to bone. The green arrow points to where the muscle attaches to skin..277

Figure 129. Imagine Kirk Douglas' chin in Spartacus and inject 2 units just on either side (but not into) the dimple. 277

Figure 130. Simple documentation diagram of injecting the mentalis with two units of BoNT on each side. 278

 Figure 131. The lateral and medial bands of the platysma are created by its edges; two edges for the left and two for the right platysma--making four bands. Photo courtesy of Yi et al. (2022); © Yi et al. (2022).........279

Figure 132. Grabbing a platysma band while the patient says, "Eeeeeee." Screen shot from a video on BoNTClass.com. 280

Figure 133. Holding the most prominent part of a platysma band with the non-dominant hand while injecting with the dominant hand (screen shot from video on BoNTClass.com). 281

Figure 134. Each green dot represents 2 units of BoNT injected sub q to treat the platysma bands. The red dots represent two units each to lift the jaw line--done less frequently than are platysma bands and described in more detail in Yi et al (2022). Diagram © by and courtesy of Yi et al (2022) under the usual open-source commons........................282

Figure 135. Sketch illustrating 10 units in all 4 platysma bands. Also, note the 4-color Bic pen. I have a few pens that cost an embarrassing amount of money. But this is the pen I prefer to use to make accurate and clear notes. It was invented in 1970, when I was 10 years old. I have used it for the past 50 years. (Available on Amazon.com). 283

Figure 136. Injection of necklace line with a sub-q bleb of 2 units of BoNT using a 30-unit insulin syringe with a 31-gauge needle. Screen shot from a video demonstration at BoNTClass.com. A green arrow points to one of the lines. 289

Figure 137. Possible treatment plan to improve the entire neck with targeting the necklace lines includes the following: (1) BoNT, (2) Vampire Facial® techniques every six weeks for three treatments, (3) Retin-A®, & (4) Altar™ (see VampireSkinTherapy.com). 290

Figure 138. The "lip," as it is commonly defined, is marked by "L". The orbicularis oris extends beyond the lip in every direction (the edges of orbicularis oris distant to the lip are marked by arrows). 291

Figure 139. Lip Flip: Injecting BoNT along the vermillion border allows the muscle fibers below the border to relax while keeping the fibers near the nose at their usual tension; the result is a pulling out of lines and a flipping up that increases the width of the lip............................293

Figure 140. Injection, from a lateral approach, into the vermillion border (green arrow) causes the BoNT to spread along the border (white line). This leaves the surrounding orbicularis oris (blue arrow) untreated— enhancing shape and softening lines. 294

Figure 141. The mouth of those of Asian or of African descent usually shows the upper lip at the same width as the lower lip (when measured in the center from the vermillion border to where the lips touch)...... 295

Figure 142. With the Caucasian mouth, the upper lip is usually near 1/2 the width of the lower lip when measured from the vermillion border (in the center of the mouth) to where the lips touch. 296

Figure 143. Understanding the usual ratios helps the injector know who to treat (and who to not treat) for a natural result.............................. 297

Figure 144. Max Planck, "A new scientific truth does not triumph by convincing its opponents...but rather because its opponents eventually die..." 298

Figure 145. This upper lip measures less than 1/2 the width of the lower lip (when measured in the center from vermillion border to where the lips touch). This mouth would be an ideal candidate for the Lip Flip (with injection of only the upper lip).. 301

Figure 146. When injecting the upper lip, the needle approaches from the side and enters the vermillion border in line with the lateral nares. After you feel the needle pop into the space, then you inject the BoNT as if you were doing an iv push. 302

Figure 147. The three injection points along the upper vermillion border. 302

Figure 148. Shorthand notation indicating treatment of the upper vermillion border with 5 units total of BoNT (2 on each side and 1 in the center)... 303

Figure 149. Holding a large ice cube (wrapped with a paper towel) on the upper lip for anesthesia and to decrease bruising. A cloth towel is draped across the chest to help with the dripping water from the ice. 303

Figure 150. If you consider the homunculus and the relative amount of brain devoted to the mouth and the hand, compared with the amount of brain devoted to other body parts (like the elbow), a reason for kissing and hand holding becomes apparent. 304

Figure 151. Injection of the lower lip with a lateral approach in line with the lateral edge of the nares. Only two injections are needed (left and right) since there is no cupid's bow on the lower lip. 305

Figure 152. Documenting a more aggressive treatment: 307

Figure 153. Syringes organized on the board for injecting the lip (screenshot from videos at BoNTClass.com) 308

Figure 154. Doctor allowing insurance to define the standard of care. 312

Figure 155. Blocking the transformation from cold emotion into warm emotion is what antidepressants do. 318

Figure 156. an idea enters consciousness (A); efferent nerves signal facial muscles to express emotion related to the idea (B); afferent nerves tell the brain the configuration of the facial muscles, emotional proprioception (C); the brain discerns the muscle configuration & cold emotion goes to warm emotion (D). 320

Figure 157. With BoNT, the efferent nerves cannot activate facial muscles to express the cold emotion (A). So, emotional proprioception keeps telling the brain "Happy" and the warm emotion of "depressed" is attenuated. (Alam,2008) 320

Figure 158. When the cold emotion of depression becomes warm, the risk of suicide goes up. 321

Figure 159. With BoNT, even though the brain perceives "sad," the muscles keep saying, "happy" --breaking the Facial Feedback loop. ... 322

Figure 160. BoNT injected into the glabellar region migrates along the afferent nerves to the trigeminal ganglion (TG) and then to the trigeminal nucleus caudalis (TNC). Both the TG and the TNC are shared by the afferent pain fibers coming from the meninges (M) surrounding the brain (B). The signals from these pain fibers are blocked at the TG and the TNC by the effects of the BoNT that migrates there. This is thought to be the mechanism by which BoNT relieves migraines. (Ramachandran,2014) Could it also have an effect in the treatment of depression? 323

Figure 161. Love, knowledge, and skill are concretized by profit. Someone's surplus (yours or another's) must buy the resources used to help others. Profit is the conduit through which your altruism passes. 325

Figure 162. Injection points for BoNT for depression (covered in more detail in Chapter 27)..326

Figure 163. Blocking the facial feedback loop by BoNT can make the brain blind to the emotional proprioception of depression while keeping it aware of happiness proprioception. Therefore, by keeping depression from changing from a cold to warm emotion, BoNT keeps depression cold..328

Figure 164. BoNT may improve migraine by blocking the transmission of pain signals of afferent nerves from the meninges--which share the trigeminal ganglion and trigeminal nucleus caudalis with the afferent nerves from the extracranial face and scalp. 332

Figure 165. A summary of where to inject all seven muscle groups as approved by the FDA for the treatment of migraines with BoNT........336

Figure 166. Injecting procerus with 5 units at the intersection of the "x" imagined by imagining two lines that go from the medial corner of each eye to the contralateral brow. 337

Figure 167. A fingertip lightly placed at the insertion site (marked by a dimple) helps with visualization of the corrugator. 337

Figure 168. Unlike with cosmetic BoNT injections (see Module 3), with the treatment of migraines, you simply inject 5 units in the center of the muscle belly (10 units on your syringe)..338

Figure 169. If you see an active "dot" of blood, if it looks like you need a BAND-AID, you are making a bruise; so, hold pressure. 338

Figure 170. The "U" shaped dip in the superior edge of the frontalis indicates a split frontalis. 339

Figure 171. For migraines, inject 4 locations, each injection site receives 5 units, for a total of 20 units..339

Figure 172. Occipitalis (Occipitofrontalis, Fronto occipitalis) receives 15 units divided into three locations, where my fingertips rest. Notice my very short fingernails--clipped short to (1) look cleaner, and (2) to avoid scratching patients. 340

Figure 173. The occipitofrontalis will extend from a centimeter or so medial to the center of the occiput to just posterior to the ear (at about 2 centimeters above the ear)..341

Figure 174. Occipitofrontalis is deep; insert the full length of your needle. No need to give them a shampoo or cleanse with alcohol--just go through the hair down to the scalp..342

Figure 175. My index finger rests on where temporalis resides. The dots mark the rhomboid-shaped injection points. The "z" marks the zygoma. 343

Figure 176. Find the temporalis by finding the zygoma and then inject 4 injection points in a rhomboid configuration. Each injection point is 5 units (10 units on your syringe). 343

Figure 177. If you grasp the "cheekbone" with your index finger and thumb, your index finger will touch the temporalis. 343

Figure 178. Injecting temporalis from screen shot of video on BoNTClass.com 344

Figure 179. For the trapezius, use three injection points of 5 units per injection on each side; 15 units per side; a total of 30 units. 344

Figure 180. Splenius capitis (arrow) attaches the mastoid process to C7, T1, T2, & T3. Injecting BoNT into the mastoid notch and then medial and inferior to the notch will relax it. 345

Figure 181. Red points to the mastoid process; blue to the mastoid notch; T labels the temporalis; M-masseter; OF-occipitofrontalis 346

Figure 182. An alternate injection pattern for BoNT for migraines (uses only 2 instead of 4 injection points for the temporalis): A, procerus, corrugators, and frontalis; B, temporalis; C, occipitalis; D, splenius capitis; E, trapezius. 347

Figure 183. An alternate map of the injection sites for the treatment of migraines. D shows injection sites for the splenius muscle (paraspinal muscles); A shows sites for the procerus, corrugators, and frontalis; B, temporalis; C, occipitofrontalis (occipitalis), shows an extra row of injections; D, splenius capitis, & E, trapezius (Zandieh, 2022) 348

Figure 184. Index finger placed lightly on the mandible and the thumb on the anterior edge of the masseter (easily palpated when the patient clenches her teeth). 352

Figure 185. The woman on the left demonstrates a cheek (c) that is wider than her jaw at the masseter (m). The woman on the right demonstrates a jaw that is wider than the cheek; therefore, if she is Caucasian, she demonstrates Runels Sign and likely suffers from bruxism. I do not know a similar sign that applies to other ethnicities. This sign is sensitive but not specific. 353

Figure 186. Cheek wider than jaw and Caucasian—she does not demonstrate the Runels Sign; thus, she is less likely to suffer from bruxism.. 354

Figure 187. Injecting 15 units into the masseter muscle to help with bruxism. Use a simple bolus of cosmetic BoNT (mixed with 1 cc to a 100-unit vial). 355

Figure 188. To find the injection point for bruxism, imagine a line from the corner of the mouth, horizontally to the back of the jaw; a needle inserted into this line in the center of the masseter muscle will deliver the BoNT in the correct place. 356

Figure 189. "The greatest obstacle to discovery is not ignorance—it is the illusion of knowledge."—Dr. Barry Marshall.................................. 359

Figure 190. Erectile dysfunction treatment algorithm: Exercise helps; cigarettes, marijuana, & alcohol hinder. Diet can help or hinder. PDE5i (phosphodiesterase type 5 inhibitor); ICI (Intracavernosal injections); VED (vacuum erection device); P-Shot® (specific method for the preparation and injection of PRP); BoNT & other Neuromodulators (NM). (Cayetano-Alcaraz, 2023), (PriapusShot.com/research) ©2023, Charles Runels, MD 365

Figure 191. Diagram of possible sequence of events after the injection of botulinum toxin. (a) The toxin becomes fixed to the motor nerve terminal (blue cross hatching); (b) axonal sprouting from the terminal, supported by Swann cells (S) which form the axolemma (al); (c) the bound toxin is diluted, and the axon forms new contacts with the muscle fiber at some distance from the site of the original end plate; (d) the contacts develop subneural folds of the sarcolemma—the result is an expansion of the innervation network. (Duchen, 1972) 367

Figure 192. Research supports the improvement in erection by BoNT in a variety of ways: smooth muscle relaxation and decreased sympathetic tone increase blood flow; blocking end plates triggers neurogenesis; increased hypoxia inducible factor-1α (HIF-1α) and increased vascular endothelial growth factor (VEGF) triggers neovascularization; decreased collagen I and III production triggers decreased fibrosis and remodeling of scar tissue. 368

Figure 193. I use the Purasyn® brand of hypochlorous solution (sold on Amazon) to cleanse the penis before injecting. 372

Figure 194. The patient is supine with the injector standing on the patient's right. The right (dominant hand) retracts the foreskin. Then, the left (non-dominant hand) grasps the glans. A gauze pad is used to help secure grip and provide more comfort. 373

Figure 195. Imagine the penis divided into thirds. Inject into the dividing lines at 2 O'clock and 10 O'clock. If the penis is less than 3 inches erect, inject only at points (a) and (b)--the other two injections are not needed. A total of 100 units is injected: if four injection points, then each injection site receives 25 units (0.25 ccs); if two injection points, then each injection site receives 50 units (0.5 ccs). 374

Figure 196. The needle & barrel of the syringe should be at 90 degrees to the axis of the penis. Changing the angle changes the depth of the injection...375

Figure 197. For depth of insertion, for most men, when using a 1/2 inch needle, (a) if the hub is hovering above the skin, the needle will likely not be fully inserted into the corpus cavernosum; (b) when the hub of the needle lightly touches the skin, and the angle of the needle is correct, the lumen of the needle will be in the corpus cavernosum in the best position for injecting; (c) when the needle is advanced until the hub depresses the skin, the lumen will often be too deep—decreasing accuracy and increasing pain...376

Figure 198. Cross section of the penis: (a) skin; (b) superficial (Dartos or Colle's) fascia; (c) areolar tissue; (d) deep (Buck's) fascia; (e) tunica albuginea; (f) corpus spongiosum; (g) urethra; (h) corpus cavernosum; (i) deep artery; (j) dorsal nerve; (k) dorsal artery; (l) deep dorsal vein; (m) superficial dorsal vein. A ½-inch needle advanced at 2 O'clock until hub lightly touches skin, at a 90-degree angle to the long axis of the peins, will position the lumen of the needle in an ideal position to inject the corpus cavernosum. 377

Figure 199. Securing a tourniquet at the base of the penis (blue line) before injecting the corpus cavernosum would prevent diffusion of the material injected into the more proximal penis (black arrow).............378

Figure 200. Charles Runels, MD...413

INDEX

1Password, 286

acne, 196, 295, 296, 298, 300

afferent nerves, 321, 323, 331, 336

afferent neurons, 322, 366

African, 295, 299, 354

Alabama, 21, 24, 27, 46, 50, 84, 86, 110, 116, 163, 284, 295, 413

alcohol, 62, 66, 67, 148

Allergan, 83, 102, 117, 142, 165

alprostadil, 358, 360, 364

Amazon, 62, 73, 105, 115, 116, 222

anatomy, 21, 161, 191, 193, 219, 336, 338, 341

angiogenesis, 368, 369, 389, 390

Asian, 253, 295, 299, 301, 353

axons, 368, 370

bacteriostatic saline, 62, 63, 163, 165, 166, 168, 266, 280, 294, 334, 335, 336, 372

bait, 55, 56

Barry J. Marshall, 382

Barry Marshall, 359

beer bottle opener, 335

Birmingham, 24, 84, 110, 284, 295, 413

Botox board, 59

Botox Emergency, 174

Botox parties, 37, 38, 46, 47, 52, 53, 55, 65, 71, 75, 85, 93, 99, 191, 307

bottle opener, 72, 73, 166, 167, 335

Brad Pitt, 356

brow lift, 71, 80, 81, 82, 93, 96, 185, 189, 236, 238, 243, 348, 349

bruxism, 22, 82, 96, 233, 311, 312, 314, 322, 352, 353, 354, 356, 357

bubbles, 44, 180

bunny lines, 80, 82, 96, 185, 260

C.S. Lewis, 40

California, 36, 50, 309

cappuccino machine, 175

Carruthers, 3

cash, 65, 84, 85, 86, 87, 102, 111, 116, 117, 121, 142, 147, 161, 313, 314, 333, 349

Caucasian, 96, 295, 299, 301, 353, 354

Cellular Medicine Association, 3, 26, 50, 105, 106, 107, 108, 326, 413, 414

Charles Darwin, 316

Checklist, 58

cold emotion, 317, 318, 319, 320, 322

connector, 32, 33, 34, 35, 37, 38, 41, 42, 50, 54, 129

connectors, 33, 69

consent form, 67, 76, 78, 79, 87, 88, 94, 97, 334, 371

conversation, 78, 146, 152, 153, 174, 188, 199, 222, 227, 354

cooties, 40

corpus cavernosum, 372, 373

corrugator, 71, 75, 76, 81, 167, 185, 190, 191, 192, 210, 228, 229, 231, 338, 355

crow's feet, 71, 80, 81, 82, 93, 96, 167, 172, 185, 189, 238, 239, 240, 241, 243, 349

Cupid's bow, 295, 303, 305

DAOs, 269, 270, 272, 273

Darlene, 46, 47, 48, 85

depression, 22, 93, 199, 223, 233, 311, 312, 314, 315, 316, 317, 318, 319, 320, 321, 322, 323, 324, 325, 326, 327, 328, 329, 332, 339

dilution, 22, 23, 165, 168, 182, 183, 266, 272, 280, 281, 282, 294, 344, 348, 355

Dysport, 1, 22, 23, 28, 382

ED, 297, 358, 359, 360, 362, 363, 364, 365, 366, 371, 373, 379, 381, 382

educate, 51, 56, 108, 117

Elon Musk, 43

email, 26, 36, 38, 48, 49, 79, 84, 87, 88, 103, 104, 119, 120, 126, 130, 131, 132, 133, 135, 136, 284

Emily Dickenson, 28

endocytosis, 322, 331, 366

erectile dysfunction, 22, 26, 45, 108, 109, 297, 311, 314, 358, 370, 371, 381, 382, 383, 387, 388, 414

Erectile Dysfunction, 310, 327, 358, 382, 383

Facial Feedback Hypothesis, 319

Facial Feedback Loop, 320, 321

FDA, 106, 107, 109, 322, 332, 333, 336, 350, 362

fillers, 25, 44, 69, 70, 93, 95, 97, 99, 106, 135, 159, 198, 214, 221, 268, 269, 270, 284, 289, 294, 299, 301, 335

frontalis, 71, 80, 82, 83, 93, 94, 95, 96, 185, 189, 215, 230, 232, 233, 234, 235, 237, 244, 245, 246, 247, 248, 249, 250, 251, 252, 317, 339, 340, 341, 347, 348, 349, 355

frown lines, 358

ganglion, 322, 323, 331, 336, 366

George Winston, 67, 68, 158, 159, 160, 221, 222, 226

glabella, 80, 81, 82, 95, 190, 230, 313, 320, 322, 323, 326, 333, 337, 338, 340, 379

Gladwell, 33, 39

grateful, 22, 24, 212, 252, 255, 267, 287, 300, 347, 353

Guiding Principle, 188, 189, 190

gummy smile, 80, 82, 96, 185, 263, 264, 265, 266, 267, 352

hair salon, 35, 40, 41, 42, 44, 61, 84, 88, 91, 97

hand mirror, 63

Hollywood, 297, 356

Homunculus, 304

hostess, 32, 33, 34, 35, 41, 67, 68, 69, 79, 94, 97, 98, 99, 100, 129, 152

husband, 36, 243, 285, 354

hypoxia-inducible factor, 369

ice cubes, 58, 73, 74

index card, 77, 78, 79, 84, 231

India, 38

insurance, 21, 110, 112, 115, 116, 127, 132, 150, 283, 311, 312, 313, 324, 333, 349 internist, 21, 24, 25, 36, 46, 112, 157, 160

Intracavernosal injections, 361

iPad, 217, 231, 283

iPhone, 64, 67, 87, 202, 276

ivory temple, 44

Jeuveau, 1, 22, 23

John Travolta, 40

Journal of Sexual Medicine, 358

Kirk Douglas, 277

Kiss, 291, 292

Larry Flint, 36

Legend of the Fall, 356

Lip Flip, 291, 292, 293, 302, 303, 304, 305, 306

LiSWT, 358, 362, 364

Lizard brain, 197

MacBook Pro, 286

magic, 28, 53, 68, 122, 123, 148, 157, 158, 162, 164, 201, 202, 316

Mark Bailey, 3, 75, 308

Marketing, 25, 54, 105, 141, 174, 178

massage, 112, 115, 149, 150, 153, 162, 227, 230, 338, 340, 379

masseter, 199, 353, 354, 355, 356, 357

mastoid process, 345, 346

Max Planck, 298

meninges, 322, 331, 332, 336

mentalis, 275, 276, 277, 278

migraines, 22, 233, 311, 313, 314, 322, 323, 325, 331, 332, 333, 334, 335, 336, 337, 338, 339, 340, 344, 345, 347, 348, 349

motor end plate, 368

multi-level marketing, 31, 69, 141

multilevel marketing, 35

multilevel marketing, 141

multilevel marketing, 142

myasthenia gravis, 92, 326, 367

nasalis, 260, 261, 262

National Center for Education Statistics, 315

necklace lines, 80, 279, 280, 288, 289, 290

neovascularization, 365, 366, 367, 369, 390

neurogenesis, 365, 366, 367, 368

norepinephrine, 366

number 11, 93, 220, 317

occipitalis, 340, 341, 342, 347, 348, 349

occipitofrontalis, 341, 342, 348

Occipitofrontalis, 340, 341, 350

occiput, 341, 342, 343

Omega Melancholicum, 317, 320, 321

opening the eye, 253

orbicularis oris, 278, 281, 291, 292, 293, 294, 295, 301, 302, 304

O-Shot®, 3, 25, 36, 38, 55, 56, 59, 64, 85, 90, 107, 128, 144, 156, 161, 413

package insert, 52, 163, 218, 245, 266, 335

paper, 64, 67, 77, 107, 115, 130, 139, 155, 156, 160, 161, 216, 217, 231, 283, 284, 285, 287

parasympathetic, 258, 323, 366, 367

parole board, 175

party, 31, 32, 33, 34, 35, 36, 37, 38, 40, 41, 42, 43, 46, 47, 48, 49, 50, 51, 53, 56, 57, 58, 59, 60, 61, 62, 64, 66, 67, 68, 69, 70, 71, 72, 76, 77, 78, 79, 80, 81, 82, 83, 84, 85, 86, 87, 88, 89, 90, 91, 95, 97, 98, 99, 100, 103, 129, 130, 131, 135, 136, 146, 155, 176, 179, 181, 185, 217, 292

PC., 285, 286, 287

PDE5Is, 360, 365, 366, 367, 369, 371

peau d'orange, 275

Penile implant, 361

penis, 26, 108, 109, 127, 358, 360, 361, 362, 363, 364, 366, 370, 371, 372, 373, 374, 375, 377, 378, 379, 388

Planck Principle, 298

platelet-rich plasma, 25, 105, 106, 288, 362, 363, 381, 386, 387, 388, 389, 390, 391, 392

platysma, 279, 280, 281, 282, 287, 288

pleats, 94, 189, 190, 239, 268, 292, 338

primary care physician, 20, 112, 132, 147, 150, 175, 325

procerus, 71, 76, 80, 81, 82, 83, 167, 185, 188, 190, 193, 220, 222, 223, 224, 227, 229, 230, 231, 232, 248, 249, 260, 261, 312, 313, 321, 323, 326, 333, 337, 338, 347, 348, 349, 379

PRP, 25, 26, 38, 50, 95, 106, 107, 108, 109, 133, 177, 288, 289, 359, 362, 365, 370, 380, 381, 387, 389, 390, 391, 392

P-Shot®, 3, 26, 36, 38, 45, 109, 127, 144, 156, 363, 364, 365, 369, 370, 378, 380, 386, 413

pull-down muscles, 83, 95, 96, 232, 233, 249, 251

Purasyn®, 373

Retin A, 289

secret, 31, 53, 69, 112, 114, 134, 146, 250, 284, 333

sensory afferents, 331

Seventh-Day Adventist, 36

Sharpie®, 294

shock wave therapy, 362

sketch, 77, 78, 79, 81, 84, 86, 87, 130, 216, 231, 283, 284

SketchWow, 284

skull, 189, 190, 224, 235, 346

smoker's lines, 291, 292, 293, 301, 307

Snap Test, 256

SNARE proteins, 332

Spartacus, 277

speaker, 35, 65, 66, 67

splenius capitis, 344, 345, 346, 347, 348, 349

SSRIs, 315, 316, 319

stem cells, 108, 362

Stephen R. Marquardt, 3

story, 34, 48, 90, 178, 299, 300

suicide, 311, 315, 316, 319

swap brains, 194

sympathectomy, 366, 367

sympathetic, 323, 366, 367

tail wagging the dog, 311

teenager, 31, 32, 40, 265, 295, 358

temporalis, 235, 278, 292, 343, 347, 348, 349

Thomas Jefferson, 374

Touchups, 252

trapezius, 344, 347, 348, 349

trigeminal nerve, 331

Tupperware, 31, 32, 36, 37, 38, 47

TV ad, 42

Type III collagen, 370

Uber, 54

Vampire Facial®, 25, 64, 95, 126, 288, 289, 290, 293

vascular endothelial growth factor, 369

VED, 358, 360, 364

VEDs, 360

Veraguth's folds, 321

Veraguth's Folds, 317, 320

vermillion, 292, 293, 294, 295, 302, 303, 305, 306, 307

vermillion border, 292, 293, 294, 295, 302, 303, 305, 306, 307

Vince Gironda, 297

warm emotion, 318, 319, 320

Warning, 85, 214, 255, 266, 278

World Health Organization, 315

Xeomin, 1, 22, 28, 327, 382

Xeomin®, 1, 7, 22, 23, 28, 327, 368, 382, 385

YouTube, 43

ABOUT THE AUTHOR

Dr. Runels worked for three years as a physical chemist at Southern Research Institute before starting medical school at the University of Alabama in Birmingham. After medical school, he completed his residency and became board-certified in Internal Medicine.

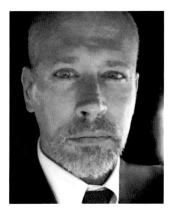

Figure 200. Charles Runels, MD

During twelve years as an ER physician, he founded the largest group of ER physicians in his state.

He then began a private medical practice and conducted research in the areas of endocrinology, urology, cosmetic medicine, & sexual medicine. He contributed to multiple peer-reviewed scientific publications in the areas of hypertension, hormone replacement, sexual medicine, and immunology.

Based on his research, he authored several popular books about sex and chapters in medical texts. In cosmetic medicine, he designed a specific way of using blood-derived growth factors to rejuvenate the face, called the Vampire Facelift®. He founded the Cellular Medicine Association to help promote further investigation in that area.

His recent work includes research on urinary incontinence and sexual function in both men and women—resulting in his development of the O-Shot® (Orchid Shot™), P-Shot® (Priapus Shot®), and Bocox™, and Clitox™, Vampire Breast Lift®, and Vampire Wing Lift® procedures. His innovative approach to sexual health and cosmetic medicine and his related intellectual properties made him a sought-after practitioner and lecturer. Over the past 12 years, he taught his methods to over 5,000 physicians in over 50 countries.

He is the father of three sons and grandfather of two grandsons. He lives in Fairhope, Alabama, with his wife and colleague, Dr. Alexandra Runels Runels, MD.

FURTHER HELP

Charles Runels, MD
1-251-648-7704

Cellular Medicine Association
52 South Section St., Suite A, Fairhope, AL 36532
1-888-920-5311

Detailed videos and updated references and tools regarding the *injection of BoNT*: BoNTClass.com

For other books and free ideas and newsletters regarding health, see the *author's personal webpage*: Runels.com

For education and research regarding the use of *cellular medicine to improve tissue health* and to treat disease: CellularMedicineAssociation.org

More instruction regarding the treatment of erectile dysfunction with BoNT: BoNTPenis.com

Books on Amazon by Charles Runels: Amazon.com/author/charlesrunels

Free information for physicians regarding the Vampire Facelift® procedure: VampireFacelift.com/physicians

Free information for physicians regarding the Vampire Facial® procedure: VampireFacial.com/physicians

Free information for physicians regarding the O-Shot® procedure: OShot.com/physicians

Free information for physicians regarding the P-Shot® procedure: PriapusShot.com/physicians

Free, 365 Health Strategies: 365HealthStrategies.com
